Classics in Psychiatry

This is a volume in the Arno Press collection

Classics in Psychiatry

See last pages of this volume
for a complete list of titles

THE PSYCHONEUROSES
AND THEIR TREATMENT

BY

PSYCHOTHERAPY

J[oseph Jules] Dejerine
and
E. Gauckler

ARNO PRESS
A New York Times Company
New York • 1976

Editorial Supervision: EVE NELSON

Reprint Edition 1976 by Arno Press Inc.

Reprinted from a copy in
The Princeton University Library

CLASSICS IN PSYCHIATRY
ISBN for complete set: 0-405-07410-7
See last pages of this volume for titles.

Manufactured in the United States of America

Library of Congress Cataloging in Publication Data
Déjerine, Joseph Jules, 1849-1917.
The psychoneuroses and their treatment by psychotherapy.

(Classics in psychiatry)
Translation of Les manifestations functionelles des psychonéuroses.
Reprint of the 1913 ed. published by Lippincott, Philadelphia.
1. Neuroses. 2. Psychotherapy. I. Gauckler, E., joint author. II. Title. III. Series. [DNLM: WM D326m 1913a]
RC530.D4413 1975 616.8'5 75-16697
ISBN 0-405-07425-5

THE PSYCHONEUROSES
AND THEIR TREATMENT

BY

PSYCHOTHERAPY

BY

PROFESSOR J. DEJERINE

PROFESSOR OF THE CLINIC FOR NERVOUS DISEASES OF THE FACULTY OF MEDICINE OF THE UNIVERSITY OF PARIS

AND

DR. E. GAUCKLER

ANCIEN INTERNE OF THE HOSPITALS OF PARIS

AUTHORIZED TRANSLATION BY

SMITH ELY JELLIFFE, M.D., PH.D.

ADJUNCT PROFESSOR OF DISEASES OF THE MIND AND NERVOUS SYSTEM, POST GRADUATE MEDICAL SCHOOL AND HOSPITAL; VISITING NEUROLOGIST, CITY HOSPITAL, NEW YORK

PHILADELPHIA & LONDON

J. B. LIPPINCOTT COMPANY

Electrotyped and Printed by J. B. Lippincott Company
The Washington Square Press, Philadelphia, U. S. A.

TRANSLATOR'S PREFACE

In translating this work, I have had in mind a very definite purpose. For a number of years, like many another, I have been struck by the immense number of minor psychic disturbances which render numerous individuals unhappy, discontented, ill, unable to hold their own in their milieu, even making confirmed invalids of many.

These individuals, variously classified as to their maladies, at different times, as suffering from functional neuroses, nervousness, neurasthenia, phobias, fixed ideas, obsessions, hysteria, psychoneuroses, etc., have been neglected for many years as objects of scientific medical inquiry. The reasons for this are obvious. They centre about the cardinal fact that the psychic life of the human being is the most complex series of phenomena in the most highly evolved creature with which human intelligence is acquainted.

The psychic problems of the individual have been left to the poet, the artist, the dramatist, and the writer.

I do not mean that the physicians of times past have not made serious attempts to understand these questions. They have, and the student of medical history may well admire the results obtained, even if to-day they may seem inadequate, if not provoking. Even taking this knowledge into consideration, however, it appears that the problems of medicine have been so many, and so difficult of solution, that the human mind has naturally and wisely grasped at those for which some adequate solution seemed practicable. It is for this reason that the comparatively simpler problems of the bodily activities, their modifications, etc., have received their wealth of study, which is one of the crowning glories of medical science in the last century.

The time came, however, when the intricacies of the nervous system commenced to be resolved, and scientific medicine arrived at a point where its hypotheses began to yield valuable results in the fields of neurology and psychiatry. With the establishment of firmer foundations, it became worth while to delve into psychic problems, with some hope of sound deductions and practical results, and within the past few generations we have seen scientific medicine take its place in this domain heretofore left to the thousand and one uninformed and quasi-scientific cults which have for centuries constituted parasitic foci in every community.

It was with the intention of furthering a knowledge of what scientific medicine could do in the domain outlined that I first translated Dubois' excellent work on the "Psychoneuroses." Its fundamental postulate was an appeal to the intelligence of the individual.

Dubois, however, was incomplete. He did not lay sufficient emphasis upon the instinctive, or, more widely speaking, the emotional side of the human machine, in its psychical situations. It is for this reason that I have, with the aid of my wife, translated the present volume, which is the product of Professor Dejerine of Paris, and one of his former assistants, Dr. Gauckler.

Herein is found that emphasis lacking in the work of Dubois. Herein Dejerine and Gauckler uncover the emotional factors which are present in all of the group of disorders under discussion. This work provides us, in the best manner at present available, the other side of the human being, which had, I feel, been somewhat neglected by former authors.

The reading of this book will show how many patients may be treated and cured without the more detailed analyses elaborated to meet more complex situations.

Just as in the domain of internal medicine a compound cathartic pill will relieve the vast majority of constipations, requiring only in a smaller percentage of cases a more intricate and time-consuming gastro-intestinal therapy, so in the domain of the psychoneuroses a prompt handling of an emotional situation, or a sound dialectic may secure for a large number of patients the relief necessary to effect an adjustment, while for a lesser number, although their number is by no means small, only a Freudian analysis will effect a cure.

With these few words we leave the work to the judgment of the individual reader. The hope, that it will prove of some service to all, patients as well as their physicians, has been the stimulus and purpose which has led to its translation.

SMITH ELY JELLIFFE.

April, 1913.

PREFACE

When, more than thirty years ago, I began to devote myself to the study of diseases of the nervous system, I was struck, from the very beginning of my practice, with the slight success which resulted from treatment of neuropaths by medicines, whether combined or not with physical measures, and little by little I was led, by personal experience, to ask myself whether it would not be wise, in the case of all patients coming under the classification of neurasthenia or hysteria, to depart from the usual therapeutic methods, and seek the cause of their disease outside of the objective symptoms which they presented.

I thus became more and more convinced that it was not the physical, but rather the moral which was the cause of all the symptoms of which these patients complained, and finally, after having practised Dr. Weir Mitchell's methods for several years, my convictions were established. In using this method of treatment, which is based practically on isolation, rest in bed, over-feeding, douches, massage, and electricity, in fact on purely physical measures, I was not long in discovering that unless the patient's state of mind improved the therapeutic results were far from satisfactory.

It was thus that I soon came to see that in order to treat neuropaths, with the hope of curing them, the first and most important thing was to get hold of their morale, in other words, to practise psychotherapy. This is what I have been doing for the last twenty-five years.

The influence of the morale on the physique has been known in all ages. It is in fact a popular belief that the health may be seriously affected by grief or vexation, but physicians have been, as a rule, the last persons to recognize that these might be connected with a very special class of affections, requiring particular treatment, based not on symptoms but on causes: and, without wishing to deny—at least in many cases—the accuracy of the old adage "*Mens sana in corpore sano,*" I nevertheless believe that, in the case of most neuropaths, whatever may be their symptomatology, the saying is not correct. With them, as a matter of fact, if the body is not sound it is because their morale is unhealthy, and because they have either suffered or are still suffering morally or spiritually.

As a method of general education, or moral guidance, psychotherapy is as old as the world. All philosophies, and all religions, above all, the Catholic religion—for the psychotherapist is nothing more than a confessor, or director of the lay conscience—have applied it, or are still applying it. Few, however, are the physicians who understand this, or who know how to make use of it, when they know the cause.

To be convinced of this, one only has to see what a large number of neuropaths are being subjected to some physical treatment, as if they had some true organic lesions. I am alluding to those patients, whose number is legion, whom I have described under the name of false gastropaths, false enteropaths, false cardiopaths, false genitopaths, sufferers from spinal disease, and false cerebral disease; who present symptoms which often seem serious, but whose origin is wholly psychic, and who are treated every day purely and solely on the lines of symptomatic therapy, with the result that the idea becomes more firmly fixed in their minds, that there is some disease localized in the organ of which they complain. I have seen thousands of these invalids.

I hold that the physicians who understand and know how to practise psychotherapy are still very few in number. I do not, however, consider direct suggestion as a psychotherapeutic measure, either when produced more or less openly in the waking state or by means of hypnosis. Such methods have the serious defect of acting only on the subconscious, and on the cerebral automatism, and are not directed to the superior faculties of the individual.

Suggestion, though much more frequently used in hysterical cases than in troubles of neurasthenic origin, whether practised in the waking state or during hypnotic sleep, is directed only to the symptom, and not to the cause; its action is only on the surface, it does not reach the depths. By this process one often succeeds more or less quickly, in certain cases, in getting rid of a paralysis, a contracture or an anæsthesia in an hysteric. But, without taking the drawbacks into consideration, and they are very numerous, the result is very uncertain, unless, by winning the confidence and appealing to the reason of the patient, or in other words by means of psychotherapy, one succeeds in making him confess his manner of living, and explains to him how and why he fell ill, and how and why he can become cured, so that he will not relapse.

Even though these methods, which are directed only to the cerebral automatism, are sometimes successful in causing some of the objective manifestations of a hysterical condition to disappear, they are absolutely without efficiency when it comes to the very complex and intricate symptoms of a neurasthenic. For here the mental condition is wholly different. One cannot cure a false gastropath or cardiopath by a brusque command. It is a case for mental pedagogy, which often requires a long time and careful development to be effectual.

It has been stated repeatedly, and with some reason, that isolation in a sanitarium is fundamental in the treatment of the psychoneuroses. In a general way this is true, but it is not absolutely imperative. In the case of many neuropaths isolation is not necessary, and the psychotherapist need not insist on it. Isolation, in fact, is nothing but a means, without which, in many cases, it would be impossible to practise psychotherapy, and which has its special indications.

A sojourn in a sanitarium is possible only to the wealthy or those who are comfortably off, and is wholly out of the question for the poorer classes of society. But the psychoneuroses are not met exclusively among the well-to-do. Neurasthenia and hysteria are, in fact, very common among the working population of Paris, and are often found in very severe forms. I have therefore tried to introduce in the hospital the suitable conditions of treatment which one would find in a sanitarium, and for fifteen years I have established in my service at the Salpêtrière an isolation and psychotherapeutic ward, where several thousand patients have been treated. The results obtained by this measure have far surpassed the hopes I had in the beginning, for they have proved quite as satisfactory, and even more rapid, than those in private practice. I will not go into the details of my methods of working in the hospital. The reader who is interested in this question will find all the necessary information in a work entitled "Isolement et Psychothérapie," published in 1904, by my pupils Camus and Pagniez. I merely make, in passing, the statement that at the Salpêtrière, as well as in the city, it is the moral treatment which is the cause of the success obtained.

According to some authors, particularly Dubois (of Berne), psychotherapy ought to be "rational," that is, based solely on reasoning and argument. I have always been of the opposite opinion, and I have frequently expressed myself on this subject, both in my courses at the Faculty of Medicine and in my clinical lectures at the Salpêtrière. If reason and argument were sufficient to "change one's state of mind," the neuropaths would find in the writings of the moralists and philosophers, and spiritual advisers, everything they would need to reconstruct their morale, and consequently their physical well-being, and therefore they would have no need of a psychotherapist.

Reasoning by itself is indifferent. It does not become a factor of energy or creator of effort; but the moment an emotional element appears the personality of the subject whose mentality one is seeking to modify, is moved and affected by it. According to my way of thinking, it is an error to consider both the judgment, which is a primitive phenomenon, and the impression or sentiment which follows it as psychological processes of the same nature. The impression and sentiment are nothing but the result of the more or less ready adaptation of our personality to the judgment which caused them, and though secondary are no less able to provoke reactions.

From my point of view, psychotherapy depends wholly and exclusively upon the beneficial influence of one person on another. One does not cure an hysteric or a neurasthenic nor change their mental condition by reasoning or by syllogisms. They are only cured when they come to believe in you. In short, psychotherapy can only be effective, when the person on whom you are practising it has confessed his entire life, that is to say, when he has absolute confidence in you.

Between reasoning, and the acceptance of this reasoning by the patient, there is, I repeat, an element, on the importance of which I cannot insist too strongly; it is sentiment or feeling. It is feeling which creates the atmosphere of confidence without which, I hold, no psychotherapy is possible, that is to say, unless reasoning produces effective action there is no "*persuasion.*" I am, in fact, convinced, and have been so for a long time, that in the moral sphere the bare idea produces no effect, that is to say, the idea alone does not move one, unless it is accompanied by an emotional appeal which makes it acceptable to consciousness and thus brings about conviction. There is something analogous to faith in this, some individual element which makes the success of the psychotherapist depend upon his personality.

This is the one and only place to refer to the ancient adage—"It is faith that saves . . . or cures."

I have been aided in the collaboration of this work by one of my pupils, Dr. Gauckler, with whom I have already published several works on psychotherapy.

J. DEJERINE.

CONTENTS

PART II.

INTRODUCTION

THIS work is devoted to the study of the psychoneuroses, and their treatment. In it will be found the ideas which have been formed by one of us who has spent thirty years in daily contact with neuropaths. In attending these patients, and noting the manner in which they have been treated, it has seemed to us that many physicians have held ideas concerning the nature of the psychoneuroses that are not only incomplete and inexact, according to our lights, but are also therapeutically dangerous. This does not imply ignorance on their part, but rather that, having been brought up on doctrines and methods which are excellent in their place, they have extended their application to a branch of medicine like the psychoneuroses, with which they have nothing to do.

All advance work in modern medicine is the direct result of progress in pathological anatomy and laboratory work. These have enabled us to get a very much more exact idea of the human mechanism, and the various troubles that may afflict it. But the fact has been quite overlooked that modifications of physical energy are not the only ones in which physicians should be interested.

All physicians rebel at the idea of any dissociation which would separate the physical organism on the one hand from the psychic and moral organism on the other. But, both instinctively, and as a result of their education, the majority of them have a tendency to subordinate the disturbances of the psychic life to those of the physical, and to always look for some initial somatic change. They refuse to even consider the existence of illnesses which owe their origin to any antecedent psychic or moral disturbance. But, there exists, according to our way of thinking, a very special nosological group, of much importance, whose symptomatology is caused solely by a primitive modification of the moral or mental state, followed by a whole series of secondary manifestations. The affections which come under this heading are known as the *psychoneuroses.*

This book is wholly devoted to the development of this point of view. It will be divided into three parts.

The first, which is *analytical,* will be devoted to the study of functional manifestations, that is, to the study of all the symptoms which are observed in the course of the psychoneuroses, whose exact nature we wish to ascertain.

In the second, the *synthetic,* we shall endeavor to make plain the general mechanism of the foundation of the psychoneuroses, as well as their variations and nature.

In the third, which is *therapeutic,* will be set forth the psychotherapeutic proceedings and helps which we feel are the only measures which should be used in the treatment of the psychoneuroses.

PSYCHOTHERAPY

FIRST PART

Analytical Study of Functional Manifestations.

We shall study, under the name of functional manifestations, all those persistent symptoms and troubles of which neuropaths complain, and which have been created in these patients without any antecedent lesion of the body.

This definition is only provisional. It is made sufficiently broad for the moment not to limit the object of our study.

As there is no mechanism, organ, or region of the body which cannot become the seat of a functional manifestation, it would seem necessary for the various parts of the organism to be involved in equal proportions. But there are numerous reasons for the variability of frequency which exists. Without dwelling, for the moment, on the part which education, whether medical or personal, plays in the symptoms felt by these patients, we must make one statement, large in theoretic consequences, which we will make good later. Some of the functions of the body are completely automatic, and never require any direction from the superior centres. Such is the function of circulation. Others, on the contrary, especially the digestive and genital, and in part the urinary, are functions which, at least in their ultimate accomplishment, depend upon various mental representations, and call the will into play. There are functions on which the action of the will is felt, but in a purely contingent manner, such as the respiratory function. Finally, even among the functions which do not come under the influence of the will, there are none whose automatism may not be more or less affected by the influence of the emotions.

But the fact is not without significance that those very functions which are the most involved are those which are most susceptible to psychic influence.

The digestive function has always seemed to us to be the one on which the greatest number of functional manifestations were localized. With it, therefore, we shall commence our study.

CHAPTER I.

FUNCTIONAL MANIFESTATIONS OF THE DIGESTIVE SYSTEM.

ALL of the successive acts of digestion are, to a certain degree, started going by an antecedent phenomenon, which at the outset is apparently peripheral, but which is accompanied by more or less vivid mental representations, which are known as hunger or appetite. It would perhaps be useful, in order to be exact, to make a distinction between these two words, hunger and appetite. They are not absolutely synonymous. The word "hunger" expresses some sort of organic need of nourishment. The word "appetite" expresses rather the psychic idea of nourishment. One can have an appetite without being, properly speaking, hungry. The appetite may be awakened by all sorts of purely psychic sensations, such as an odor, a savory taste, etc., . . . as well as association of ideas, bearing on the time, or on places which recall the idea of food, and lead to appetite. As a matter of fact, from the point of view which interests us, the two terms may be used indifferently, and the only thing to which we attach importance is the knowledge that if this first phenomenon of digestion may, so to speak, be an outside appeal, it may also be largely dependent upon the intervention of the psychic mechanism.

Disturbances of appetite will be the first which we shall pass in review. We shall then study a whole series of functional manifestations, which may be produced at different stages of digestion.

DISTURBANCES OF APPETITE.

These disturbances may be quantitative or qualitative. We shall take up successively:

A. *Mental anorexia. Quantitative disturbance of the appetite due to lack of food.*

B. *Quantitative disturbance of the appetite due to excess.*

C. *Elective anorexias, or qualitative disturbances of the appetite.*

A. Mental Anorexia.—It sometimes happens that a physician has patients—they are more apt to be women—whose appearance is truly shocking. Their eyes are brilliant. Their cheeks are hollow, and their cheek bones seem to protrude through the skin. Their withered breasts hang from the walls of their chest. Every rib stands out. Their shoulder-blades appear to be loosened from their frame. Every vertebra shows through the skin. The abdominal wall sinks in below the floating ribs and forms a hollow like a basin. Their thighs and the calves of their legs are reduced to a skeleton. One would say it was the picture of an immured nun, such as the old masters have portrayed. These women appear to be fifty or sixty years old. Sometimes they seem to be sustained by some unknown miracle of energy; their voices are strong and their steps firm. On the other hand, they often seem almost at the point of death, and ready to draw their last breath.

Are they tuberculous or cancerous patients, or muscular atrophies in the last stages, these women whom misery and hunger have reduced to this frightful gauntness? Nothing of the kind. Their lungs are healthy, there is no sign of any organic affection. Although they look so old they are young women, girls, sometimes children. They may belong to good families, and be surrounded by every care. These patients are what are known as mental anorexics, who, without having any physical lesions, but by the association of various troubles, all having a psychic origin, have lost a quarter, a third, and sometimes a half of their weight. The affection which has driven them to this point may have lasted months, sometimes years. Let it go on too long and death will occur, either from inanition or from secondary tuberculosis. However, it is a case of nothing but a purely psychic affection of which the mechanisms are of many kinds.

Sometimes we meet individuals afflicted with well-defined characteristic psychoses who will not eat. Such are the melancholics who think they can commit suicide by doing without food. There are also those with persecutory delusions, who are overcome by the fear of being poisoned. Other subjects, such as the *major deliria,* do not eat, because their delirium is sufficiently intense to inhibit — temporarily — all peripheral sensations. All these patients, once the delusional idea has disappeared, are able to be fed up immediately, and in an intensive manner. These do not come within the limits of our study. The mental representation of appetite is neither actually nor virtually lost to them.

Neither shall we consider those apparent cases of mental anorexia which we find in certain hysterics who affect anorexia in public, but who eat on the sly.

True mental anorexia consists in the progressive loss of the mental representation of appetite.

For the moment that the inhibition of the psychic phenomenon which constitutes appetite is accompanied by an inhibition of the physical phenomenon—which is the feeling of bodily hunger—mental anorexia is established.

We shall study under the name of *secondary mental anorexia* those cases where the taking of food has been restricted with the idea of relieving some former digestive trouble. We shall give the name primary mental anorexia to those cases in which originally, and often voluntarily, the amount of food taken by the individual had, for some cause or other, been diminished. The common characteristic of all these patients is that, when their affection has reached a certain stage, they get to the point where *if they should want to eat they could not,* for they no longer have any feeling of hunger.

In *primary mental anorexia* two classes of facts must be considered. Sometimes the loss of appetite is emotional in its origin. Sometimes the reduction of food has been purely voluntary at the start.

Here, for example, as an illustration of the first class, is the case of a woman, fifty years of age, who has been a widow for several months. Her children live at some distance from her, and are not of much comfort to her. Her whole life was wrapped up in her husband. She is extremely thin. She weighs seventy-nine pounds, instead of her normal weight, which is in the neighborhood of one hundred and ten pounds. This loss of weight has been rapid. It has taken place in three months. She says she is actually incapable of eating. Her food sticks in her throat. She chews it indefinitely, and cannot get up courage to swallow it. An egg, two or three cups of milk, and a few mouthfuls of bread are her daily diet. It is the typical picture of mental anorexia. How did it start? Here is a case which is purely emotional in its origin, and this is how it happened. This woman continued to occupy the apartment where she had lived with her husband. When she sat down to her meals, his image would rise before her, as would be natural from the association of ideas, bringing a whole train of emotional sensations, constriction of the throat, a feeling of weight in the stomach, lack of appetite, etc. She would get up from the table without having really eaten anything. By degrees this restriction of diet which was purely emotional in its origin brought her at last to the condition of mental anorexia.

Cases of this kind are extremely numerous. Grief, disappointment in love, or unhappiness in marriage are very often the emotional source of the most characteristic mental anorexias.

In other cases the restriction is at first voluntary and intentional. It is often due to coquetry.

A young girl, nineteen years of age, weighing one hundred and forty-three pounds, thought she was a little too heavy, so she tried to grow thin. She succeeded in losing twenty pounds in five months. In the meantime she became engaged. Her future husband thought she was too thin; so she tried to regain all, or at least some, of her lost weight, but her efforts were useless. She could no longer eat, and she continued to grow thinner. Her previous struggle against her appetite had caused her to become an anorexic.

Mysticism is responsible for a great many cases of mental anorexia. Regular fasting, instead of an occasional fast, is what induces it. Here is an example of a young lady, who hitherto had had no psychopathic taint. She had a brother who in several months was to come up for his examination in a great government school. She took a vow that she would eat nothing but the smallest portion that would suffice her.

Being very scrupulous she observed her fast qualitatively as well as quantitatively. The brother passed his examination and entered the school, and the young girl tried to eat as she had formerly done. But her appetite was no longer there, and she was obliged to spend several months in a sanitarium to cure the mental anorexia, which had reduced her to the last degree of emaciation.

Following the same idea, we once knew of a young man who intended to enter a monastery. Fearing that he would not be able to stand the fasts which this life imposed, and yet desirous of following his call, he thought that he would make a sort of test, and put himself through some privations in the matter of food. In a few months his efforts were rewarded by an attack of mental anorexia.

This case is similar to those of notable fasters who some years ago made a regular sporting profession of fasting, and who would go twenty or thirty days without eating.

Finally there are cases of mental anorexia whose origin is wholly different. This anorexia is of a social origin. It is the anorexia of poor people, who are obliged by the necessities of life to deprive themselves to such a degree that, when the illness or lack of employment which has caused these privations has disappeared, they find it impossible to take food again.

Patients afflicted with primary anorexia have this special characteristic, that in spite of their extreme thinness, they keep a good deal of their strength. We have seen, in illustration of this, young girls, who had gone down to fifty-five or sixty-five pounds in weight, continuing to live as their friends did, going for long walks and playing tennis.

Organically, these patients, as a rule, present only one important symptom, namely the suppression of the menses.

Secondary mental anorexia differs from primary mental anorexia in a certain number of ways. First of all, in this form the two sexes may be equally attacked, while, as we have already indicated, primary mental anorexia is found chiefly in women. In secondary mental anorexia, while the clinical picture is the same, as far as the loss of weight goes, the strength of the patient, on the contrary, is very much less. When they are lying down they are hardly able to raise themselves up. This is because it depends upon disturbances which have taken place very slowly. The alimentary restriction is only secondary. These are the false gastropaths or enteropaths who, either spontaneously or, alas, more often by reason of medical prescriptions, have entered upon a very strict régime, which they have followed only too well. By reason of constantly noticing themselves and classifying their foods and rejecting all kinds that they think they cannot digest, they finally manage to live on an incredibly small amount. Alimentary phobias creep in, and without showing any other intellectual disturbances, or any other modifications of character, these patients become rebellious, or make a great scene whenever anyone tries to make them eat. There are some who subsist on a quarter of an apple. For others two or three prunes form their daily rations. A certain one took two or three eggs a day. We saw another who had gotten to the point where she could live if she had a bowl of sugar water beside her. She dipped a paint brush into it from time to time, and moistened her lips with it. This was her only nourishment.

There are, unfortunately, only too many examples of cases where these conditions have been brought about by dietary regulations prescribed by some ill-advised physician. These patients, in fact, will often say to you, " It is no wonder that I eat so little, for they have steadily cut down the quantity of my food on the one hand, and on the other hand, they have put me on a diet from which they have cut out everything I like to eat."

A young girl, eighteen years of age, who had undergone much grief and emotion and anxiety, lost her appetite. A physician was consulted, and she was put upon a diet, thanks to which, at the end of six months, she weighed only sixty-one and a half pounds.

A child of fourteen who had lost her father a year before, and whose mother was left a widow with four children, was much affected by the poverty in which they found themselves. She developed some digestive troubles of whose origin the physician was ignorant. He reduced her diet to soups and milk foods, with the result that the child faded away before one's very eyes, until she weighed only fifty pounds.

At other times mental anorexia is established without any previous emotional disturbance, but simply by ill-advised medical treatment. A young girl of nineteen was sent to us from the provinces, on account of her excessive loss of weight. She weighed only sixty-two and a half pounds, and ate nothing but a little fruit and an egg each day. Until six months before she had been hearty and well, but having a sore throat she was put upon a liquid diet that was far from sufficient. Her appetite gradually disappeared, and in three months she had lost forty-four pounds.

The lack of recognition of mental anorexia is all the more serious because patients who are afflicted by it may die of inanition. The pulse then becomes very rapid and respiration difficult, fetid odors come from the mouth, and some patients slip away who could certainly have been saved by better treatment.

One of us has seen several such cases of death, in his private practice, as well as in the hospital. One of these patients, whom he saw forty-eight hours before she died, had come from a sanitarium, where she had been put upon a restricted diet.

Secondary mental anorexia occurs at all ages of life; but primary mental anorexia is more apt to be found in young girls from fifteen to twenty years of age, though it may occur much earlier or much later.

Nobécourt first and then Aynaud have studied the modifications which the blood undergoes in anorexics during the development of their affection, and during the period when they begin to take nourishment again. At the entry of a certain patient to one of our services, Aynaud found 5,000,000 red corpuscles and a normal percentage of hæmoglobin. But this blood formula is only apparently normal in consequence of the concentration of the serum. After this patient had been for three days upon a forced milk diet, the red corpuscles were only 2,800,000 and 60 per cent. hæmoglobin. The same patient, who at her entrance showed a certain degree of leucopænia, had a little later 12–15,000 white corpuscles, and later still, when her menses returned, a trace of eosinophilia.

In the same patients, the condition of the gastric juice has been examined. It has been found at times normal, and at times hypochlorhydric, which in itself explains the lack of desire for food.

A frank case of mental anorexia can be easily recognized by any physician who is at all informed. Nevertheless, we have found many severe cases of anorexia that were nursed along and aggravated in their anorexia, by physicians who were exaggeratedly devoted to dietetics and physical treatment.

On the other hand, mental anorexias that are in process of development are very seldom recognized, and there is an incalculable number of pseudo-dyspeptics and false gastropaths who by virtue of medical prescriptions are slipping gently into mental anorexia, without anyone doing anything to stop them on their dangerous way. We shall come across these patients, later on, in studying the different functional troubles which are connected with the digestive system.

Mental anorexia is perhaps the most serious of all the functional manifestations, for it endangers the patient's life in two ways; either incidentally, by diminishing his resistance to any organic disease which may attack him—particularly tuberculosis—or the mental anorexia itself may cause death. One can hardly realize, in fact, the condition of cachexia to which these patients may be reduced. Their emaciation is frightful. We have seen loss of weight running from forty-four to sixty-six pounds, and patients who normally weighed one hundred and ten pounds or more were reduced to a weight of sixty-six, sixty-one, and fifty-five pounds. We have even seen examples of patients who have lost half their bodily weight. When this limit is passed, in spite of all treatment, the case is generally hopeless. The near approach of death is generally heralded by the fetid odor given off by the patients and by tachycardia and dyspnœa.

But there is no absolute and distinct sign by which one can distinguish the patient who cannot recover from the one who will respond to treatment. We know patients who have reduced their food to a few teaspoonfuls of *café au lait,* and who had lost half their weight, but who, nevertheless, were cured. The anorexic who is cured regains her health completely; and in women the reappearance of the menses constitutes an important sign of cure. When carefully treated, according to the general treatment of neuropaths, which we shall take up later, there is no danger of a relapse.

But badly treated, they may recover temporarily, but a relapse is almost fatal. When such a relapse takes place soon, the loss of weight is much more rapid than it was in the case of the first attack. This is easily explained by the fact that the patient's reserve force lies chiefly in fat.

To sum up, whether incipient or established, mental anorexia is a fact of frequent occurrence. It is an affection which no physician has the right to let pass unrecognized. Whether he mistakes established anorexics for patients with an organic disease and treats them with medicine, or whether he permits an undeveloped anorexia to become established, he is equally to blame; for anorexics respond beautifully to treatment, while the failure to recognize such an affection leads more or less directly and more or less rapidly to the death of the patient.

The diagnosis of mental anorexia is extremely simple. It merely requires thought. It only becomes complicated when the mental anorexia is grafted on to a true organic disease. But even in these cases the history guides you, and every time that you find that the patient has gone upon a restricted diet, either voluntarily or from some emotional cause, and this has been followed by a loss of the psychic idea of appetite, you can safely assume the existence of mental anorexia, either pure and simple or associated with something.

B. Quantitative Disturbances of the Appetite due to Excess.—Neither the cravings of hunger in some psychoses, nor the true defensive processes which constitute the polyphagia of diabetics or convalescents, come within the scope of our study. It is a wholly different class of cases which we wish to describe. In these, psychic hunger corresponds no more to organic hunger than it does in the case of a diabetic. The appetite is purely psychic. It is created by a mental systematization of such a nature that mental images connected with the taking of food are awakened, and lead, as it were, to a *false mental hunger* which is quite analogous to the false hunger described in certain organic diseases, where the sensation of hunger is aroused by the repetition of peripheral stimuli, as it is in our patients by the repetition of psychic stimuli. Such cases are evidently much rarer, and much less apparent, as well as much less serious, than the cases of mental anorexias.

They deserve, nevertheless, to be noticed, on account of their mechanism. As a rule the psychic orientation of the subject is of a purely medical origin. These are individuals who have been convinced of the necessity of taking many and frequent meals. We have seen neurasthenics of this order who have been convinced that they could not dare to take even a short walk without carrying with them some refreshment to sustain them, and enable them to continue the effort. Under the influence of this psychic orientation, these patients, if they are not provided with their customary daily lunch, are sometimes seized with a veritable obsession of hunger, which forces them to retrace their steps in order to get their forgotten food.

In other cases we have to do with individuals who at some previous time, and for a definite reason, have been overfed, and who, when the forced feeding is no longer necessary, and even when they are persuaded that it is not so, cannot return to a normal régime, sometimes for months, and sometimes even for years. We have been able to follow certain patients of this kind who have continued to experience very lively sensations of excessive hunger fully fifteen and twenty years after a treatment of overfeeding—for pulmonary tuberculosis, for instance.

Furthermore, in certain individuals, a sensation of hunger being produced under normal conditions assumes an intensity which is wholly out of the ordinary. We are reminded here of the case of a young man who, in order to enter upon a certain career, was obliged to go without his early breakfast. Now, each time that he tried to do without this slight meal, he was seized with sensations of hunger, that were so acute that they amounted almost to faintness. On analyzing it, it proved to be a case of an intense exaggeration of the sensation of hunger, under the influence of purely psychic phenomena. The anxiety which the patient felt, lest he be obliged to give up his career by reason of his not being able to change his régime, was the only cause of it. It was so entirely the cause that, once the young man was assured of it, he was cured in several days, and could easily accommodate himself to this slight irregularity in his habits of eating.

These cases are often rather difficult to analyze, and such manifestations must not be confused with the phenomena which are found in certain subjects, such as congenital neuropaths, in whom the fear of not being able to follow the treatment laid down for them fully or conscientiously enough becomes the starting point of an obsession or a scruple. Here there is nothing of the kind. Our patients feel a very real hunger starting from within, but accompanied by the whole series of sensations of taste and salivary phenomena, which they would experience as the normal consequences of the sensation of hunger. Moreover, the purely psychic nature of these phenomena is further demonstrated by their rapid disappearance under appropriate treatment.

However it may be, one fact remains patent, and that is that under the influence of association of ideas, of psychic convictions, or mental interpretations, it is possible for acute sensations of hunger to arise, and to be accompanied by all the physical peripheral reactions, both normal and abnormal, which such a sensation is liable to produce.

Let us call attention, on the other hand, to the existence of sudden attacks of real hunger, following some more or less lively emotion, and which are brought back upon the repetition of the emotion. We have never seen such phenomenon give rise to persistent troubles of the kind which we have just been considering; but we shall not dwell upon this, but will now pass to another kind of digestive trouble.

C. Elective Anorexias.—When, just now, we were studying the mental anorexias, we found many patients who refused vaguely to try any food whatsoever. This is by no means the same affection, and is infinitely less serious; in fact, the subjects which we really have in mind may get food in a variety of ways, but though there is no longer a quantitative restriction, there is a qualitative restriction in their food.

Mr. M., fifty years of age, a manufacturer, having had numerous business perplexities, a family to provide for, and a sick wife, was at a certain time attacked by gouty symptoms. His physicians conceived the idea of putting him upon an absolute milk diet. He stood the treatment remarkably well. But when the symptoms had disappeared and the patient was advised to return to a normal diet, it was absolutely impossible. With every other food except milk the patient acted like a true anorexic. He would chew his meat and vegetables indefinitely, and would swallow them with the greatest difficulty. In fact, the attempt to go back to a normal diet resulted in a very rapid and considerable loss of flesh, so that after having lost twenty pounds the patient returned to his strictly milk diet.

In the psychological analysis of the case, it was brought out that the patient for whom the milk diet had succeeded so well, either from causal relations or by simple coincidence, was afraid that by going back to his normal food he would again experience his gouty symptoms, and in consequence his commercial activity would be interrupted. Hence the phenomena observed. This patient was treated by one of us only for a very short time, in the course of which it was impossible to make him take any solid food whatsoever. On last hearing from him the patient was still upon a strictly milk diet, and, not finding himself any the worse for it, absolutely refused to try to go back to more normal nourishment.

For the same reason we often find people giving up certain dishes which have disagreed with them, though perhaps it was mere coincidence. Thus regular *food phobias* are created. We shall find plenty of them in studying the large and complex group of *false gastropaths.* Certain people, who are able to digest food which is supposed to be extremely indigestible, will reject from some purely psychic cause such and such a dish, for which after a time they acquire a feeling of positive disgust, which will bring on, simply by a mental attitude, the most varied disorders.

There are other disturbances of appetite which frequently depend upon purely psychic phenomena. The capricious appetite which is so common among young girls and young women, may often be psychic or emotional in its origin. We could cite numerous examples of such cases.

In fact, it is a very common thing to find that the sensation of appetite is susceptible to modifications of degree and in kind, according to the patient's psychic condition. Either a definite mental representation or an emotion is capable of inhibiting a phenomenon which is normally purely reflex. This is the ultimate conclusion to which we are led by the study of this first series of functional manifestations.

Disturbances closely allied to those we have just been considering are developed by neuropathic modifications of thirst. To avoid unnecessary repetition, we shall study these disturbances when we take up the subject of the modification of the amount of urine in connection with the psychoneuroses.

Functional Digestive Manifestations Properly So-called.

Normal physiology recognizes a certain number of steps in the process of digestion, which are as follows:

The taking of food; buccal digestion; mechanical and secretory phenomena (mastication and salivation); passage through the pharynx and œsophagus; deglutition; stomach digestion; passage through the pylorus; intestinal digestion; passage through the ileocæcum; cæco-colon digestion; defecation.

There is no one of these stages which may not be, either directly or indirectly, influenced by neuropathic phenomena. For convenience in description, and because such a division corresponds better with the clinical types, we shall study them in four distinct chapters as follows:

A. *Functional disturbance of the first three stages of digestion.*

B. *Gastric disturbances in nervous patients;* a study which we have already taken up in previous works ("False Gastropaths and False Gastropathies," 1906).

C. *Functional modifications in elimination.* Nervous diarrhœa and nervous constipation, and their consequences.

D. *Intestinal modifications properly so called.*

A. Functional Disturbances of the First Three Stages of Digestion.—An educated man of thirty-eight years of age, well informed in medical matters, and formerly syphilitic, had seen several persons of his acquaintance die of general paresis. He knew that difficulty in speech, trembling of the tongue, and trouble in swallowing were frequently in the list of symptoms of the disease with which he more and more believed himself to be threatened. From that time on he examined his mouth and his tongue many times a day. Soon he thought he felt a certain stiffness in the muscles of his face and cheeks. He continually made chewing movements, and it seemed to him—to use his own words—that he had a piece of rubber in his mouth. All these movements could not help but stimulate an excessive flow of saliva, which rendered his speech somewhat difficult. He constantly had bubbles in his mouth. It was not long before difficulty in swallowing made its appearance. All these disturbances were purely phobic in their nature. The patient did not dare to swallow. He chewed his food a long time before making an effort to swallow, and in this way, by progressive auto-suggestion, there was created a characteristic syndrome of difficulty of mastication, rather abundant salivation, and slowness in the act of swallowing, to which were added some speech disturbances which we shall meet with elsewhere.

Analogous syndromes are formed under the influence of incidents fixed in the mind of the patient. A workman, an engraver, came in March, 1909, to consult one of us. He was a bachelor thirty years of age, of an emotional temperament, but having had during the development of the symptoms of his disease no emotional cause exterior to it. He came to us in a very emaciated condition, having lost forty pounds, and declaring that he could no longer swallow anything except, with the greatest difficulty, a little milk and bread which had been soaked a long time in it. Six months before he had accidentally swallowed something the wrong way. The fact was trivial, but the patient had been so painfully affected that from that time he had not dared to swallow. Every time that he took a mouthful that was a little larger than usual he thought that the same thing would happen again, hence his condition of growing apprehension—augmented rather by a local treatment which a physician had made him undergo, thereby causing progressive restriction of food, and bringing the patient to the point where he was when he was seen at the Salpêtrière. There we made him eat small meals with one of us present. At first it took him several hours to eat what another person would have consumed in several minutes. Before making up his mind to swallow, he would chew for a very long time. Then he would stop for a while, and one would see him as if hesitating before swallowing. He would thus start chewing three or four times before being able to make up his mind. Under these conditions a state of voluntary contraction was produced in the region of his pharynx which made swallowing painful. This was the reason that the affection continued, as well as being encouraged by various suggestions of a medical nature.

In this particular case the patient, who quickly exhausted his powers of salivation, by his prolonged mastication, complained of dryness of the mouth in connection with eating, and was obliged to drink very often and in rather large quantities, in order to get through his meal. This patient was cured in a few days.

We have had occasion to see an absolutely identical series of symptoms in the case of a factory worker. His emaciation was so extreme, that at first sight one would have taken him for a case of organic disease. He had gone down to a weight of one hundred and eight pounds from a normal weight of one hundred and sixty-five pounds. The cause in his case was slightly different. One day he had swallowed a mouthful that was a little too large, which had gone down with difficulty, and not without causing him some twinges of pain and a transitory spasm of the œsophagus.

Here, on the other hand, is a history of a young woman thirty-seven years of age, who, at the age of twenty-one, after a year of married life, was left a widow with a child. She had promised her husband at his death-bed never to re-marry. The struggle with herself, which she had gone through in order to keep this promise, had made her exaggeratedly emotional.

One day, while eating fish, she swallowed a bone which stuck in her throat. They sent for a physician, who was not able to find the offending object until after repeated efforts. The impression had lasted long enough to become fixed, and the patient, becoming dysphagic, had gotten to the point where it took her five or six hours a day to swallow the smallest quantity of liquid. This condition lasted for seven years, and the woman was really in a cachectic state. Her symptoms disappeared in a few weeks.

A patient in comfortable circumstances furnished us an example of analogous phenomena, called into existence by a rather different mechanism. While she was at the table she arose, and her brother, in fun, seized her by the throat to make her sit down. She swallowed the wrong way. She was afflicted with trouble in swallowing for seven months. She could only manage with the greatest difficulty to swallow purées and liquids, and her meals took an infinitely long time. In six months she had lost twenty-four pounds. We must add that in her case her emotionalism was caused by material anxiety and unhappy conjugal relations, and that the underlying cause of this particular symptom was the fact that she had read in one of her children's books, the statement that one could be in danger of choking to death if one swallowed the wrong way.

There are other cases of patients who, by swallowing a liquid that was too hot, which slightly burned their throats, had got the idea into their heads for months that nothing could go down their œsophagus except liquids or broths.

Spasm of the œsophagus is caused by a mechanism analogous to these. As a pure and isolated symptom it is very rarely found, and the patients whom we have been able to study are much more apt to have the syndrome which we have just described, due to one of the following causes: An accidental phenomenon in the region of the pharynx or œsophagus; a secondary psychic fixation; consecutive phobias which are partly real, as a result of fixing the attention upon phenomena which are usually automatic.

Disturbances of the same kind may occur by a very curious mechanism. They occur in individuals who are troubled with slight rhinopharyngitis with granulations of the throat, and who have been treated by cauterization, or by repeated applications, and who thus have their attention continually directed to the region of their pharynx. They are always thinking about their swallowing, and finally get to the point where they experience in different degrees the whole series of symptoms which we have just described.

It seems to us that by an analogous mechanism might be explained in many cases that peculiar trouble, which may be fraught with various consequences. We refer to aërophagia or air-swallowing. This difficulty is developed in proportion to the number of movements in swallowing, each movement bringing with it a certain quantity of air, especially when one swallows nothing, so to speak, on top of a mouthful of food or a very small quantity of liquid.

It occurs in subjects who have their attention slightly but not intelligently focussed on their pharynx. To this class of individuals, in particular, belong those patients so well known to all physicians who cannot swallow pills or capsules. The patients continually swallow their saliva and thus create a type of interprandial aërophagia, that is to say they develop their trouble between meals. But there are also in certain individuals similar difficulties which spring from another mechanism, identical to that which creates these troubles we have described above. Following any accident whatsoever to the act of swallowing, these people, instead of not daring to swallow at all, no longer dare to take normal mouthfuls. They will only swallow very small quantities at one time, and thus the whole series of aërophagic phenomena are developed in them. Aërophagia, as one knows, makes itself worse, and the expulsion of gas often leads to the swallowing of a larger quantity of air.

We shall meet these patients again further on, amid the false gastropaths, whose study we shall now take up.

B. Gastric Symptoms in Nervous Patients.—Gastric disturbances are so common among nervous people, and particularly among those suffering from neurasthenia, that they have come to be considered an integral part and almost as a necessary element of the symptomatology. In reality it would not be fair to make such a sweeping generalization, for there are very many neurasthenics, who, to tell the truth, however, fix their attention on some other part of their body, but whose digestive tract is in admirable condition. Nevertheless, gastric troubles are extremely frequent, and need to be studied very carefully in detail, because their mechanism is extremely varied.

In the long nomenclature of gastric semiology, there is no objective or subjective symptom but that can be felt by a nervous patient, without any real organic affection to cause it.

One may find in them symptoms which are evidently objective, such as nausea, or even vomiting, as well as symptoms of true dilatation of the stomach closely corresponding to those of a very real, although purely neuropathic distention.

Semi-objective signs of various natures, such as pain caused by pressure, and finally the whole gamut of subjective sensations, from a simple feeling of heaviness to the most acute burning sensation, may very frequently be observed.

The pathogeny of all these troubles is varied. A part is played by real modifications of the gastric secretion, following anorexia, which suppresses the juice psychically, according to the mechanism which Pawlow has demonstrated.

Diminution of the tonicity of the gastric muscle, which in exhausted and emaciated neurasthenics bears the same relations to their stomachs as their muscles do to the strength of their limbs, and aërophagia which often occurs in neuropaths form the factors, in a certain way organic, in that they are of nervous origin, which determine a certain number of the troubles which are experienced.

The part which the psychism plays is none the less important. It results entirely from the patient settling his attention on his stomach, and on his digestive functions. Sometimes the patient's attention is drawn to his stomach by some passing difficulty, following too hearty a meal; sometimes it is a gastric trouble, such as those that occur in the later stages of pregnancy, which fixes the patient's psychism; sometimes it is the loss of several pounds weight following excessive physical exertion, such as night vigils, etc., which draws the attention of the patient to his functions of nutrition; sometimes, again, it is through articles in the newspaper, or advertisements of pharmaceutical preparations; sometimes, and *much more often,* it is medical advice that has given impetus to a series of phenomena which by mechanism of auto- or hetero-suggestion will go on developing themselves. A line of treatment has been laid down, medicines prescribed, and examinations made which have centred the patient's attention upon his digestive tract, and which keep him by reason of medical direction in a continual state of auto-observation. In fact, it is possible to start up a false gastropathy every time that a patient, for real or for fancied reasons, has had his attention directed to his stomach. Then one may see the development of a very interesting phenomenon, namely that each examination, each consultation, each new prescription, starts up some aggravation, or some extension of the troubles observed. At other times, and it not infrequently happens, it is an emotion, and especially a repeated emotion, which clutches the throat, makes one's stomach feel like lead, and takes away one's appetite, and which serves not only as a starting point, but as a means of development by reason of the bodily sensations which it creates.

The influence of the morale on the functions of the stomach is commonly accepted. Everyone knows that when he is in a temper or has a sin on his soul his appetite falls off, and his digestion is bad. Yet, notwithstanding, physicians have never properly recognized the importance of this fact.

But now let us take a case where there are real gastric disturbances, following nervous troubles, occurring in some region connected with the digestive tract, such, for instance, as constipation. As to the persistence and the encouragement, so to speak, given to digestive manifestations in nervous patients outside of all foreign intervention, they come from a psychological mechanism, which seems very simple to us. As a matter of fact the digestive function holds a leading place in our physical life, not only from the point of view of its importance, but also as to the time it occupies. It is psychically associated with a whole series of ideas and perceptions. The day is laid out according to meal-times, certain rooms of the house are given over to the preparation or consumption of food. One is obliged to order meals, and to plan one's life by them in such a way that the number of ideas which are associated with the digestive functions is very considerable; and once a digestive systematization is created in a patient, the facts and impressions of the day will continually serve to re-create or reinforce it.

Returning to the classification which we have already adopted, we shall study successively:

1. *Simple dyspepsias of neurasthenics.*
2. *Gastric phobias.*
3. *Characteristic pseudo-gastropathies.*

Finally a chapter will be devoted to the study of:

4. *Dilatation of the stomach in nervous patients.*
5. *Vomiting as a neuropathic manifestation.*

1. *Simple Dyspepsias of Neurasthenics.*—Appetite, if we are to believe the teachings of modern physiology, is the best stimulant to digestion. The neurasthenic is never hungry; therefore, he digests badly. As a matter of fact, the sensation of slow and difficult digestion, with a heavy feeling after meals, is very frequent in neurasthenics. Digestive disturbances have their objectivity in the active modifications of the gastric functions, but are none the less pathogenically and therapeutically of a purely psychopathic nature. Their mechanism lies in a very mild form of mental anorexia, to which the majority of neurasthenics are subject.

As for this anorexia itself, several elements combine to create it. The act of taking food requires, in fact, some effort, and one knows how distasteful effort is to the neurasthenic, whether it be intellectual, physical, or alimentary in its nature. The bother of getting himself fed starts an anorexia, and that kind of anorexia which especially avoids all kinds of foods which would require any kind of effort to prepare or eat. Very frequently, on the other hand, the neurasthenic is obsessed or preoccupied with some idea. Obsessions and preoccupations are in themselves capable of neutralizing to some degree the sensations of physical life, among which the sensation of appetite occupies a place in the front rank. Very frequently, moreover, obsessions and preoccupations act by the intervention of a state of unintermittent emotions which they occasion, leading to a whole series of impressions which take away the appetite.

The first class of facts is only interesting on account of the mechanism from which in such cases the digestive symptoms arise. Clinically the gastric symptomatology is usually swallowed up in the great number of phenomena of which the patients complain. Generally they are themselves aware of the contingent and accessory nature of these troubles. As they are the most common, they are also the least interesting of the functional gastropathies.

2. *Gastric Obsessions and Phobias.*—A neurasthenic is afflicted with vague dyspeptic troubles. He has no definite symptomatology; neither vomiting, regurgitations, pains, nor heart-burn. Sometimes he even has no special dyspeptic symptoms, not even those which we have just noted in our first class of patients. He has an excellent appetite, he digests well; being of an emotional type and easily depressed, he is liable to have obsessions. Sometimes spontaneously, and because he has heard it said that analogous conditions to his could be the forerunner of a poor state of digestion, but more often because his attention has been medically fixed on his digestive tract, he will become the victim of a true gastric obsession, combined with food phobias. Paying the strictest attention to himself, he will begin to classify foods. This one has no perceptible effect upon him, that one he cannot digest at all, while, on the other hand, another agrees with him remarkably well. Taken by themselves, certain foods are easily digested, but eaten together, they do not agree with him at all. The patient's whole life is regulated by an incalculable number of restrictions, all of which have to do with the digestive functions, and which, in proportion as his affection becomes established, grow more numerous and more complicated. If you question any of these patients at the beginning of their trouble, you will be astonished at the very slight symptoms of which they complain. Further, it may be noted that the majority of the difficulties from which they suffer, and for which they hold their food responsible, have only the remotest connection with the digestive tract. It is in this class of patients that you will find individuals who

do not eat in order that they may do better work; in this class also you will find a whole category of people who, having read books upon dietetics, have begun to put themselves through a regular course of experiments. It is the form of functional gastropathy in which, among society people, the elements of fashion and snobbery play their rôles. The well-served and bountifully provided tables of our fathers have been turned, as it were, into veritable dietetic tables. Mr. X. has his régime, Mrs. Y. has hers. We must hasten to add that often their régimes are wholly conventional, and that they do not refuse the appeal of a well-served appetizing dish, or that, when followed most rigorously at meal-time, they cease to exist at the confectioner's or at a late supper at some social affair. The matter might be taken very lightly, as worth nothing but a passing word of ridicule, if it were not that people who are predisposed by obsessions, phobias, and scruples sometimes go so far that they meet disaster.

We have seen patients of this kind who, by reason of insufficient food, and extreme malnutrition, have become so excessively thin and weak, that they have fallen prey to organic affections, and although such cases with grave physical consequences are not very numerous, the moral and social effects are, on the other hand, very frequent, particularly in the middle and poorer classes of society. While in the majority of cases stomachic phobia is grafted on to a more or less acute gastric condition, it is also often the case that it is the gastric psychosis which makes the patient neurasthenic, by reason of the moral and material preoccupations which it begets.

Slowly accumulated savings are melting away at the doctor's and druggist's. The constant watching of the state of his stomach diverts the individual from his daily business. The inevitable outcome is social and business failure, which finally leads to a serious and lasting neurasthenic state, due to the lack of the essential elements required to resume normal life.

And why should all this be? Because the unfortunate person in whom a gastric obsession has been set going has never come across a physician who could determine the exact nature of his trouble, and put him on his guard against all the consequences which might result from it; and because, on the contrary, it generally happens that the physician who has cared for him has not been sufficiently warned himself of the extreme impressionability of such persons, and has unconsciously done all that he could to set him definitely upon his downward way.

Such patients are purely nervous or purely mental cases. The pathogeny of their condition is evident, and scarcely needs discussion. It only needs a few well-directed questions to bring it out sharply.

Do you want examples? Here are a few taken from a class of patients in society.

Mr. X., fifty-two years of age, and a high dignitary, of large fortune and very well known in the Parisian world, has lived for the last twenty years upon poached eggs, boiled potatoes, broiled meats, and cooked fruits. His diet has been limited exclusively to these four foods. Mr. X. often dines in town. On these occasions he fasts, because his rule is strict and absolute, and he will not allow himself a single exception. For twenty years he has never once tried to evade these dietetic obligations. And what was the origin of all this? A few vague dyspeptic troubles, without any logical cause, and of no duration, which happened to follow an emotional depression caused by some family troubles. Grafted onto these troubles was a doctor's prescription, which resulted in so fixing the patient's mind in this direction that for twenty years he has nursed a stomach, which otherwise would have cheerfully tolerated a bottle of good Burgundy at every meal.

This case is simply amusing, for the patient, by the way, eats an enormous amount, is very active, and his morale is excellent.

We might cite the case of a certain patient who could eat nothing except bread; of another who could eat eggs in the morning, but could not touch them at night. It would make an extremely curious chapter, and one full of surprises, if one were to note all the dietetic selections practised by such patients. But, as a matter of fact, as long as the restrictions in food are simply qualitative, and the modifications of diet nothing but a habit, and the patient's morale remains sound, such doings are not at all serious. Nevertheless they sometimes turn out unfortunately after all. The following case is an example:

It concerns a man thirty-six years of age, an officer of infantry in a town in Northern France. He had been ill for eleven years. Having failed at St. Cyr, he enlisted. He succeeded in being admitted to Saint Maixent. There he worked tremendously hard, was constantly overtaxed, and left the school absolutely run down. He then found himself confronted by a whole series of difficulties in the way of his career which overwhelmed him morally. Becoming thinner and thinner, and having lost thirty pounds in a few months, he began to pay attention to his stomach.

He then went to see one physician after another. Some examined his gastric chemistry, others put him upon a diet; there was one who made him undergo treatment by static electricity. From that time on he had a fixed idea; the unfortunate man took no notice of anything else but his stomach, and neglected his calling. *Without ever having had the slightest characteristic gastric symptom,* he was continually trying to find out what foods digested easily, and which did not digest so well. Following all his own personal observations, as well as the various régimes which had been laid down for him, he continually restricted his diet more and more, both as to quantity and quality, until it was extremely reduced. His condition becoming graver, he gave himself up to doing nothing. To the preoccupations of his career were added those of material cares. In this very emaciated condition, he was dragging out a pitiful and apparently hopeless existence.

As a matter of fact, this patient is completely cured, has returned to his former way of living, and takes no more interest whatsoever in his stomach.

We could cite thousands of examples of this kind. There is not a week but at the Wednesday consultation at the Salpêtrière at least half a dozen such patients present themselves, and tell this stereotyped tale: "I have grown very thin; I no longer eat anything. I have been obliged to give up my work, or my profession. I had to do it, for they say I have stomach trouble." This procession is all the more lamentable because the patients have nothing the matter with them except purely psychic difficulties. Their affection belongs by definition to the category of avoidable diseases. All their physical, material, and moral failings would never have occurred if they had been cared for at first by a physician who paid some little attention to their mental hygiene and psychic prophylaxis, and who knew by what mechanism this alimentary restriction had been established in them. It is this mechanism which we now wish to develop a little.

The Psychic Mechanism which Leads False Gastropaths to Adopt Certain Régimes.—In the great majority of cases the patients whom we have had to treat have not been gastropaths from the start. More often, at the beginning of their trouble they were neurasthenic, or depressed, and experiencing troubles of a general nature, among which a lack of appetite, or, to express it better, a feeling of not wanting to take the trouble to eat, occupied an important place. The disturbance which was to follow was in reality born at that moment by an *error of interpretation.* The patients, either spontaneously or more often as a result of therapeutic intervention, attributed everything that they felt to gastric troubles, when more often the whole fault lay in their morale, and the intensity of their suffering was measured by the degree of their depression.

From this moment the first psychomotor, or psychosecretory manifestations appeared, and with them the whole well-known series of sensations of pressure, heaviness, flatulency after meals, which nearly all of these patients will enumerate as a regular thing. They very naturally try to remedy these troubles by changing their diet. In this way they plunge right into the downward path of choosing and rejecting certain foods.

How, and according to what laws, do such suppressions and elections become established? It is very certain that the means will be purely mental. In regard to the general lack of appetite of the patient, the process is more often apt to be of a negative order. The patient will keep upon his list of foods, not those which please him the most, but rather those which are least distasteful to him. The problem, therefore, presents itself in the following manner. According to what mechanism is one food better tolerated than another by this special class of patients?

This mechanism, in order to be brought out clearly, ought to be studied in patients of the poorer class, or at least in the less well educated class of society. With those who, being more intelligent, have their own ideas, which are often totally wrong, on the degree of digestibility of any food, the matter becomes complicated. The more or less preconceived ideas which they have of food values, and of the length of time which it takes to digest such or such a product, guide them in laying down their dietary. But even among these latter, the mechanism, at bottom, remains the same and is revealed by a little careful study.

The food which would be the best tolerated would be that which will necessitate the least effort to take and which by its qualities would awaken to the least degree the psychic idea of eating.

This, on analysis, seems to us the principle which unconsciously serves as the guiding therapy to most false gastropaths in the elaboration of their régime.

This is why, at the very beginning, they eliminate from their foods *all which are hard to chew or difficult to swallow.*

It is well established that, among such patients, a food may be excluded from the daily diet because *it sticks in the throat.* Such was the case with a patient whom we had to care for, who had no constriction of the œsophagus whatever, but who could not eat bread unless it had previously been soaked in water or milk.

It was for similar reasons to this, and because it was difficult and took a long time to chew them, that these patients with gastric phobias always cut meats out of their diet in the order which corresponds precisely to the degree of difficulty that they have in masticating them: first, beef and mutton, then chicken, fish later, when it had not already been off their diet list at the start, for one or other of the reasons which we shall examine a little later.

It practically means that, if the patient refuses to make the effort which the taking of rational nourishment implies, all foods which by their taste or odor remind him that he ought to take nourishment, will one after the other be crossed off his food list. These are the foods which "turn the patient's stomach," and take away the little appetite which he may seem to have. After having taken a mouthful of them, the patient believes himself to be, *or feels,* nourished. At least, such are the expressions which we have almost constantly heard our patients use.

Still another factor comes in, — the idea of quantity. Here is a patient whose chosen diet was established. If small quantities at a time of one of his chosen foods were presented to him he would take them, and would manage in the end to get enough. Try, on the other hand, however, to make him take a considerable quantity of this same food at one time, and he would say: "*Never, I could never eat all that.*" He would immediately be frightened at the effort he had to make, and this food from that time forth would not agree with him. If it did not agree with him once it would be sharply and definitely cut off from his daily diet.

That is to say, in fact, that every time that the psychic impression of being obliged to make an effort to take food occurs, whether by reason of the difficulty of mastication, or swallowing, or whether on account of the taste, or odor, or quantity of the food presented, the patient will examine himself, analyze his feelings, and seek to establish —and on this head he will always manage to establish—some unpleasant result. This is the true foundation of the mechanism of alimentary restriction in false gastropaths.

Among those who, being better educated, have been in part influenced by theoretic ideas, and among those also who, under the guidance of physicians, have been put upon various régimes, the outcome is the same, thus verifying the mechanism of this phenomenon that we have just explained.

In the end these patients get to the point where they can take *nothing but soft food, semi-liquid or liquid, and only in the smallest quantities.*

As a matter of fact, in the majority of our false gastropaths, who had been suffering for a sufficiently long time, their regular food allowance would oftenest consist of milk (in quantity rarely more than a quart in twenty-four hours) and one or two eggs. Sometimes they added to this diet some patent pre-digested food or vegetables in a purée. The very rare exception would be when they could take a little finely chopped meat fairly floating in a broth.

We must hasten, however, to add, that all these restrictions are not necessarily regularly progressive. According to the moral condition of the moment our false gastropaths may arrive at this ultimate régime, which we have just described, either very rapidly, or slowly and surely, or by successive starts, separated sometimes by periods of great improvement.

This study, which shows just how far these subjects who have simple phobias of the stomach may go in the matter of dietary restriction, leads us to the third class of patients.

3. *Established False Gastropathies.*—Nervous gastropathies with complex symptomatology may be established at the outset. More often these affections are only the end results of the forms which we have just described. Here the patients whom we are now considering show distinct signs of recognized gastric affections. Vomiting of food, late vomiting, occurring several hours after eating, or even in the morning before breakfast; heart-burn, faint feelings of regurgitation, frequent

eructations, pains at the pit of the stomach, occurring spontaneously or after taking food; tardy pains with heart-burn, sharp pain on an empty stomach soothed by taking food or hot drinks; pain to the touch in the region of the stomach: all these are found variously combined. Here, you would say, is pyloric stenosis with stasis; there you would say hyperchlorhydria; here you would believe there was a gastric fermentation; sometimes even the thought of an ulcer, or a cancer in the early stages of its development will come to you, so definite is the symptomatology, and so changed sometimes is the general condition as to seem to imply the existence of an organic affection of the stomach.

Before entering into the discussion of these cases, we wish to relate a certain number of observations:

Mr. C., forty-two years of age, an engineer, has been, for ten years, nursing himself for a gastric affection characterized by the following symptoms: heaviness; distention and feeling of weight after meals; three or four hours later, feelings of heart-burn; sour regurgitation, and frequent eructations; almost complete loss of appetite; vomitings, rather frequent and copious, occurring several hours after meals, and even in the morning before breakfast; very marked emaciation and insomnia.

The affection has very evidently had its starting point in alcoholic excesses, and, although for ten years the patient has completely ceased to drink, the original trouble has nevertheless persisted. Our patient, who is a foreigner, has been in all the world-famed sanitaria. He has been in Berlin, in Paris, in Switzerland. The results, obtained by means of therapeutic methods based exclusively on régime and pharmaceutic medication, have been absolutely nil. He came to us in exactly the same condition that he was in ten years ago, except, however, that his mental state had grown progressively worse. He felt extremely exasperated in not being able to lead the life that everybody else led, and he found himself limited in his activities by his gastric trouble, and his feeling about his condition had gone to such lengths that sometimes he thought of suicide. Now in a month's time this patient was put upon his feet by psychotherapy, and his gastric troubles have absolutely disappeared.

Madame B., forty-eight years of age, a very nervous woman, living in Paris, and having led a life of considerable excitement, has been cared for for the last two years by stomach specialists. They told her that she had an attack of hyposthenic dyspepsia, with secondary fermentations. As a matter of fact, she presented all the classic signs of this affection, distentions, pains, regurgitations, gas, anorexia, biliousness and constipation. She was put upon a reduced diet by one of her physicians, and lost considerable weight, while the phenomena, sometimes objective and sometimes subjective, only grew worse. Then she was subjected to bismuth treatment of the stomach, and again there was no result. In addition she was ordered to take absorptive powders, combined with nux vomica. The results were wholly unfavorable. She was a purely nervous woman whom the proper means cured in three weeks.

Here are a certain number of cases, taken from our hospital practice:

The first is that of a woman, fifty-seven years of age, cared for in the Pinel Ward, bed number 16, in the isolation service, which one of us organized at the Salpêtrière. She stayed there from the 28th of March to the 7th of June, 1905. I give her history in her own words.

"Having suffered with my stomach for twenty-five years, as the result of an emotional disturbance, I had completely lost my appetite. I never felt the slightest need of eating, and I felt aversion to the sight of food, especially of meat. I consulted more than fifty physicians. They all prescribed a milk diet. I could never take more than two quarts of milk and one or two eggs a day, oftener nothing at all.

"In all the hospitals where I went for consultation, they looked at my yellow skin, and everywhere with the same thought: 'Oh! nothing can be done for her.' They were convinced that I either had a cancer or pyloric lesions. Two years ago they wanted to operate upon me. The physician who was taking care of me in the last place, becoming discouraged, sent me to a specialist, who kept me under observation for eighteen months.

"They always put me upon a milk diet, but finally I could take almost none, as I suffered too much from pains in the stomach and intestines. I continued to grow thinner, and I was completely discouraged. They tried lavage of the stomach, plasters, gavage; but nothing did me any good."

This auto-observation needs to be amplified in several points, and in particular as to the starting point of this affection which brought the patient to us.

Twenty-five years ago, she had a husband, who has since died of general paresis, who was brutal to her, and who one fine day, reversing the proper order of things, wanted to lock her up in an asylum. She was intensely frightened, and felt her stomach close as it were. Since that time the same sensation would come every time that the patient experienced any emotion. And emotions were of daily occurrence, being caused by her son, who was lacking in regard for her. She used to wait in anguish for him to come into the house. But the moment that she saw him come, she would experience a sensation of restriction, and could no longer eat. Thus were developed and encouraged the evidences of this gastropathy, whose symptomatology was at one time so characteristic that surgical intervention was deemed necessary.

We have nothing particular to note concerning the residence of the patient at the hospital. The first day she took three quarts of milk, at the end of the week she was taking five, and by degrees she was put upon an ordinary diet. Weighing eighty-eight pounds when she came in, she weighed one hundred and fourteen when she went out,—she had therefore gained twenty-six pounds. She went away completely cured. She has been seen several times, and again this spring (1910), and she has kept in excellent health for five years.

This was a case in which a casual examination, owing to the cachectic appearance of the patient and the gastric symptomatology, would suggest the diagnosis of a neoplasm. In reality it was nothing but a case of a gastropathy, the functional nature of which appeared when questions as to its etiology were carefully put.

Another patient, aged thirty-six, entered the Pinel Ward, bed number 11, on March 22, and went out completely cured on June 5, 1905, having gained eighteen pounds in weight. Here is what she wrote us before leaving, on our request that she should relate her own history:

"I am a natural child. My mother married, and had two children. I have always been treated as a stranger. As I was by nature very affectionate I experienced great grief on this account, which increased as I grew older. When I became old enough to work they gave me no leisure. I had to work without any recreation. Sometimes six weeks would go by without my having a chance to go out of the house. I became anæmic, and had three hemorrhages from the lungs. After that my mother had a long illness and then I had to work day and night. Then I had a mucous fever. In consequence I became very nervous, and could neither eat nor sleep. I was always wanting to cry, and instead of being encouraged, I was repulsed. I led this sad existence until I was twenty-nine years of age, when I married. Having a good husband I was better. At the end of the year, I had a child. He died in a single day. My condition was then aggravated anew. I went several months without being able to eat. I suffered extremely with my stomach. Three years ago one of my children was nearly killed. My condition then became somewhat serious, so that I could not take more than a quart of milk a day. I consulted ten physicians, who treated me for gastric dyspepsia, and dilatation of the stomach, but no treatment did me any good."

On questioning this patient on the stomachic symptomatology of which she complained on entering the service, this is what was found: heart-burn, very sharp pains after meals, and particularly when she had taken meat; a sensation of tension and distention after meals, with very slow digestion; pain brought on by pressure in the region of the pit of the stomach. It was more than could be expected that physicians who were not sufficiently alert should fail to be led to believe in the real existence of a gastropathy.

But, eight days after her entrance, the patient took five quarts of milk in twenty-four hours. It was, nevertheless, very difficult to make her take meat. During the month of April she consented to try it for the first time, then she refused it again. At that time it was necessary to be rather determined in this matter. She decided to try meat diet again, and in ten days she succeeded in taking and digesting a beefsteak every other day, when formerly a single mouthful caused her intolerable pain.

By the time she left the hospital, her stomachic psychism was completely under control. "She digested without knowing it." Moreover, it seemed that, under the influence of her sojourn in the Salpêtrière, she had succeeded in curbing her emotional tendencies somewhat, and had herself pretty well in hand.

Here is then a second instance where a stomachic symptomatology, that was sufficiently pronounced to deceive several physicians, proved to be in fact only a false gastropathy. The mechanism of the progressive psychic localization showed itself clearly. Of an emotional temperament, and having undergone a series of small shocks when she was overworked, she became first a neurasthenic. Then little by little, largely due to the different diagnoses of physicians, her stomach first came upon the scene and then occupied the whole stage. She felt all the symptoms which the doctors had tried to find in her case. The proof of this lies in the very diversity of the established diagnoses.

A woman forty-eight years old entered the Pinel Ward in June, 1905, in whose case many physicians would have made a diagnosis of pyloric stenosis, or Reichmann's disease.

We shall let her, also, tell her own story.

"You have asked me some of the details which brought about the condition in which I arrived here. When I was very young, I was obliged to work extremely hard, but, as I had a good constitution, several hours of rest would suffice to keep up my strength.

"During the siege of 1870, I underwent a great many privations, but they had no effect upon me. It also seemed to me that work and privations never hurt me. It was only mental worries that in the long run were able to break down my energy and my will. I could have been very happy, but I had the unfortunate idea of wanting to keep my mother with me in my household, and in spite of all my efforts I never managed to make my mother and my husband agree. I only succeeded in making all three of us horribly miserable, and that lasted ten years. In these ten years of friction and tears I became very irritable and very nervous.

"In the month of September, 1896, I had attacks of vomiting, with a feeling of aversion for all food. At night I would throw up water and bile and in the daytime I vomited nearly everything I took. My weight went down to only ninety-six and a half pounds. This state lasted three years and a half.

"In the month of May, 1902, I lost my mother. The vomiting and pain which I had experienced came back. As this condition, which I was helpless to overcome, caused me great moral discomfort, I decided to go to the hospital. I first went to Dr. Barth, at Necker, who sent me to Dr. Dejerine at the Salpêtrière, assuring me that I would be cured."

On the fifth day, this patient took five quarts of milk. Her weight increased rapidly. At the end of three weeks she was put upon regular diet. She digested with the greatest ease all the food that was given to her. She no longer knew that she had a stomach. She had gained twenty-two pounds, when at the end of July, 1905, she left the hospital.

Here is the case of a young patient, whom we have had in the Pinel Ward for three months. Although she was very stubborn during the first weeks about her treatment, nevertheless, she ended by being cured. Hers was a case of painful gastropathy, simulating those that are described under the name of hyperchlorhydric attacks.

She was twenty-seven years old, and had suffered since she was twenty-one. When she was a little girl she was not very strong, and being very sensitive, she had had her feelings wounded by unfeeling relatives, who reproached her for the care and expense which her health caused. As she would have liked to have earned her own living, the state of her health weighed on her mind, till it was really an obsession. Suffering first from simple digestive troubles, she soon had characteristic gastropathic symptoms, heaviness, pains, heart-burn, vomitings, each time after taking food, and the impossibility of taking milk, which "curdled on her stomach"; nothing was lacking. This patient left the Pinel Ward, on the 12th of January, 1905. In September we had news of her. Everything was going almost as it should. From time to time she still felt attacks of depression, during which she suffered with her stomach, but she knew "that she could, and that she ought to take the upper hand," and she succeeded in doing so.

Here is the history of a young girl, nineteen years old, who spent three months in the Pinel Ward in 1905. She complained of very sharp pains in her stomach which came on two or three hours after-meals, with acidity, burning sensations, feelings of tension and abdominal distention, heaviness and sleepiness. Here again the epigastric region was painful and the patient would hardly let herself be touched, when they tried to palpate there.

In this case also, therapeutic treatment was the cause, and the words—weighty words for a young and impressionable mind—dilatation of the stomach, hyperchlorhydric dyspepsia and gastric fermentation had been pronounced, and taken at their full value.

The mechanism of this gastropathy took a long time to trace, but at the end of several days we succeeded in gaining the patient's confidence, and learned from what it arose. It was an attempt upon her virginity which had given rise to all her ill-health. Entering the hospital weighing ninety-nine pounds, the patient left weighing one hundred and twenty-three pounds, and was no longer concerned about her stomach. We have had recent news of her, and her health continues to be excellent.

Here is another history of a woman forty-five years of age, the mother of a family, whose life has been very hard. She was reduced to penury after having lived in comfort. For several years she had had the care of an invalid sister. Her husband died six months ago. One of her sons was about to be married against her wishes.

For some years she had complained that her digestion seemed slow and difficult. But, after the death of her husband, it took on quite a different aspect.

Vomiting, even in the morning on an empty stomach, cramps that were relieved by food, elective anorexia for meat, waking in the middle of the night with a sensation of emptiness in the stomach, such were the symptoms of which she complained. There were no acid regurgitations, and no marked eructations.

This patient entered the Pinel Ward the first of November, 1905, and the second day after she was there she took five quarts of milk. By the 15th of November she had gained nine pounds.

She was soon put upon regular diet, which agreed with her perfectly, and she left the Salpêtrière cured at the end of six weeks. She had gained twelve pounds, and when we saw her last she was in excellent condition.

Before entering the Salpêtrière she had seen nine physicians, who had treated her for a gastric affection, the name of which changed with every physician consulted. It seemed in her case almost as if the whole stomachic psychosis might be of medical origin. Complaining vaguely of her digestion, she had had her attention fixed on her stomach by medical questions and examinations which had preceded any of the active symptoms which had been previously sought.

A case bearing on this subject is that of a young woman, twenty-eight years of age, who, having formerly been rheumatic, had a mitral lesion of the heart, that, being badly compensated for, caused her to pant when she made any effort.

In her the gastric troubles were noticeable chiefly after meals, and especially when she made any movement. They consisted in slight regurgitation, with frequent eructation, and a sensation of heaviness and weight and distention after eating. When she walked, as she did from time to time, these first phenomena would grow worse, and vomiting set in.

This patient at the end of fifteen days had gained four pounds. She no longer had any pains, nor did she vomit. It took two months to accomplish her cure.

What in her case was the mechanism which produced these gastric troubles? She had had a pregnancy which had ended six months before, in the course of which she had had a number of gastric phenomena, and in particular very frequent vomiting. It was in this way that her attention had been drawn for the first time to that part of her body. But her pregnancy had also influenced her heart condition, and when afterwards she wanted to walk, she would immediately begin to suffer from shortness of breath. She attributed the whole thing to her stomach, and from that arose this strange gastropathy, which was exaggerated when the patient walked, and grew less when she rested, with regular variation.

In this particular case there certainly was a somatic lesion, but it was of the heart, and not of the stomach, and it was this previous psychic orientation of the patient which was the cause of the false gastropathy.

Here finally is our last case:

Madame M., forty-nine years of age, entered the Pinel Ward on the 4th of January, 1906. She was suffering from a gastropathy, which dated back to 1870, a gastropathy with recurring attacks, which grew worse at intervals, but which did not become definitely established until 1890. At this time she had a very bad influenza, which left her much exhausted for some time. As she was indispensable to her husband, whom she helped in his little business, the inactivity which she was forced to endure was extremely hard to bear. While thus morally upset and weakened, she was seized with very marked gastric disturbances,—with vomitings, sometimes with mucus, sometimes with bile, but never of food. She exhibited great interest in the advice of her physician, and paid close attention to the character of these vomitings, so much so that they continued until her entrance to the hospital.

She went away on the 17th of February, completely cured, having gained ten pounds in weight. She was seen quite recently. The vomitings had never returned, and everything pointed to the conclusion that they had disappeared. The patient was convinced of this as well as ourselves.

When we tried to find the exact point of departure in this patient's affection, it was quite easy to settle the origin, and to determine the mechanism.

It was during the privations of the siege of Paris that she felt her first gastric disturbances. One can only too easily picture the condition of a little anæmic girl of fourteen under these circumstances. She was taken to a physician for a consultation, but he treated her for her stomach, and with powders and other medications which were freely dispensed to her, she plunged headlong into a functional gastropathy. A few digestive troubles which she had felt as a consequence of the unusual food during the siege was the origin of her sickly condition, but therapy established her troubles upon a firm basis, and having oriented the patient's psychism made a definite thing of what from its nature should have been merely transitory. Thus the functional gastropathies also are the offspring of the siege . . . and of the physicians.

These are a few facts. We could multiply them almost indefinitely. But they must be interpreted. To start with, there are a certain number of definite ideas which we have gained as a direct result of our observations.

The first is, that there exist gastropathies, having all the clinical appearances of what are called organic gastropathies, and which are susceptible of cure without any kind of special therapy, by the general processes of treating the psychoneuroses.

The second is, that in all these cases the psychic factors, which appear to have intervened, are the indefinite psychic prolongation of acute conditions by the phenomena of auto- or hetero-suggestion, particularly by medical education, and finally emotional manifestations.

The third is, that the symptomatology of our patients was sufficiently acute, and the objective phenomena sufficiently numerous to dispel from the start any question of error of interpretation on the part of observers, or of simulation on the part of the patients. The problem, therefore, presents itself to us in the following manner: Just to what point is emotion, error in mental interpretation, medical education, suggestion, capable of creating gastric symptoms? And, on the other hand, to what degree is there any identity between these manifestations, shown to be of a neuropathic nature, and the recognized gastric affections?

First of all, it is very certain that we may be reproached for not having supported our observations by chemical examinations of the gastric secretions. Why have we not made such examinations? Because, first, we consider them as only secondary in value, from the point of view of diagnosis, and then—we say it frankly—because we regard them as irreconcilable with a psychotherapeutic treatment, which logically depends upon itself.

What we have just said upon the subject of examining the gastric juice, we might repeat word for word apropos of the radioscope, or of radiography of the stomach, a method which also has, as its principal result, the further establishment of the patient in ways contrary to those in which one is trying to, and in which one ought to lead him.

But, although we ourselves have not made it a rule to examine the gastric juice, we might be permitted to add that a very great number of our patients, either at the hospital or private clinic, have given us the results of the chemical examinations which had previously been made upon them by the most competent physicians and chemists; and these analyses have not always disclosed a remarkable modification of the normal chemistry. This argues nothing against us. What is of much interest in itself, and shows the slight value of this examination of the gastric juice, from the diagnostic point of view, is that in the majority of these patients, and in particular those in private practice —who frequently examine into the condition of their gastric chemistry —the results were most variable. Sometimes in fact there was hyperchlorhydria, and sometimes hypochlorhydria, sometimes again a normal chemistry. And this shows us that even when there are considerable modifications in gastric chemistry, there is no reason to state that one has to deal with an affection not amenable to the ordinary treatment of the psychoneuroses.

On the other hand, what is there astonishing in the fact that these various psychic modifications just enumerated by us, such as moral shocks, grief, preoccupation—on the etiological importance of which we have so lengthily insisted—should be able to bring about a very considerable number of gastric manifestations?

Nobody doubts that an emotion is capable of producing gastric disturbances. Vomiting is a phenomenon which can very frequently be created by emotion. Psychic impressions, such as disgust, inspired by a certain food, or even simply by the memory of a food, are able to interrupt digestion, and bring on nausea, even vomitings. Is not anorexia, created by gastric obsessions, able to directly cause the psycho-secretory modifications with which we are familiar? Have we not just seen mental anorexia, a psychic phenomenon, bring about, in the gastric functions, such secondary disturbances that it was sometimes very difficult to learn to take food again?

Under these conditions, it seems to us legitimate to hold that in very many cases there is a substitution of a psychic pathogeny for a peripheral pathogeny, without denying the real existence of motor or secretory modifications, which, however, we consider as being created directly by emotional factors, such as education, error in mental interpretation, auto- or hetero-suggestion.

And, if one is willing to admit, on the other hand, what is only too evident, that all trouble that is susceptible of being cured by persuasion is a neuropathic trouble, the demonstration of the existence of affections of the stomach, organic in appearance, but psychic in cause, would seem to us to be unquestionably established.

It remains for us to ascertain what is the proportion of cases in which a peripheral pathogeny is imposed. Most certainly we do not seek to deny the existence of alcoholic or drug gastropathies. We are quite convinced that there are hyperchlorhydric dyspepsias of which ulceration may be an accompanying factor, and which have developed without any neuropathic cause. There are gastric troubles in connection with other organs, the liver, peritoneum, intestines, kidneys, etc. It is none the less true that, if we refer to our personal statistics, among the persons whom we have treated, and who complained of dyspeptic troubles, more than four-fifths were purely and simply nervous. Nearly all those in this last category had been, we ought to add, considered by others as gastropaths properly so-called, and had been futilely treated for a long time—often for years. We repeat again—for just here lies the question of difference and misunderstanding—that we do not deny the actual existence of symptoms verified by stomach specialists; only, instead of referring them to some primitive disturbance of the solar plexus, or gastric innervation, we say that it is necessary to go back to the generating psychic cause of all these observed phenomena.

The evolution, the progress, the diagnostic study of these functional gastropathies all tend, however, to confirm a certain interpretation of things. Do we not find that these affections are variable, and dependent to a certain extent upon the mental state of the patient, or his degree of obsession? Do we not see symptoms, hitherto non-existent, appearing because they have been looked for? And the symptomatology presented by our patients always keeps pace with their education, which is most often medical. Sometimes certain of these patients, under the influence of some violent emotion, or of a change in their lives, completely forget their gastric affection from one day to another. What physician has not seen young girls of a marriageable age, who had dyspeptic attacks, completely get rid of all their troubles after a happy marriage? The organicists, it is true, attribute everything to the modification of the ovarian secretion; but, how common it is, when a child is seriously ill, or the household is not running smoothly, for all these dyspeptic troubles which had been forgotten—that is the word—to reappear.

It is, therefore, the variability of the affection in its intensity, in relation to moral causes, its genesis at the time of some shock or crisis of life, as well as its too rich symptomatology, as a result of the most diverse suggestions, which characterizes for us the pseudo-gastropaths, and permits us to make a diagnosis.

4. *Dilatation of the Stomach in Nervous Patients.*—The history of dilatation of the stomach in neurasthenics is of great interest. This is because dilatation of the stomach, associated or not with visceral ptosis, has been for some time considered an important factor in neurasthenic conditions, by reason of the fermentations which it causes, and the auto-intoxication of which it is the starting-point.

As a matter of fact, dilatation of the stomach, with all its physical characteristics of percussion and succussion, appears objectively with some degree of frequency in neuropaths. Under what circumstances, and by what means?

It is met, first of all, in cases of major neurasthenia with exhaustion and emaciation. We have sometimes seen in such persons such extreme dilatation of the stomach, that this organ descends almost to the pubis. This dilatation seems to us to be the result of the general atony of the patients. There is no question in such cases of pyloric stenosis or primitive organic affection of the gastric muscle. The proof of this is seen directly from the fact that the dilatation of the stomach disappears very rapidly, as fast as the patient's weight increases, and that this occurs in spite of a diet which, in accordance with general ideas, would appear absolutely paradoxical from the large quantity of liquid which is represented by the four and a half or five quarts of milk taken each day. There is, therefore, a dilatation of the stomach in nervous patients, that is dependent on their general condition, and in which gastric atony is only a result of the emaciation, and the loss of tone of the muscles of the organ itself as well as in its relation to the body as a whole.

This form is by far the most frequent, but it is not the only one. In fact by the mechanism already explained, the nervous patient may be an aërophage, where a purely passive dilatation of the stomach is characterized by extreme variability, and by all the objective signs of aërophagia.

But in other cases different mechanisms come into play. We have seen patients suffering from marked constipation, who presented at the same time a very considerable dilatation of the stomach. It is true they were very much emaciated, but not to the same degree as the major neurasthenics whom we have just described. In such cases it was often sufficient to give a slight purgative, and to pay a little attention to educating the functions of the bowels to be regular, and one would find that the gastric dilatation had suddenly disappeared. It has seemed to us that some people who are relatively weak might be described as having a sort of retro-dilatation of the stomach.

Finally there are dilatations of the stomach due to a complex mechanism, in which the atony of emaciation, constipation, and aërophagia may, for various reasons, all come in as associated factors.

It is no less true that in certain subjects, if one tried to improve the symptoms that are felt, by restriction of food, as is only too often done, we would be apt to aggravate the local as well as the general symptoms.

As to the pathogenic rôle played by these conditions of stomach dilatation in the genesis of the whole symptomatology, it appears to us absolutely nil. The proof of this lies in the inconstancy of the phenomenon, and in its rapid disappearance under proper treatment. Many patients may remain neurasthenic for weeks and weeks after the dilatation has disappeared; while, on the other hand, unkind as it may be to point it out, the fact remains that many neurasthenics have never shown the slightest sign of such an affection.

In short, dilatation of the stomach is only a secondary manifestation in neurasthenic conditions. From the therapeutic point of view, except for the causes which engender it, it ought to be passed over without comment.

5. *Vomiting as a Neuropathic Manifestation.*—Although vomiting occurs more often, in the course of the psychoneuroses, in connection with a whole series of other troubles, which go to complete the symptomatology, yet it may also in some circumstances constitute the only objective symptom presented by the patients. For this reason it deserves a special description, as well as for the reason that the various mechanisms which can produce it are very interesting and very suggestive.

Vomiting in general pathologic physiology is a reflex phenomenon, produced by various peripheral stimuli, of which the starting-point may be found in the pharynx, the larynx, the stomach, the peritoneum, etc.

In neuropaths one may distinguish, *a priori* from the point of view of pathological physiology, three kinds of vomiting, namely, vomiting created by emotion, and emotional states, vomiting created by the exaggeration of the peripheral sensibilities, and finally, outside of all peripheral excitation, vomiting in simple relation with mental representations of any kind.

Emotional vomiting is a fact which we are no better able to explain than we are any of the other emotional reactions. It is a particular way that certain subjects have of expressing their emotional condition. Their emotion, as we might vulgarly say, takes them in the stomach. The vomiting may be the only objective emotional reaction, as also it may be accompanied by phenomena of cardiac depression, with or without a tendency to faint, or vertigo, etc. However it may be, the curious thing about it is that those subjects who have once reacted to an emotion by vomiting, will react consecutively in the same manner to all the emotions which may happen to come to them.

Mrs. X. is a lady seventy years of age, who for a certain number of years has complained of gastric disturbances which consist exclusively of vomitings, which come on every time she experiences any emotion whether it be great or small. Being of a very emotional and sentimental nature, she has not found in certain of her children those sentiments of affection which she would like to see. Very often, when she comes to take a meal at the house of one of them, she finds herself chilled and upset by the attitude which they show to her. That is enough, she is obliged to leave the table, and begins vomiting.

These symptoms date back five or six years. They were produced the first time on the occasion of a violent emotion, but at the time they did not make any impression on the patient, who, being very intelligent, took into consideration their emotional cause. It was not until much later that she paid any attention to it, when, although the memory of this great emotion of her life had disappeared, she found herself, in spite of everything, reacting in the same inconstant manner to all her little emotions.

That suggestion played its part with this lady, not only at the actual time, but in the too frequent reproductions of her symptoms afterwards, is not only possible, but probable; but, at the beginning, all the circumstances of the psychological condition of the patient would have seemed to be against the purely suggestive interpretation of the phenomena.

Emotion, it would thus appear, can play an autonomous pathogenic rôle in the onset of vomiting, as well as in its persistent recurrence.

Vomiting once started, or at least made too easy and too frequent, by the exaggeration of the peripheral sensibilities, corresponds to known clinical facts.

There is, first of all, a whole series of individuals who cannot swallow a powder, or a pill without throwing it up. A little cream in the milk, for some people, is sufficient to produce the same phenomenon. Here it is a question of quasi-constitutional irritability, for one sees the thing happen even in little children. Along the same line of ideas, there are subjects who react by vomiting to certain sudden movements, such as swinging, see-sawing, etc.

We must add, however, that often these subjects encourage themselves to become progressively worse, and become more and more sensitive by a regular education of their reflexes, but it seems, nevertheless, in all such cases there must be something that is partly constitutional.

The cure is by no means the same for those patients who are afflicted with neuropathic disturbances of their upper digestive tracts (dysphagias of all kinds, and spasms of the œsophagus), and who have frequent attacks of vomiting whenever they take any food that is in the least degree solid, or not sufficiently masticated. It is evident that here the intervention of a mental representation of some kind may be held responsible for the phenomena. Nevertheless, it has seemed to us as if certain patients must really have an exaggerated reflectivity, which is the result of their attention to this disturbance, and of the secondary education induced by it, for they actually are sometimes taken with vomiting at the moment when they are least thinking about it.

In fact, the great majority of neuropathic vomitings are due to mental representations which are produced without any peripheral stimulation. The most healthy individual will often find that any vivid or definite idea which brings about a feeling of disgust for some food that he has taken is enough to make him begin to vomit or at least feel a sense of nausea.

It is, in fact, usually through the intervention of mental representations which are exaggerated and unlikely, that neuropathic vomitings occur in the case of neurasthenics who have no appetite or in anorexics who feel the sensation of disgust at the sight of all food.

Under other circumstances, by keeping in mind the idea of the impossibility of digestion, or even simply in an automatic manner, due to habit (merycism), some patients voluntarily set out, more or less consciously, to make themselves vomit. They get the result more or less easily at first, but as vomiting is susceptible to education, it is apt to be the case that at the end of a certain time these vomitings become very easy, as easy as they are frequent.

Disgust, the mental representation of digestive incapacity, whether or not due to gastric or digestive symptoms of any kind, or the establishing of some custom at a certain time which has fixed the psychism of the patient, all these are the mechanisms which are present in establishing vomiting in the course of mental anorexias, false gastropathies of every kind, merycism, or rumination, and which may also complicate the pathogeny of vomitings due to emotional attacks or to exaggeration of the peripheral sensibility.

To conclude, a résumé of the pathogenic study which we have just made might be set forth in the following classification:

I. Emotional vomitings.

II. Vomitings caused by exaggeration of the peripheral sensibility. (*a*) Constitutional, (*b*) acquired.

III. Vomitings caused by mental representations. (*a*) By disgust, (*b*) by representation of inability to digest, (*c*) by habit.

We therefore consider vomiting as a symptom in a great number of neuropathic conditions. It may in itself give rise to secondary symptoms. Sometimes, for instance, vomitings may be so frequent that they prevent all assimilation, outside of any question whatever of insufficient food.

We thus see how what may be called uncontrollable vomiting may be established. It is quite possible that certain of the uncontrollable vomitings of pregnancy may be put in this class of neuropathic vomitings. We have not wholly made up our minds on this point, but there certainly are cases of uncontrollable vomiting which are purely neuropathic, particularly in the case of hysterics. They cannot naturally occur without involving considerable loss of nourishment, which in itself is very serious. They may also give rise to nervous anurias.

On account of the condition of syncope which it can bring about, vomiting may become a factor in a whole series of consecutive troubles, false cardiopathies, production of vertigoes, etc. We shall come across all the phenomena further on, when we shall also dwell more fully upon certain descriptive or pathogenic points which, in order to avoid repetition, we have only briefly noticed here.

To sum up all that has gone before, concerning the presence of gastric symptoms in the course of the psychoneuroses, we will state that a certain number of gastric symptoms are found among neurasthenics, and that whether objective or subjective, they all have their cause, either in the emaciated condition of the patients, or in their more or less developed anorexial condition, which brings with it a whole series of gastric obsessions, and alimentary phobias. If the symptoms can be localized in the stomach, their true cause lies in the psychism of the subject. The patients are, to put it briefly, false gastropaths.

C. Functional Troubles Connected with Defecation, and Their Consequences.—M. X. is a very distinguished ecclesiastic. Madame Z. is a society woman, the mother of a family. The observations made on these two patients are exactly analogous. Neither the one, nor the other, had ever had any serious neuropathic symptoms. With the one, as with the other, the same trivial accident was the starting-point of numerous troubles, which for a long time completely upset their lives.

It was a question, purely and simply, of a slight "accident," which had soiled their linen, and necessitated a brusque interruption of their occupations to hurry into the house and repair the mishap caused by the passing of a burst of wind. Ever since, these two patients lived in constant dread that the same accident would happen again, and place them in a ridiculous position. They did not dare to go out of the house, without first having had a movement of the bowels. By degrees, under the dominion of this obsession, or phobia, they got to the point where their social activity was greatly diminished, so much so as not to be able to leave their rooms without terrible apprehension. It is hardly necessary to add that both of them became noticeably depressed, although, as a matter of fact, the accident which they both dreaded so much never occurred again.

A similar case was that of a young woman, who became neurasthenic after a period of great stress and emotion, which she spent at the bedside of her husband, who was suffering from typhoid fever.

While taking an elevator to make a visit, she had had an attack of diarrhœa and soiled her underclothing. When one of us saw her she had lived a most distressing life for some eighteen months; and for an accident, which as a matter of fact had only occurred once, she had completely given up making calls.

These were cases of a primary form of trouble where the psychism alone was the cause, and serve as an introduction to our next subject, for in the same way that we have described the phobias of the stomach, we shall, apropos of such patients, take up the study of the diarrhœa phobias.

There are also constipation phobias. These occur most often in individuals who, on account of some organic trouble, have been advised that they must never allow themselves to become constipated. Such are patients with hæmorrhoids, arteriosclerosis, people who have been threatened with cerebral hæmorrhage, and who, when left to take care of themselves, sometimes exaggerate, in the most fantastic way, the medical advice which has been given to them. We have known one patient of this kind whose whole existence centred around that function of his daily economy. He spent about four hours every day in the toilet. He was not constipated in the slightest degree, but he was always fearful lest he might not have completely emptied his intestine, hence his exaggeratedly prolonged sittings. It can readily be understood that this very special trend of his life could not help but lead to a series of disorders. The patient was, of course, hampered in his social life as well as in his business, which he necessarily neglected, and finally sank into a serious neurasthenic condition.

It may be noted that before this time he had not shown the slightest sign of hypochondriac preoccupation.

Our first class of patients then is made up of those who suffer from neurasthenic manifestations of diarrhœa or constipation. But, along with this first group, there exist active diarrhœas of psychopathic origin.

Nervous Diarrhœas.—One knows that among the many phenomena, for which the emotions may be responsible, diarrhœa is by no means the least frequent. There are classical examples of men who have been obliged to give up political life, as the excitement which they felt whenever they addressed crowds took this very special form. The diarrhœa of armies is an emotional manifestation equally well known. We have often seen emotional people in whom frequent or continued emotions would always cause the same trouble. In such cases there would be a primary form of nervous or emotional diarrhœa, which would be severe in proportion to the intensity of the emotion, then the phobia of the diarrhœa itself would also play a pathogenic rôle, and prove as important a factor as the emotion.

Here is an example: A young woman, twenty-eight years of age, and the mother of three children, was treated for four years for an intestinal disturbance. She was put upon all sorts of regimens, and particularly on an exclusive farinaceous diet. They claimed that in that way they could stop a persistent diarrhœa. The only result was to make her lose thirty-one pounds. No physician ever concerned himself with her mental conditions. Now what was the real trouble? She was the daughter of a man of prominence, occupying an important post in a foreign country. One day when she was driving with him in an open carriage, they were fired upon, and she was exposed to the shots which were intended for her father. She threw herself upon him to protect him. Fortunately, neither she nor her father was hurt, but she was taken at that moment with an attack of emotional diarrhœa, the memory of which became a regular obsession. She found herself the victim of a perpetual diarrhœa, which, however, was not so persistent but that it would stop when her attention was called to other things, which, however, happened very rarely to her. The case of this patient was diagnosed as a pseudomembranous enterocolitis, and every day she examined her stools to see if there were any false membranes.

She was very much upset over her condition, and became profoundly neurasthenic.

When treated therapeutically, in isolation, this patient saw her intestinal troubles disappear in a few days. Starting at the first with ordinary diet, in three months she regained her lost weight, and was able to return to a perfectly normal life.

Outside of any kind of emotion, diarrhœa may also be produced in nervous people by a very different mechanism. The need of going to the toilet is, in fact, nothing more than a mental interpretation of a sensation localized in the region of the rectum and anus. It is a phenomenon which we believe is very susceptible to education.

Mr. X., a merchant, forty-nine years of age, had two years ago a serious attack of gastro-intestinal poisoning which caused profuse diarrhœa, obliging him to go to the toilet as many as sixteen or eighteen times a day. The attack was so depressing to him that since that time the patient's attention seems to have remained fixed, as it were, on his lower bowel, and when we saw him he was still going to the toilet six times a day at least. The diarrhœa remained, and his stools were quite unformed, and all the dietetic treatment to which he had been subjected was without effect. Large doses of bismuth and opium alone were able to give him temporary relief. But this patient was cured rapidly by the simple prescription of making himself voluntarily increase the interval between his stools. In order to avoid any of the effects of obsession, we advised him to stay at home, and to lie down during the hours when he was obliged to go to the toilet, and to try and occupy his mind by reading or conversation. In this way he managed to go to the toilet no more than four times, then three times, then twice a day. His stools became formed, and the cure which resulted has continued for the last six months without any other incident.

How are we to interpret such a case? Has it anything to do with an organic affection?

The very mechanism of the cure renders such an hypothesis unlikely. It seems to us that here was a patient who had, so to speak, been constantly educating himself from everyone who had attended him, ever since the first acute attack, which had been brought on by some sort of a "psychic impression." On the other hand, it is certain that the fact of going frequently to the bath-room, by reason of the efforts made at such a time, and the intestinal contractions which they provoke, would be likely to hasten the passage of the intestinal contents, and to prevent the large intestine from thoroughly emptying itself. Thus a permanent diarrhœa might be established without any organic reason for its existence. This is the way by which what we might call diarrhœas due to education become established.

Neuropathic Constipation. — Nearly all the nervous constipations are due to a mechanism analogous to that which we have just attempted to explain. They are constipations due to education. They may develop under very different circumstances. Sometimes they occur in individuals who, until that time, had had a very good digestion, but who have had an attack of some anal affection, such as hæmorrhoids or fissures. As defecation is extremely painful to them, they voluntarily try as far as possible to put it off. They thus finally get to the point of inhibiting, so to speak, the sensation of needing to go to the toilet, and even after the hæmorrhoidal attack has disappeared, or the fissure is cured, they remain, and will remain constipated, until by inverse education they teach their functions to resume their regularity.

Other individuals, and this is the usual cause of constipation among women, forget, for some reason or other, to go to the toilet, or else they will not make the proper normal effort to attain a favorable result. They thus get to the point where their digestive tract is completely upset, and we have seen some cases, particularly among women, who, without suffering any apparent inconvenience, were apt to go from one to two weeks without having a movement.

Other persons educate themselves in a different way, and form a habit of having a movement by artificial means only, such as enemata, or inserting suppositories into the rectum, etc. In these cases artificial defecation is often practised without the slightest preliminary attempt to have a normal passage.

Certain individuals reach the point of no longer experiencing the slightest need of defecation. It is an absent idea. We once saw a patient of this kind who, from the time that he was three or four years of age, when his mother, in accordance with a medical prescription, had given him enemas, had been completely ignorant of what it meant to go spontaneously to the toilet. He had never even tried it. When we saw him, he was fifty-two years of age, and had taken—we amused ourselves by making a computation—about fifteen thousand enemas.

Finally there exists a whole class of individuals whose constipation is due to persuasion, and in fact, in the case of nearly all the patients whom we have just seen, their constipation was due to their laziness. These latter, being convinced that they were afflicted with a stubborn constipation, would go, it is true, to the toilet, but being wholly persuaded that it was no use they would occupy the time by reading the paper or a magazine.

There are others in whom a cramp occurs almost immediately when they call up the idea of constipation. How many times have we heard patients tell us that when they went to the toilet, although it seemed to them at the time that the need was urgent, yet the moment they got there their "inspiration" failed them. They had an impression of a cramp, which at some other time had actually occurred, but—and this is a matter of by no means small importance—under a psychic influence. If ten minutes or a quarter of an hour later these patients would return to the bath-room, when their attention was distracted by something else, the normal effort would be attended with success. But, though there is little danger that any more serious phobic manifestations would become established, or that the patient would have obsessions, yet a serious and obstinate neuropathic constipation is apt to set in.

It goes without saying that a constipation due to education may become, after a certain time, a real constipation, having as its starting-point nervous symptoms of a different nature, which we shall take up further on.

Along with these constipations of education, there exists, in many neurasthenic patients who are extremely emaciated, a form of constipation due to intestinal atony, which is the result of the general low tone of the patient's body. It arises through a mechanism analogous to that which we have seen creating a certain form of gastric dilatation in neurasthenics. Here the psychism does not act directly, but the fact remains that the general weakness of the organism, of which the gastro-intestinal atony is but a symptom, bears a direct relation to morbid disturbances of a neuropathic nature. It is none the less true that to treat these patients as if their whole trouble were centred around their constipation would be quite irrational, and fraught with many dangers.

Neuropathic Constipation and Diarrhœa; Their Immediate and Ultimate Consequences.—The neuropathic origin of a diarrhœa, and more particularly of constipation, does not render these troubles any less liable to bring about a whole series of symptoms which are apt to follow in the course of a constipation or a diarrhœa of organic cause. If we consider, in addition, that nervous patients are very apt to voluntarily use every kind of artificial means, such as enemata, purgatives, etc., for their constipation, because they, more easily than others, are apt to be obsessed on the subject of their constipation, and are always looking for some means of overcoming it; we are able to conceive what a large number of secondary disturbances might be added to these neuropathic phenomena. Intestinal cramps, profuse mucus secretions of the large intestine, or intestinal catarrh, if one so prefers to call it, may be the direct results of a purely neuropathic constipation.

As for the diarrhœa of neuropaths, it too is apt to have less effect upon the local condition than upon the general state of health, for as it hurries the partially digested food along too quickly, not enough can be absorbed, and even on a sufficiently hearty diet, there may be emaciation which is sufficiently pronounced to be noticed by the patient as well as the physician.

We shall not dwell upon this point, but, according to our opinion, this is the mechanism in part, at least, of the origin of many of the intestinal disturbances which are found among neuropaths. These are the troubles that we now have to consider.

D. Intestinal Manifestations of Neuropaths.—Here again, as in our preceding studies, we shall have two classes of patients to study. On the one hand we have the phobics, who are obsessed about their intestines. On the other hand, those who present intestinal symptoms of a purely neuropathic nature, or which are connected with some nervous trouble localized elsewhere.

As far as the first class of these patients is concerned we must state at once—for this is a question which we shall take up elsewhere—that they are not hypochondriacs. The principal characteristic of hypochondriacal manifestations lies in their diffusion, and in their variability. Here we have individuals who are systematized, and whose intestines have become the source of obsessional preoccupations. As for the mechanisms which have brought about the intestinal localization, they are numerous. Sometimes it is an attack of colic which the patient has never been able to forget, sometimes it is something which he has read, or conversations which have turned his mind upon his intestines. Is it not a peculiar thing to see to how large a degree intestinal manifestations have developed during the last twenty years? We know, only too well, that a large number of the cases that we hear of are cases of purely neuropathic symptoms. Innumerable medicines and an infinite variety of diets have been laid down for the treatment of intestinal affections, and people who have never had the slightest local trouble of this kind, as well as those who have some trifling complaint, "try" the medicine, or the much lauded diet under the vain pretext that "at least it can do them no harm." But alas! by fixing the patients' minds upon their physical organs, it does "do them harm," and one sees patients going from one step to another, palpating their abdomens, examining the nature of their stools, and finally ending by really feeling positive symptoms in the locality of an intestine that only wants to be allowed to perform its functions. These are the false enteritides, the psychics of the intestine. Their number is legion.

There are also false appendicites. These are patients who have had some intestinal pain in the right groin. Knowing that this is the way in which appendicitis often appears they go in search of a physician. He naturally finds nothing the matter, and not taking the patients' mental condition sufficiently into account, he advises them to keep a watch upon their intestines, and not to neglect consulting a physician the moment a pain of the same kind appears again. "Your life," he tells the patients, "may depend upon it." We have seen individuals of this kind living for years in the expectation of an attack of appendicitis, which never came, and which never had any reason to come. While waiting for it, their lives have been spoiled. Matters have sometimes gone even to the point of an operation for an appendicitis which did not exist.

The second category of cases is formed of patients presenting some real trouble in the locality of the intestine, but trouble which seems to us to have every reason to be considered as being of a neuropathic nature.

At this point we might write the whole history of membranous enterocolitis. Here is an affection which thirty years ago was almost unknown, or at least, was so little known that one could easily count the cases. Now, in these later years it has become so widespread that in many watering places, as well as in a considerable number of sanitaria, they treat this trouble almost exclusively. Such rapid growth is, to say the least, singular. Moreover, the patients afflicted with this disease are, for the majority, neuropaths, characterized as such even by those specialists who are determined to refer the symptoms to an organic origin. There are no physicians who do not recognize that mucomembranous enterocolitis is almost certain to develop on a neuropathic soil.

Characterized essentially by glairy and mucus stools, sometimes accompanied by false membranes, by alternative attacks of diarrhœa and constipation, by painful sensations in the region of the large intestine, just how can one tell whether or not the symptoms which constitute such a diarrhœa are likely to be nervous in their origin?

So far as the mucus hypersecretion of the intestine is concerned, it may be due to different factors. The intestinal secretion may be a true phenomenon of defence against constipation, this being very frequently created, as we have seen, in neuropathic soil. Moreover, the various means employed, by the patients, to get relief are not without a possible irritating action on the intestinal mucous membrane. Finally, we may add, that the glairy secretions and false membranes are extremely frequent in people who have never had any trouble with their intestines. In women, particularly at the time of their courses, it is a very common phenomenon, and one which has no significance, unless the attention of the subject has become fixed upon it.

But in what degree, on the other hand, may the nervous system be susceptible of directly engendering difficulties in the region of the intestine? We have already seen that emotion creates diarrhœa. It would be trite to state that constipation frequently occurs in the psychoses, properly so-called, and especially in melancholia. We believe that the fixing of the patient's attention on any part of his body whatsoever is apt to produce some disturbance in that region, whether an error in mental interpretation may be considered as a cause of functional disturbances, or whether one considers the emotion with which the patient has been preoccupied as the starting-point. At all events, there is no reason why the psychic secretory manifestations which have been physiologically demonstrated in connection with the stomach should not also exist in the intestinal region.

The whole make-up of the painful disturbances which enter into the symptomatology of mucomembranous enterocolitis are too subjective in their nature for the nervous system not to be liable to play an important part. On the other hand, we cannot believe that an over-lively imagination may of itself be the cause of such troubles; and as far as the painful symptoms of which the patients complain are concerned, we are of the opinion that they really feel them. According to our ideas, the fact is that there may be developed an exaggeration of the visceral sensibility, which has been in some way educated by the attention of the patient being constantly brought to bear upon that special part of the body. It must not be forgotten that through apprehension and fear, impressions may be felt as very painful, which under other circumstances would pass by completely unperceived. We have seen patients in whom painful symptoms of an enteric nature would suddenly disappear under the influence of psychotherapy. This was probably because the normal functioning of the intestine had been somewhat painful to them. As to the phenomenon of cramps which often accompany the manifestation of a mucomembranous enterocolitis, and which may constitute the painful element, they may be explained in very different ways. Constipation—this is a self-evident fact —brings about spasm of the large intestine. It is in this case a form of mechanical defence. But, on the other hand, the condition of spasm is the condition of all the organs, and all the painful muscles, and whether the pain be of peripheral origin, or of central origin, or purely psychic in its essence, the spasm cannot be other than a common result.

However it may be—and we shall find all these theoretic questions taken up later on—we have seen a great many patients attacked by symptoms described, not only by us, as mucomembranous enterocolitis, who were rapidly cured by the ordinary methods of treatment of the psychoneuroses.

A few years ago, one of us had occasion to see a young woman whose husband was in one of the liberal professions, and who for the last ten years had been treated for symptoms of enterocolitis. Naturally she had been put upon very reduced diet, of which the first result had been the loss of thirty-five pounds of her weight. Her enterocolitis was really of emotional origin, but she had also nursed it along and aggravated it extremely by unwise therapeutic measures.

After three months of treatment this woman regained her normal weight and went back to her regular life apparently cured. But, as a matter of fact, the cure was not realized, because, as it was inferred by the reticence of the patient, her pathological convictions had not completely disappeared. As a matter of fact this patient, when seen a year later, had had a complete relapse, and was suffering more than ever. We then got her complete confession. Her physician who had always treated her was ill-advised enough to tell her that nothing would be done for her intestines. "He cannot treat you for your enterocolitis," he said to her, "for he does not believe in it." The conviction that this woman felt, that her own ideas were being opposed merely by another purely theoretic set of ideas, was what had kept her from giving up her belief in the reality of her affection. Once having confessed, she rapidly grew well, and this time definitely.

Here is a case that is very interesting, because the psychotherapy that banished the symptom came about spontaneously. It was the case of a woman, forty years of age, who had been separated from her husband for some years, and who came to the Pinel Ward during the service of one of us, at the Salpêtrière, to be treated for functional manifestations of the bladder. The examination of our patient revealed this truly pertinent fact—that the vesical pain dated back eleven months, but that for two years before that the patient had had characteristic symptoms of enterocolitis, constipation, glairy and false membranes, sharp pains in the iliac fossa, and fæcal matter in the form of little balls. The diagnosis of enterocolitis had been made, moreover, by several physicians. We ought to add that this patient, who was in a serious nervous condition, having had a great many material and moral cares to engross her, did not derive any benefit from the various treatments that were prescribed for her at that time. But suddenly on experiencing real suffering, the whole symptomatology of enterocolitis had disappeared from the moment that the patient's attention was localized upon her bladder.

Another example of the same kind is furnished us by a patient who had suffered for three years from enterocolitis. This patient went to consult a physician who attributed her series of intestinal symptoms to her gastric condition. In a few weeks she had developed a false gastropathy, but her enterocolitis had disappeared.

These are nervous metastases, and one can apply the old proverb to them,—"One nail drives out another." There exist numerous examples of such cases. We shall have occasion to mention others. They serve better than any theory to confirm the purely neuropathic nature of symptoms which need only distraction, in the etymological sense of the word, to make them disappear.

We have now analytically set forth all of the neuropathic manifestations which may affect the digestive tract. In general these manifestations appear under the form of phobias, or obsessions, localized in the viscera, which may be complicated by psychomotor or psychosecretory phenomena, as well as by secondary symptoms resulting in some way from the vicious habits formed in those parts of the body which we have just studied.

We have described separately each of the manifestations which we have come across in our practice, but it is very evident that morbid associations may be created leading to neuropathic syndromes, resulting from the simultaneous appearance in the same subject by diffusion, as it were, of several of the phenomena considered.

CHAPTER II.

FUNCTIONAL MANIFESTATIONS IN THE URINARY ORGANS.

BY REASON of their frequency these manifestations are no less important than the digestive or genital disturbances. But, as they are so closely allied to the latter, we find it better to place their study before those of the last mentioned localizations.

We shall study successively—

A. *Floating kidney in connection with the psychoneuroses.*
B. *Modifications of the urinary secretions.*
C. *Difficulties in micturition.*

A. Floating Kidney in Connection with the Psychoneuroses.—Floating kidney in all its variations, is found very frequently in neurasthenics. We naturally do not think of pretending that this phenomenon constitutes essentially a neuropathic symptom. But we believe that in the majority of nervous people, if not in all, it is brought about by the simple mechanism of losing flesh, which causes the fatty capsule of the kidney to disappear, and becomes the factor of its abnormal mobility. A floating kidney in neurasthenics is, therefore, only a secondary manifestation, and to attempt to use its more or less frequent occurrence, to establish a pathogenic theory of neurasthenia, seems to us dangerous at least. Of course we do not wish to be understood as speaking of a floating kidney which has really become displaced, which is a manifestation independent of all previous or consecutive neuropathic phenomena, when we say that the floating kidney of neurasthenics does not need treatment. When patients get back to their original weight, they do not complain of it objectively. Subjectively, however, they continue to complain of it, for fear that having spoken of it may put them in a false position mentally. In fact, we have seen, in a great number of patients, false floating kidneys following a true floating kidney, which persisted subjectively for a long time after the phenomenon itself had disappeared. In this way it creates renal or lumbar pains which are sometimes the starting-point of errors in diagnosis. These patients are thought to have appendicitis or so-called stones, especially when, as it often happens, the symptomatology is complicated by urinary phenomena. The floating kidney in fact, whether persisting or cured, may be the starting-point of numerous neuropathic manifestations by diffusion, and, above all, when ill-advised therapeutic treatment has intervened.

From this point of view in particular, the various kinds of girdles and corsets or bandaging, which are definitely indicated in cases of true floating kidney, cannot help but constitute a real danger to the neuropath, by constantly calling his attention to it, and thus creating obsessions concerning it.

B. Modifications of the Urinary Secretion.—We shall only study under this title the quantitative modification of the urine secreted. It is true that this quantitative modification can be more or less associated with disturbances of micturition, which we shall glance at in the following paragraph. It is none the less true that the quantity of urine secreted, which is a renal phenomenon without any immediate bearing on vesical or urethral symptoms, may be modified by purely neuropathic influences.

First of all, we shall describe nervous polyuria. This manifests itself under many different conditions. Sometimes it is a question of a purely transient phenomenon, consisting of the emission of large quantities of clear urine, which might be described as nervous urine. This is a trivial phenomenon, without any ill consequences or significance, which may occur after any stirring emotion. The only reason for noticing it is because, although its intrinsic importance is slight, it may nevertheless, under some circumstances, become the starting-point of fixed ideas and secondary phenomena. In the majority of cases which interest us,—that is to say, in those in which the polyuria is persistent,—it is a question of an habitual mechanism, or of the education, so to speak, of the organism. It gets to be polyuria, by polydipsia.

Mrs. B., fifty-nine years of age, has suffered from a polyuria for five years. She passes at least from six to seven quarts of urine every day. Her urine is clear. The analysis shows no pathological element, and, if one did not take the quantity of liquid into account, one would find in their usual proportions all the mineral and organic elements of normal urine. In spite of the quantity that she drinks, the arterial tension is very close to the normal, and does not pass 17 on Potain's sphygmomanometer. With the exception of the polyuria there is no objective disturbance. Subjectively, the patient complains of a whole series of troubles,—dryness of the throat, difficulty in salivation, etc., which occur the moment that she goes for any length of time without drinking something.

What has happened in this particular case? The history of the patient explains the mechanism of the phenomenon very clearly. Six years ago she nursed, both night and day, a son who was afflicted with pulmonary tuberculosis. Being very emotional, each time that her child had an attack of suffocation, she herself felt contractions in her throat, and would drink abundantly to relieve herself. She thus got into the habit of taking a large quantity of liquid every day, and more particularly at night. Her son died and she was overcome with grief. She did not sleep at night, and, haunted by the memories of his death, was overcome by the same emotional phenomena which had been produced by his sufferings.

The habit of drinking a large quantity was in this way kept up. Since then the emotional symptoms had disappeared, but the polydipsia and polyuria persisted. We must add that apart from her emotional disturbance the patient has never shown the slightest neuropathic trouble. She was of slightly weak mentality, but did not in the slightest degree show the mental make-up of an hysteric. She had made great efforts for some months to lessen the quantity of liquid that she drank, she tried to cheat her thirst by the usual methods, but could not succeed. It was necessary to proceed very slowly with her, by imperceptible reductions, in order to obtain any perceivable improvement.

In other cases it is a question of subjects who in the course of convalescence from some acute illness, typhoid fever for example, had been accustomed to drink liquids in great quantities, and who had continued for weeks, and even months, to keep up the same kind of liquid food, less from any organic need of it than from the establishing of a habit which made them feel the need at regular and specified hours of drinking large quantities of some liquid. This last class of patients are cured very quickly. It is often only necessary to make them understand the nature of their polyuria for them to be relieved of it in a few days.

In other cases, again, there are patients who, for some reason or other, have been put upon a milk diet of four or five or six quarts of milk a day, and who, when their normal régime was prescribed again, continued, if they were not carefully watched, to drink in excessive quantities for some months. We have seen some in whom the phenomenon lasted for years.

Here is still another mechanism. It is the keeping up of the emotional polyuria to which we have just made allusion. It is curious that it should be so, but it very frequently happens that the same individuals nearly always externalize their emotionalism in the same manner. Then there is also such a thing as emotional polyuria due to the repetition of extrinsic emotions, as also the polyuria itself may become, in an impressionable patient, the starting-point of preoccupations and emotional phenomena which encourage it to continue.

In short, in all these cases we must take into account two mechanisms,—the emotional mechanism, coming directly by the intervention of a polydipsia, and the mechanism of education; and we must never lose sight of this fact,—viz., the direct action which emotional phenomena have upon the renal secretions.

These are the true nervous polyurias, which must not be confused with pollakiuria of the same nature, which we shall study later. It goes without saying that they are more apt to be met in patients who are hetero- or auto-suggestible,—who, for example, easily persuade themselves of the necessity of drinking large quantities, or who are easily impressed and obsessed by an accidental polyuria. It is none the less true that the question of simulation, whether conscious or semi-conscious, does not enter into the question. In these troubles the will is not brought into play. This does not mean that there may not exist simulated polydipsias and polyurias. But they have nothing to do with the true nervous polyurias.

This last mechanism of simulation, possibly combined with suggestion, we admit most readily in what we have called major hysterical polyuria. Here the quantity of liquid that may be drunk and urine emitted passes all limits of imagination. Patients of this kind have been known to pass from fifteen to twenty and even thirty quarts of urine in twenty-four hours. That a certain number of these patients are up to tricks and resort to fraud to fill the urinals is a fact not to be doubted, and agrees perfectly with the mentality of the patients who are subject to such an affection. They are, as a matter of fact, usually degenerate men, alcoholics, hospital rounders, and wilful simulators. It is none the less true that very often the mechanism of education from an antecedent polydipsia may be brought into play, and it is a fact that a polyuria often sets in after long and frequent alcoholic bouts. But in these latter cases it is rather a question of a true dipsomania, a mental condition which is outside the bounds of our studies. For in these intensive polyurias the action of emotion as well as of traumatism have been called into play. We, therefore, feel that these are doubtful conditions that we would hesitate to consider as true functional manifestations,—that is to say, according to our conception, as phenomena where the conscious will of the patient does not come into play, and which are to be distinguished, on the other hand, from mental manifestations due to pure psychoses. As a matter of fact, these patients are extremely rare at the neurological clinic of the Salpêtrière, and we would be rather inclined to believe that simulation plays an important part because they are apt to avoid the clinics for special nervous diseases, where, according to their opinion, one does not pay sufficient attention to their malady, and are more inclined to frequent the clinics in general medicine.

But quite the opposite phenomenon is to be observed in ischuria, or the anuria of nervous patients, in which the quantity of urine secreted is abnormally reduced almost to nothing. As a rule, scanty urine is closely allied to the small amount of liquid consumed. This may occur as a consequence of mental anorexia, where, as we have seen, liquids and foods are only taken in infinitesimal quantities. It often arises from an elective anorexia for beverages, from true nervous sitiophobias. How do these latter occur? Very often the sitiophobia is of medical origin. A patient with a dilated stomach, or afflicted with obesity, has received the advice of a physician to drink as little as possible. Persecuted by the idea of the dilatation, or obsessed by the obesity, and desirous of being rapidly cured, such patients cut down the amount that they drink to unbelievably small quantities. They finally develop a fear of drinking, and push this fear so far that they will refuse foods which are rich in water, such as vegetables, fruits, etc. We have seen, in illustration of this, a cachectic young girl, a false gastropath with dilatation, who managed to get into this state in one month's time and is still in it, where she absolutely suppressed every kind of drink, and got to the point where even the idea of drinking caused a real sense of anguish analogous to the condition of anguish which is felt by our polyurias at the idea of not being able to drink. Under these conditions such patients get to the point where they pass the most insignificant quantities of urine,—from one hundred to one hundred and fifty grams at most, during twenty-four hours, of thick urine, which is extremely turbid in certain obese cases. Such a disturbance may go on for a long time, while the health remains almost normal.

Such cases are what one might call ischuria by adipsia, which represents a primary category.

To what extent, on the other hand, may emotion or suggestion be susceptible of decreasing or suppressing the renal secretion?

Two forms of anuria, or hysterical ischuria, have been described. One is simple anuria, characterized by the simple suppression or diminution of the urinary flow; the other is hysterical anuria, with uncontrollable vomitings, where there is established a sort of balance between the amount of the vomiting and the quantity of urine passed. Others do not agree about this last form. Some consider that the vomiting forms a sort of supplementary flow; others think that it is a question of conditions of gastric intolerance, and that the suppression of urine really depends upon the non-alimentation of the subject. We ourselves are more inclined to throw our opinion on the side of this latter interpretation.

We have seen elsewhere how many gastric manifestations of neuropathic origin there may be, and how the gastric reflectivity was influenced by the phenomenon of emotion and hetero-suggestion. In fact, in the case of anuria with uncontrollable vomiting which we have outlined, the patient was perfectly convinced that her stomach could not tolerate anything. As for her anuria, she considered it a purely secondary phenomenon. She had not even paid any attention to it. It is very certain that, under the influence of her conviction of gastric intolerance, she ate only with feelings of repulsion on account of the nauseas and vomitings arising from a purely psychic cause. One can conceive how in these conditions psychotherapy can easily get control of these states.

So far as pure and simple urinary suppression is concerned, it is a phenomenon which has often been observed in hystericals, following an attack or an emotion. This is usually a purely transitory anuria, lasting from twenty-four to thirty-six hours. As to the prolongation of the phenomenon for a very considerable time, although we know to-day that the retention of calculi in the ureter is compatible with life for a rather long space of time, it leaves us rather sceptical. And here we would be very much disposed to admit the intervention of simulation. As a matter of fact, these patients can scarcely be said to flock to the special clinics for nervous diseases, and, as far as we ourselves are concerned, we have never observed a single example of urinary suppression in hysteria.

To sum up these functional manifestations which lead to the reduction of the urine, we see that total or elective anorexia and gastric intolerance play a part. If sometimes an emotion may come in in a direct manner, it does not seem to us any less true that the majority of these modifications of the urinary secretion are due to modifications of absorption. And this conforms pretty generally to the idea with which we started at the beginning of our study,—namely, that the functional manifestations properly so called, outside of the phenomenon of strong emotion, require the intervention of mental representations, and that the functions which, like the secretion of urine, have no mental representation must intrinsically be but slightly affected.

C. Disturbances of Micturition.—Disturbances of micturition, whether isolated or associated with genital troubles, are extremely frequent in nervous people, and particularly among neurasthenics. They occur almost exclusively in men.

In order better to understand them, it seems to us necessary to offer a few preliminary remarks upon the physiological mechanism of the excretion of the urine.

The bladder, owing to its muscular development, forms an elastic reservoir which dilates in proportion to the amount of urine secreted by the kidney and brought into it by the ureters. This wholly passive dilatation is made possible, on the one hand, by the fluted beak arrangement of the urethral orifice, which permits the urine to flow in, but prevents it from flowing out, and, on the other hand, by the presence of the smooth sphincter. The sphincter, in its condition of elastic, and perhaps tonic, contraction (whether reflex or not), is still further reinforced in men by the prostate, which presses elastically upon the urethra.

When the bladder has attained the limit of its normal elasticity, its sensory nerves are stimulated, and transmit, to the vesicospinal centres of the spinal cord, an excitation which is reflected on the motor nerves, and thus the muscular walls of the bladder are caused to contract. Some drops of urine then involuntarily overflow the smooth sphincter, from the neck of the bladder, and come in contact with the mucous membrane of the prostatic region of the urethra. They there provoke the peculiar sensation known as the desire to urinate. If one resists the desire, the striated and voluntary sphincter of the prostatic and membranous regions contract and hold back the urine in the bladder for a time. Then the desire reappears, and finally becomes irresistible. At last the voluntary sphincter relaxes, and the contractions produced by the bladder and helped by those of the muscles of the abdomen little by little force the urine, which is ejected in the form of a continuous stream at first, but which becomes intermittent, and goes in little spurts at the end. These spurts are due to the contraction of the bulbocavernous muscle, which expels from the urethra those last drops of liquid on which the contractions of the bladder and abdominal pressure could no longer act.

In short, in micturition the intervention of superior centres is manifested several times,—namely, in the sensation of wanting to urinate, in the interpretation of the sensation, in the voluntary contractions of the striated sphincter to hold back and the contraction of the abdominal wall and the bulbocavernous muscle to hasten and terminate micturition. The vesical contraction itself, by the intermediary of spinal centres of arrest, may in a certain measure be inhibited by the will.

In these conditions of normal micturition, which presuppose the intervention of the psychism, it is quite easy to understand that it may often be disturbed in neuropaths by the psychic fixation of the patient upon his bladder and his genito-urinary organs. The first problem which presents itself to us has to do with the mechanism itself which causes this fixation.

It often happens, and we shall find these facts a little further along, in connection with the study of functional genital manifestations, that the urinary symptoms are only secondary, and are derived from localized genital troubles. But often also there has been fixation on the bladder and urethra from the start. It sometimes occurs in patients who, having had urethritis, are haunted by the fear of stricture. They consult a physician, he passes a sound, but he may assure them in vain that their urethra is normal; the nail has been driven in, and the patient's preoccupation grows more intense every day. Under other circumstances the starting-point is quite different. A patient, for example, has been known to develop the whole symptomatology of a false *urinaire,* because, having one day gone too long without relieving himself, he had a slight attack of false incontinence or, on the contrary, considerable difficulty in voiding the urine.

The rôle of emotion, on the other hand, may play an important part. Everybody has experienced pollakiuria, a frequent and repeated micturition, amounting often to a mere trifle, and causing one to hurry for nothing at all, which one experiences when under the stress of an emotion. Such a condition offers, either by the continuity of the emotion or by secondary psychic fixation, a mechanism which could produce functional urinary symptoms.

Moreover, there are physiological phenomena which will aggravate the matter. There is a slight prostatic congestion which occurs in the morning, from an overfull bladder, which by lessening the force and size of the jet can become the starting-point of an erroneous interpretation.

Under other circumstances again it is a question of real urinary modifications. The passing of a little sand or urinary phosphates, or, on the contrary, the exceeding clearness of the urine, will preoccupy the patient and make him fix his mind on his urinary functions.

Sometimes patients will be subjects suffering from some heart trouble who know that the quantity of urine bears some relation to their cardiac contractions and who will thus have their attention drawn to the organs of urinary secretion. It is not only the accidental polyurias by taking of diuretic liquids or following a migraine, but also comparative anuria which may be created by energetic purgation or very abundant perspiration, all of which, though trifling causes in themselves, may produce great effects in this domain of functional manifestations.

However it may be, we shall take up successively retention of urine, incontinence, pollakiuria, pains in the urinary passages, and all the modifications (properly so called) of micturition.

True *urinary retention*—that is to say, the impossibility of voluntary micturition—is a rare symptom. It has, however, been noted in hystericals, who can go twenty-four or even thirty-six hours without urinating, following an emotion, a traumatism, or an hysterical crisis.

What, however, is extremely frequent, is the inhibition in various degrees which certain patients have of the sensation of the desire to urinate. Sometimes it is connected with phenomena which are wholly foreign to the urinary tracts, and one sees people who are under the influence of an obsessive idea or a preoccupation or lasting emotion forgetting to urinate for a greater or less length of time. Sometimes these are prostatics or have phobias concerning their urinary tracts, and voluntarily hold back their micturition as long as possible, and who manage in this way to educate themselves to go without voiding urine more than once or twice during the day, less from need than by reasoning. Among these patients there is created, under the direct mental influence, a spasm of the striated sphincter of the urethra, and this sphincter may become subjectively and objectively painful.

Urinary incontinence may be met with under very different conditions. First of all, one must remember that there is a false incontinence which may be observed in hysterical patients who are retaining their urine and who urinate because their bladder overflows. This, however, is a phenomenon rarely observed. True partial or relative incontinence is of very frequent occurrence in women, and we know that certain women when the bladder is full are unable to laugh heartily or make the slightest violent effort without voiding at least a few drops of urine. The phenomenon in itself is nothing, but may become serious by the obsessive preoccupation which it may cause. We have seen one lady of this kind shut herself up completely for fear of causing an accident, which, however, had never occurred with her outside the bounds of physiological possibilities. We knew another woman who was so preoccupied with the subject that she got to the point where she had involuntary micturition so abundantly that she wet her clothing and undergarments, although the micturitions were created solely by the mental representations which she had.

In certain neurasthenic men one sees phenomena of the same kind. They are, however, very rare, and are generally allied to pollakiuria.

The nocturnal incontinence of children or of youths is a functional trouble which does not have anything to do with the manifestation of psychic origin which we are studying here. As to true and absolute incontinence, we for our part have never met any examples among neuropaths.

Frequency of micturition is a common phenomenon among neurasthenics. It is directly caused by urinary obsession. The patient, thinking too frequently or continuously upon his urinary tracts, invites by his mental representation contraction of the bladder, and experiences as a consequence the desire to urinate. We see, moreover, analogous mechanisms in normal life, for a desire to urinate is essentially contagious, and individuals who are not in the least neuropathic will rarely allow their companions to go alone. It is for this reason that in our urinary neurasthenics everything that is likely to call their attention to their urinary tracts becomes the starting-point of a desire to urinate. It cannot be other than the fear of not being able to satisfy their pollakiuria which is the starting-point of their imperious desire, which sometimes amounts to real agony.

One of us treated in his service at the Salpêtrière a woman, twenty-eight years of age, who became pollakiuric as a result of emotions, and who for eighteen months did not go out of her apartment, for, whenever she did go out, she was haunted by the idea that she was going to urinate and would be obliged to relieve herself no matter where. In her own home, however, knowing that the toilets were in close proximity, she did not pass urine any more often than would a normal subject. She was cured after six weeks of isolation and psychotherapy.

These patients are profoundly unhappy, for all social life is impossible to them. They go from one physician to another and from one drug to another. They abstain from drinking or, on the contrary, they take great quantities of liquid, and create additional troubles. Psychotherapy is the only thing that is able to cure them.

An unfortunate laborer, a mushroom raiser, came to us in an intensely neurasthenic condition. He was a false *urinaire.* He experienced pains in the perineal region and was attacked with very marked frequency of micturition. The origin of all this was nothing more than a slight eczema of the penis which had appeared four years before, but which had been the starting-point of his psychic fixation through medical encouragement. As the patient was not very young, the doctors thought it would be a good idea to make him undergo a course of massage of the prostate, the latter being by some pronounced large and hypertrophic and by others small and sclerotic! It must be noted, and this is important from a diagnostic point of view, that this pollakiuria was purely diurnal and that it disappeared entirely during his sleep.

Sometimes his frequency of micturition was accompanied by partial incontinence, due to the too imperious demands upon the patient, which he believed did not give him time to relieve himself in a rational manner. But this is a very rare case. More often the patients who at this time feel themselves wet are so not through urine, but on account of an exaggerated secretion of the bulbourethral glands, whose presence is recognized by a few drops of colorless liquid trickling from the meatus and resembling submaxillary saliva. At other times they believe themselves attacked by spermatorrhœa for the same reason. It is not difficult to convince them that this liquid is not the spermatic fluid.

Under certain circumstances frequency of micturition is apt to lead directly to a more or less marked degree of polyuria: whether the renal secretion is directly solicited by the continued emptiness of the bladder creating a sort of appeal or whether, by a mechanism already described, the subject drinks a great quantity of liquid to overcome his pollakiuria. But these polyurias caused by pollakiuria are never very abundant. The quantity of urine rarely passes two quarts or two quarts and a half.

Pains are extremely frequent, either occurring alone or associated with other manifestations. They bear no direct relation to micturition and are more generally located in the region of the membranous urethra. They are apparently connected with the painful contraction of the striated sphincter. They are felt subjectively in the form of a sensation of tension and fulness. Objectively they are augmented by pressure and the passage of a sound in the region of the membranous urethra.

But urethral pains are not the only ones which may be experienced by these patients. There are various shooting sensations, sometimes in the lumbar region but more often in the subumbilical region. Sometimes they also produce true vesical pains. In certain of these patients even the bladder itself may under some circumstances become painful to pressure. This is generally true in pollakiuric individuals who have, so to speak, educated their vesical sensibility, and whose bladder has become more and more intolerant and more and more painful by a purely mental mechanism. This association of the vesical phenomenon with pollakiuria creates the false cystitis of which we have had the opportunity of seeing a certain number of examples. It was thus that during a number of weeks we had in the Pinel Ward, in our service, a patient who complained of this association,—imperative pollakiuria and vesical pains. The starting-point was medical in its nature. This patient, being preoccupied with the condition of her genital regions, on account of marital reasons, had consulted a physician, who, before examining her, and suspecting an anteversion which he could not have established objectively, had questioned the patient upon the frequency of her urination. This was sufficient to make the patient fix her attention upon the region of her bladder. She at first experienced simple pollakiuria, then imperative micturition, and finally painful sensations in the lower abdomen. It is useless to add that the examinations of the urine, being completely negative, confirmed the purely functional nature of the manifestations experienced.

We have often noted phenomena of the same kind in women who, suspecting their husbands and living in fear of being contaminated by gonococci, experience in regular progression the whole series of symptoms which we have just indicated.

In the same way with men, we have seen them, after suspicious contact and without any urethral discharge, work up symptoms of the same kind, the patient fearing, he tells us, that he has directly infected his bladder. This in fact is a type of false urinosis which is not rare, but which is very little known and which one finds in men as well as in women.

The *disturbances of micturition,* properly so called, on the contrary, are exclusively the prerogative of men.

Mr. X., fifty-two years of age, a pronounced neurasthenic, complained of urinary troubles characterized by the emission of urine in a continually interrupted stream. All his micturitions as long as they lasted acted in the same way as would be normal for the last few drops. Our patient had had urethritis. He was afraid, before any symptoms appeared, of being threatened with a stricture. What had happened in his case? Careful observation enabled us to trace the mechanism of the phenomenon. Obsessed by the idea of having a full and normal stream of urine, our patient contracted with extreme intensity. He contracted not only his abdominal walls but also his membranous sphincter, and the result was such that his urine would only run when the contraction ceased by the exhaustion of the muscular contraction. The same thing would begin again and the jet stopped, to go on again when it was again exhausted, and so it would continue, whence the prolonged and spurting micturitions, which had more and more firmly rooted in the patient's mind the conviction that he was attacked by some unknown urethral affection which they did not want to tell him that he had.

We have seen patients of this kind the victims of errors of diagnosis. As the phenomena were naturally more marked when the bladder was full, it followed as a result that the patients complained chiefly of difficulty on awaking in the morning. They were therefore treated as prostatics, while they were, in reality, false prostatics.

We have seen, however, a very great number of another kind of *false prostatics.* They were, it must be confessed, the victims of medical therapy. They were patients of a certain age who had shown some one of the urinary functional manifestations which we have just described. The physician naturally thought of hypertrophy of the prostate and treated it accordingly. More particularly have we seen patients who imagined that they could not exist without regular massage of their prostates. As a matter of fact, these patients were purely prostatic phobics, made so as a result of medical suggestion.

We have described separately the different symptoms which false *urinaires* may present. It goes without saying that these manifestations may be associated one with another, to constitute the most varied as well as the most variable syndromes. It is all a question of attention, of interpretation, of medical suggestion and auto-suggestion, or again a question of education. If we bear in mind that under the effect of an emotion all these elements constitute the factors of urinary functional localizations, and that, on the other hand, a mental representation is quite as susceptible as an emotion to lead up to spasmodic phenomena, we shall have finished with the study of false *urinaires* having treated the subject rather briefly because the majority of the phenomena which are met in it have already been described in the masterly study of Pr. Guyon (1889).

CHAPTER III.

FUNCTIONAL MANIFESTATIONS OF A GENITAL NATURE.

MANIFESTATIONS of this kind are extremely common in both the sexes. According to our personal experience, they are almost as frequent as the digestive manifestations, whether the genital localization is of first importance in the neuropathic condition, and is predominant in the symptomatology constituting what has been called sexual neurasthenia, or whether it is associated with other preëminently morbid manifestations.

As a matter of fact, it is comparatively rare for a neurasthenic, when questioned about this matter, not to confess to some troubles of this nature if willing to unbosom himself at all. But it must be added that very often one must tactfully draw from the patient a confession of the existence of these manifestations, which, from a sort of feeling of shame or mistaken self-respect, he is often reluctant to tell about. And if this is true for men, it is still more often true in the case of women, in whom sexual functional manifestations are much more frequent than is generally supposed, but which are also generally very carefully dissimulated.

This question of genital troubles in men and women does not seem to have hitherto received sufficient attention from physicians. Too often they do not concern themselves with it at all in questioning neuropaths, and too often also they dismiss the subject as a negligible quantity or even as a subject for passing pleasantry. Nevertheless, when one sees the unhappy homes, and the ruined health and depressions sometimes ending in suicide, which are the consequence of these troubles, physicians ought, we insist, to pay the most careful attention to them.

We shall study successively—

A. *Genital troubles of men.*

B. *Genital troubles of women.*

Finally we shall study in a special paragraph—

C. *Pseudo-gynæcological manifestations of a neuropathic nature (false uterine or false pelvic cases, etc.)*

A. Genital Troubles of Men.—The starting-point of all functional manifestations of this nature lies in the psychic fixation of the subject on his genital organs. The very mechanisms of this fixation are extremely variable. And, without pretending by any means to give all of them, we shall attempt to review the principal among them.

Very frequently the attention of the individual is attracted to his genital organs by what might be called venereo- or cyprido-phobia. These are patients who, for one reason or another, are in terror of having contracted some venereal disease, sometimes because they have had suspicious coitus, and sometimes because they have noticed an herpetic eruption on their genital organs or a small eczematous patch, or, because they have not been sufficiently taught in matters of necessary cleanliness, they have had a slight balanitis. Sometimes, without any physical reason whatsoever and merely because they have felt some general disturbance, they imagine that they must have contracted syphilis, and from that time on they examine themselves daily for any genital manifestations. One sees chaste young men really obsessed in this way, sometimes suffering perfect agony by imagining that they may have contracted syphilis by contact with an unclean seat or vessel.

From that time on these patients pass their time examining themselves. If they fear urethritis, they have themselves sounded if they pass either a drop of urine after micturition or a little urethral or prostatic fluid. And just as such men will later pass easily over into false urinosis, they can also develop sexual neurasthenia properly so called. If they fear syphilis, they often succeed, by repeated examinations and lavages, in creating irritative lesions which still further fix the idea in their minds that they are syphilitic, and then they conjure up a whole series of ideas concerning the exhausting effects of syphilis. Believing themselves to be contaminated in some way, they are afraid of contaminating others. Then every genital symptom may follow in the wake. These patients are legion. Urinary specialists and syphilographers know them well. They form a large part of their customary clientèle.

Onanism also plays an important part in the fixative mechanism. Its rôle is by no means physical, for, taking it all in all, masturbation, if not practised by the very young, of course, nor too frequently, has only psychic consequences. Sometimes there are patients who, through practising masturbation, have taken a sort of distaste to the sexual act. Sometimes, and much more often, individuals who have masturbated, even though very rarely, have become convinced that they have done their body some incurable damage, and that they will be henceforth and forever weakened and impotent. The cause of this lies evidently in the education intended to warn the young, which has put into the patient's mind a whole series of erroneous ideas on this subject. But it is sometimes these very ideas which spoil their lives for them.

But much more often, by virtue of moral or religious training, they have felt a sense of disgrace from the beginning of their masturbation, and this perpetual state of self-reproach has finally produced in them a depressed condition which, of itself, is the true cause of their sexual impotence.

Neither the loss of a certain quantity of spermatic fluid in masturbating nor the nervous exhaustion which a young man experiences will weaken him, it being of course thoroughly understood that the act is not too often repeated, if he does not combine with it the idea of moral reproach or a fear of physical exhaustion, a fear which is at present quite too common and which is encouraged by conversation or by reading the vast literature on onanism and its dangers. We have seen cases of this kind in men from thirty to fifty years of age, and even still older, living with this impression that by reason of having masturbated in their youth they had dwarfed and devitalized their organs in a definite manner, and that they were still paying the consequences of their bad habits.

By reason of having convinced themselves of their general inferiority, these patients are very apt to be persuaded concerning their special inferiority, and in this way become sexual neurasthenics. We have seen lamentable shipwrecks of this nature, men who have given up the idea of marrying because they were convinced that on account of their masturbation they would be unable to procreate or that their children would not be born living or normal.

By an analogous mechanism, *sexual excesses* may come in as factors of sexual neurasthenia. At some period in their life certain individuals may have indulged too repeatedly in coitus. As a natural consequence, they have experienced a certain normal fatigue. But, according to the degree of their impressionability, they begin to consider themselves irreparably weakened, as much in their general health as in their special vitality. We saw a man of this kind who was fifty-two years of age, of a remarkably good constitution and in perfect health, but who suddenly fell into a state of sexual neurasthenia as the result of a conversation with a physician. This man had had daily coitus since he was young, but his physician gave him to understand that it seemed to him rather excessive to maintain his genital activity with the same degree of energy in his sixth decade. And this individual, hitherto in perfect health, became neurasthenic, with genital manifestations, because he feared that he might have exhausted himself and have unwittingly compromised his old age, and also because he thought that his careless excesses of other days could not have been without special deleterious influence upon his genital functions.

It sometimes happens that a man has at some time in the course of his existence indulged in sexual excesses. Years may have passed without his having felt any consequences of them. He would not think of them again did not some sexual trouble arise, but he then begins to remember these excesses, systematizes his symptoms around them, and attributes his trouble to their far-off effects.

At other times emotion alone is the cause of it. This is the case, for example, in certain chaste individuals who on marrying "know nothing or dare nothing." These are they whom Montaigne describes as being as helpless as a tongue-tied orator.*

* Montaigne's witty simile, "l'aiguillette nouée," is meaningless in a literal translation.

In other cases genital symptoms are brought about by means of mysticism or remorse.

Then again a simple nocturnal pollution, which could perfectly well be explained as a result of absolute continence, is the starting-point of the symptom. The patient is filled with remorse because he has had a rather voluptuous dream accompanying his pollution. He imagines himself to have taken a more or less voluntary part in it. We have seen patients of this kind who were most miserable, leading an impossible existence and suffering the deepest contrition for facts of this kind. Sometimes the patient has more definite reasons for reproaching himself. He has not been able to resist a very strong temptation, and he becomes obsessed because he has broken the rules of chastity.

In other circumstances matters become more complicated. The person has more or less deliberately made up his mind to yield to the "temptations of the flesh." But at the psychological moment the intervention of religious ideas has exerted an inhibitory action. Sometimes he looks upon the intervention of this idea as providential, but at other times he will add to his feelings of reproach and remorse the conviction that he is impotent, and he will become subject to a sexual obsession with all the consequences of such a mental condition.

Now we come to the long category of patients in whom sexual neurasthenia is established as a result of transitory impotence, which in itself is related to obsessive preoccupation or an emotion or sometimes even a simple state of fatigue. The desire to succeed too well, the fear of failure, or some association of ideas which refuses to be banished, give us the whole mechanism by means of which patients may fall headlong into sexual neurasthenia, for the reason that, if they have once failed in the act, they will henceforward in all successive acts remember it and be troubled by it. The emotion of the first attempt, any rather considerable excitement, the nervous dread of being surprised, the fear of scandal and its consequences, the fear of pregnancy, the memory of a former mistress, or of a dead wife whom the present one with whom he is having the experience recalls too vividly,—any one of these may serve as a means by which the initial genital localizations are established. Sometimes, again, it will be the too overwhelming desire to awaken a little warmth in a partner who is too cold. We have seen numerous examples of every one of these conditions.

By an analogous mechanism, under the influence of real physical malformations or those which are purely theoretic, another large class of patients may develop sexual neurasthenia. Here, for example, is the case of two young foreigners living in a country where the boys were accustomed to bathe naked. The idea came to them to examine one another, and they found that they were not formed in identically the same fashion. It was a question of size and dimension. From that they hastily concluded that, not being strictly alike, they were probably both of them malformed. They both became sexual neurasthenics.

Sometimes the existence of a phimosis, and sometimes the influence of a more or less careless circumcision that has left a slightly painful cicatrix, will serve as the starting-point of psychic fixation.

Under other circumstances it is as a result of a real genital disease, a blennorrhagia, an orchitis, or any other venereal affection, that the idea of possible sexual incompetence gradually penetrates the mind of the patient. The symptoms soon follow.

Unwholesome conversations or reading may also play the same rôle, and draw the attention of an individual to some genital pseudo-anomaly. In addition to these we have seen sexual neurasthenia develop in men who were comparatively old, in whom the loss of power, being purely relative, was quite normal. They could not, however, get rid of the idea that they were failing, and symptoms of depression with genital localizations followed.

Finally, other individuals, though feeling themselves more or less weakened, still retain an instinctive desire for the sexual act, combined with a reflex fear. They look upon the sexual act as depressing and fatiguing, and when they yield to it are conscious of a feeling of the danger connected with it, and from that may result under some circumstances functional difficulties which fix the patient's mind on his genital organs.

Genital localizations, whatever may be the psychological mechanism in any particular case, always result from the same pathological physiology. The series of reflexes of which copulation and ejaculation are the goal may be put into play by simple mechanical excitation. But the part that the psychism plays is considerable, for we know that without any peripherical excitation an erection may take place under the influence of a desire, a story, a conversation, the association of ideas, a memory, etc. Under these conditions the ejaculation itself may be provoked by simple mental representations. Inversely, there exist numerous psychic images which are able to inhibit genital reflexes. Emotion has a very distinct inhibitive action of this kind. One can thus conceive how, if preceding or during the sexual act there should intervene any emotional manifestation or psychic obsession which should in some way divert a person's mind from the act, it might be rendered impossible. Reciprocally one can see that under the influence of excitement or too great psychic tension the successive reflex phenomena of the sexual act might be hurried along too quickly, and that numerous disturbances might result.

These various considerations bring us to the clinical study, properly so called, of genital fixations.

These symptoms occur in all ages, but they are more especially met with in young men at the beginning of their sexual life, and in comparatively old men at that period which one might describe as the masculine menopause. In other words, it is at the time when the functions begin and at the age when they are disappearing that, for reasons which are very evident after what we have just said, those conditions are more apt to be found which permit the genesis of genital fixation.

As to these genital disturbances, they are of extremely diverse nature. We shall study them first analytically.

The most common of all the functional genital manifestations is undoubtedly spermatorrhœa. It generally passes through a series of successive stages. A description of the following case will enable us better to understand its mechanism.

X. is a soldier twenty years of age whose family persuaded him to become engaged. He was in this way separated from a mistress to whom he had been a most faithful and devoted lover. At first he began to practise masturbation, during which the mental representation of his mistress would serve as the psychic stimulus. Then, under the influence of dreams reproducing the images which he had voluntarily tried to evoke by his practice, he had nocturnal pollutions. These disturbed him considerably as they became progressively more and more frequent. Accompanied at first by voluptuous sensations, they got to the point where they could be produced without any mental representation. Later still, the patient had diurnal pollutions, consisting of the involuntary loss of a few drops of seminal fluid in the day. These physical phenomena were accompanied by a psychic syndrome, characterized by a great general depression, and chiefly by a real obsession over his seminal losses.

This spermatorrhœa—which must not be confused with prostatorrhœa, and above all with the discharge of urethral mucus, which is a very frequent phenomenon in urinary phobias—finds its motive for continuing, within itself, by the obsessive impressions which it causes, and which become in a more and more subconscious way the starting-point of a very great exaggeration of genital reflectivity. In these patients an ejaculation takes place at the slightest mechanical stimulus. We have seen, as an illustration of this, an officer who got to the point where he had to give up riding horse-back because the friction of the saddle in the course of a ride of a few hours' duration would give rise to several pollutions. Another of our patients could not ride in a carriage or a street-car without an ejaculation.

It is rare that these local phenomena do not become diffuse, and that the neuropathic manifestations do not extend beyond the genital region and pervade the general state of health, leading, by the conviction under which the subject is laboring, that his spermatorrhœa depresses and weakens him, to a condition of general asthenia and more or less marked depression.

Another form of genital functional localization is established by what we might call partial impotence.

Mr. X., aged fifty-six years, was attacked with a very peculiar form of impotence. He is a married man but extremely inconstant. During the last two years his legitimate relations have been natural and normal, and it has become quite impossible for him to have any extra-conjugal relations. What has happened in this particular case?

When the symptoms started, our man was extremely taken with a woman to whom he had been assiduously making love for more than six months. This lady showed signs one day of weakening her resistance, but gave a rendezvous at her own home to her would-be lover. The latter, fearing to be surprised, and overcome with emotion at the success for which he had not dared to hope, found himself inert.

One can conceive of the despair of the unfortunate man, who, beginning to grow old and fearing definite impotence, rushed off to professionals. But his efforts never amounted to anything, because the moment that association of ideas recalled to him his recent lack of success he was seized with a peculiar state of anxiety which inhibited the sexual act, and which grew progressively more intense in proportion as his fear of permanent disability became more fixed. Nevertheless, during this whole period his legitimate relations, which it is true were few and far between, remained normal, thus proving, in an almost experimental way, the psychic nature of these manifestations.

We have been able to observe another case of the same kind, under slightly different conditions.

A man, forty-eight years of age, married to a woman only a little younger than himself, and who had reached the period of her menopause, perceived that in their conjugal relations his wife, who had hitherto been rather voluptuous, was gradually growing more and more indifferent. Instead of attributing this phenomenon to its true physiological reasons, he believed himself responsible for it, and in order to convince himself on the subject he tried to prove himself elsewhere. Naturally he could not do this without arousing a whole series of emotional phenomena, which we might easily attribute to distraction by observation. Hence his impotence, which was also partial, because at home his sexual relations remained normal. Matters did not progress very well with this last patient, who was somewhat of a philosopher, for owing to the indifference of his wife he simply gave himself up to absolute chastity. But cases of this kind are rare, and in this instance the man could not bear to admit any falling off in his powers and put himself under unnecessary restraint. Sexual obsessions frequently follow, and the condition, as a rule, becomes complicated.

Another manifestation consists of premature ejaculation. This is a phenomenon very often observed among neurasthenics. It consists in the production of a very rapid ejaculation, often before there has been any chance of intromission, the latter being, moreover, frequently hindered by insufficient erection. We have had a great many patients complain of this phenomenon, either alone or associated with other genital manifestations. It is very rare to find it at the beginning of any trouble. More often it follows some symptom or other of the sexual life, and particularly an accidental failure. Tormented by the fear of another failure, and obsessed by the desire for a normal sexual relation, these patients work themselves up into a great state of sexual excitement. They prepare themselves for coitus a long time in advance. They produce in themselves as it were a sort of psychic coitus, and the first venereal contact is enough to set off the ejaculatory reflex. This is apt to be a symptom in a progressive process which sometimes ends in absolute impotence.

Absolute impotence is, as a matter of fact, very rare as a neuropathic manifestation. There exist, it must be admitted, cases where the subjects cannot effect any sexual relation, because it is impossible for them not to associate with it some phenomenon of emotion or obsession. These patients are capable of having an erection under the influence of psychic excitement, but they are unable to profit by it, because the very idea of the sexual relation in itself or with any particular person is enough to make it fall. The following cases will furnish us examples of these troubles.

Here is a young man who had become engaged, but who nevertheless was accustomed to go to prostitutes. He was overcome with self-reproach, which followed him to the very night of his wedding and rendered him helpless. When after several months of medical treatment he found that his condition was in no way improved, he became desperate and was ready to commit suicide, for no one had ever thought of inquiring into the moral cause of his condition.

Here is another, and it is a very common case, of an accidental weakness followed by continuous impotence. One day one of us met, rushing into his office like a whirlwind, a vigorous young man whom he had treated a few years before for a slight attack of neurasthenia. "I am lost," he cried. "I have no longer any manhood; I can no longer have conjugal relations. I have a very good erection, but the moment that I am in position I see by my wife's face that she is convinced that I cannot continue, and immediately my erection falls. I am profoundly unhappy." This condition, which had lasted for several weeks, came as a consequence of a failure in coitus after a fatiguing day. A cure was very easily brought about by advising the patient to practice coitus in complete darkness.

A workman, a house decorator, who was young and vigorous, was called upon to exercise his pictorial talents at the house of a kept woman, who, finding him to her taste, proposed to him certain occupations which though possibly quite as arduous were undoubtedly more pleasurable than his own. Finding himself thus in luxurious surroundings, with a lady whose underclothes were more fussy and complicated than anything he had known, our man was thrown into a state of nervous incapacity. That was all that came of it, except as a result he became intensely neurasthenic, with vague ideas of suicide.

A young man who, being a bachelor, had never had any reason to complain of his genital functions, married. Everything went well the first few days, then in the third week he became absolutely impotent. His wife was the cause of this, for she expected of him nothing short of the labors of Hercules. She had listened to her young married friends, who had persuaded her that a husband's affections could be measured by the number of proofs of his love which he was capable of giving daily. Somewhat credulous, she had reproached her husband, who nevertheless had conducted himself very well, of not loving her often enough in the twenty-four hours. No sooner had she uttered the remark when her husband found himself absolutely helpless.

Here is a man who has been impotent for six years, because he was operated upon for a phimosis too short a time before his marriage, and the first approaches were painful.

Here is another who can do nothing because his wife at the beginning of their genital life showed excessive resistance. Another has been impotent since the beginning of his marriage,—that is to say, for ten years,—because his wife suffered too much at the first approaches. His erection collapses at the moment of intromission. The family of his wife demanded a divorce because she had remained virginal. To show that he was not impotent in the true sense of the word and not wishing a divorce, the husband practised coitus with a prostitute before witnesses.

A third, a widower, became impotent because the mistress whom he had chosen bore an astonishing resemblance to his first wife. When he was near her he would have erections, but at the moment of practising the act his erection would fall, even though on the same day he could practise coitus with a prostitute. That was because with the latter he had no inhibitory obsession nor remorse.

The following case demonstrates very plainly how strong may be the influence of remorse. A man thirty years of age, who is very vigorous, and who had often proved that he possessed normal genital power, asked the hand of a girl with whom he was deeply in love. The engagement lasted for several months, when one day being overcome by his need he went to a prostitute, but, feeling that he was behaving very badly, he could do nothing. Haunted by this first failure and believing himself impotent, he tried with others, and quite naturally one failure succeeded another. Disgusted with life he came to consult one of us with ideas of suicide. He was told to hasten his marriage; but he could only decide to do so when he had been convinced that, in marrying a young girl who was ignorant of everything and who could not make comparisons, there was no necessity of his being successful the first night, while if he married a widow it would be different. The advice succeeded perfectly.

Another rather rare form of functional manifestation is established, in the absence of any other trouble and in spite of a good erection, by the impossibility of intromission. In these cases there is generally to be found some slight organic trouble.

We were very much astonished one day by the confession made to us by a sexual neurasthenic. "Doctor," he said, "I must be malformed; I must have a conical penis which naturally cannot enter a woman's cylindrical vagina. It is impossible for me to have more than a slight intromission for I am immediately caught." The man in question had been circumcised, and showed at the margin of the frænum a slightly painful scar. It was the passage of this scar which, causing a slightly unpleasant sensation, stopped his intromission and had become the starting-point of all his symptoms.

Such cases may be very infrequent, but they ought nevertheless to be known, because they are not always easy to diagnose.

There is still another genital disturbance among neurasthenics to which we desire to call attention. It is the absence of complete ejaculation in spite of a good erection. We do not mean by this its delay, which may be sometimes more and sometimes less, according to the psychism of the subject,—a phenomenon that is by no means common in neurasthenics, who, as a rule, have a rapid ejaculation,—but its total absence. This is a difficulty which we have had a chance to observe on only one occasion. It occurred in a man thirty-eight years of age, in perfect health, who, having remained chaste on account of his religious convictions, married at the age of thirty-seven. He practised coitus quite normally, but never succeeded in having an ejaculation, and, after having made every effort, often for an hour at a time, he would withdraw still in erection without having succeeded. The starting-point of this had been a vaginal hyperæsthesia of his wife at the beginning of their marriage. The husband would begin coitus, then at the end of a moment would withdraw without having had time for an ejaculation. When the vaginismus had disappeared, the habit of not achieving had become fixed. A month's separation of this couple caused the phenomenon to disappear.

Finally, there is a large class of patients who become impotent by a wholly different mechanism. Here, properly speaking, it is a question of manifestations of a very special kind, belonging rather to mental difficulties than to neuropathic troubles properly so called. We allude to the whole category of sexual inverts who by abnormal mental representations succeed in incompletely inhibiting, by means of the distaste which they gradually acquire for the normal sexual act, the whole series of reflexes which produce it. These patients do not come within the scope of our study except when occasionally they are impressed beyond all measure with their very special impotence, or when they develop some abnormal manifestations of sexual life. We have seen extremely severe neurasthenic conditions develop in sexual inverts of this kind.

Along with these patients we have seen others in whom the sexual relations cause only the very faintest voluptuous sensations. Such a phenomenon seldom exists alone, but is generally associated with other functional manifestations. More often the voluptuous sensation is inhibited by the preoccupation of the subject concerning the mechanical conditions of his sexual relation.

And this brings us to inquire how these various manifestations which we have just described group themselves or follow one another in the same individual.

As a rule, patients develop sexual neurasthenia in two different ways. Sometimes it is by the mechanism of spermatorrhœa; sometimes, and more often, it is because an attempt at coitus has ended in failure. But when one takes up the question of the condition itself, one finds oneself in the presence of a morbid syndrome of which spermatorrhœa is often an element. Urinary manifestations are frequently associated with this condition, and especially all the troubles of micturition as well as the painful symptoms which we have described in a preceding chapter. As for the symptoms of impotence which are associated with an antecedent or consecutive spermatorrhœa, they are progressive. Although at the start it may be only a question of psychic phenomena by emotional obsessions which have temporarily inhibited the reflex genital functions, yet the erections rapidly become inadequate and accompanied by extremely rapid ejaculations.

Concerning the relations of the genital functional manifestations with general neurasthenic conditions, two classes of facts may be observed.

When limited to the too rapid ejaculations, associated or not with spermatorrhœa, genital localizations are very frequently met with in individuals who have become neurasthenic for reasons which have no relation to the genital sphere. The genital manifestations may in these patients become the starting-point of preoccupations, and superimposed obsessions, which continue to develop and aggravate their condition; but their rôle as a pathogenic factor is nil.

In many other circumstances the case is quite different, and the genital trouble is the initial phenomenon from which a consecutive neurasthenic state is developed. It is difficult, in fact, to realize how much upset many individuals are when they believe that their virility is attacked. There is nothing that disturbs them more. We have seen patients by whom material losses and very deep grief were treated as hardly worth considering in comparison with the importance which they attached to their genital afflictions. It would seem that the sexual function—which is in fact the chief function, the function of reproduction and perpetuity of the race, and above all an instinctive function—could not be touched without the entire personality of the individual being affected by it. Thus, we cannot too strongly advise the necessity of always examining the neuropath to learn the condition of this function. These patients are sometimes so ashamed of the troubles which they present, because they feel as if they were in some way humiliated by them, that they are very apt to try to hide them from the physician. This is a characteristic which is not without some value, because, as a rule, the opposite is true, and the patient is only too disposed to attribute an often complex symptomatology to his genital localizations alone.

B. Sexual Manifestations of Women.—The sexual life of a woman, although it is, to be sure, less external than that of man, may, however, be none the less intensive for that. For, if in earlier times physicians attempted to establish a relationship between the female genitals and the phenomenon of hysteria (a more than doubtful relation), it must have been because they considered as frequent in women certain manifestations bearing some resemblance to those which in a man constitute sexual neurasthenia. Was it a certain reserve on the part of the authors, not wishing to expatiate upon so delicate a subject, was it because physicians discreetly forbore to inquire too frequently concerning these things, for fear of offending the easily awakened modesty of their patients, or was it dissimulation on the part of the patients, who wilfully refused to explain any phenomena of this nature which they might experience?

For our own part, from our personal experience, we have for a long time been convinced not only of the great frequency of these troubles, but of their extreme importance as pathogenic factors in a great variety of neurasthenic conditions. This is the more easily explained because in the life of a woman the sexual function holds a most important place, for upon it depends the phenomenon of maternity.

In all that concerns the psychic mechanism itself connected with these localizations, a very important part must always be attributed to education. We have seen that in man chastity was one of the frequent causative conditions of the psychoneuroses of a sexual nature. The fact of in some way symbolizing the sexual acts or of subordinating them to moral or religious conditions has as a consequence the result that in the consummation of the sexual act the psychism occupies a too important place, and is capable of singularly modifying physical manifestations. It must not be forgotten that the sexual act is the most instinctive phenomenon of organic life, and that all the psychic manifestations which are added to it are supplementary, useless, or dangerous. Therefore, it is very certain that as far as woman is concerned any education touching on her sexual life is essentially anti-instinctive. Every effort is made to cultivate in her a sense of modesty, and to make her consider her sexual manifestations as something mysterious, we might almost say shameful. A young girl is often ignorant, even at the moment of her marriage, of what the sexual relations really are. She is often frightened by the revelation and the education which she has received is frequently of such a nature as to start up, apropos of these relations, a whole series of emotional and psychic phenomena which are peculiarly liable to upset her.

We by no means think that free course should be given to the instinctive tendencies, nor do we consider abnormal those restrictions which moral and social considerations bring to bear upon instinct. Quite the contrary. But we do hold that there is no high moral strength where there is ignorance, anxiety, or emotion. There is no morality without conscious knowledge. And if we are persuaded on the one hand that all the methods of education which may disturb a young girl's mind are bad, and if we know on the other that in certain subjects ignorance is the best prophylaxis, yet we are none the less convinced that many of the sexual disturbances which have spoiled the life of more than one woman could have been avoided by rational education. Should not the object of a wise education be to harmonize the instinctive tendencies of individuals with the rules of sound, healthy morality? Those methods of education which try in some way to annihilate an instinct, to consider it as non-existent, and to make one think that all its manifestations are immodest, have seemed to us to occur frequently as factors of the genital obsessions which we have had the opportunity to observe in certain women.

The whole subject resolves itself into a question of tact, perception, and the right moment. It is very certain that a so-called "liberal" education may, from this point of view, be extremely one-sided, if not dangerous. If certain teachings which tend to take no notice of an instinct that ought to be normally exercised in life are unhealthy, those teachings which exalt it and pervert it are still more to be feared. An excessive repugnance or a too marked taste are the opposite poles, each of which, according to our way of thinking, is as dangerous as the other.

It is a fact that women very frequently develop sexual neurasthenia when they first begin their sexual life. The part which *defloration* plays in the development of genital localizations is really very great. Sometimes the fault belongs wholly to the partner, who is clumsy, either through ignorance or brutality. Sometimes it is the ignorance of the woman which causes it and her education which makes it repellent to her. She is horrified with everything that has anything to do with sexual relations, and finally gets to the point of having sexual phobias. With her the instinct has been inhibited by her education, unless the peculiar circumstances of her defloration have annihilated, for a greater or less time or even completely, the natural tendencies. Sometimes the instinct or desire of maternity exists even when the coitus instinct has disappeared. One can then imagine the complication in her psychic life which this may bring about, and the moral break-down which may follow. On the other hand, the latter may be the direct result of the disturbed matrimonial relations to which such manifestations almost inevitably lead. It sometimes happens that the union is brusquely broken; it also happens that the wife, loving her husband, tries to hide her feeling of repulsion. She may succeed in doing this, but will live in continual anguish, which cannot be without more or less immediate influence upon her moral state. In the most fortunate cases she may, after a certain number of months or years, accustom herself to it after a fashion. It is no less true that even under these circumstances the entire course of her life may have been misdirected in consequence.

In a similar way, it is very frequent that violences inflicted upon a woman become the only too legitimate starting-point of very serious genital disturbances.

Violation as an accomplished fact, or simply attempted, and even simply touching the organ may sometimes make such a strong impression upon the victim's mind that vigorous mental representations may spring up which are susceptible of completely modifying the sexual life of the woman.

Incomplete coitus, we hold, is a very frequent cause of sexual troubles in women. Whether it be a question of real physiological disturbance accompanying abnormal practices, or whether it be due to the intervention of the phenomenon of attention in an act which theoretically ought to be free from it, or whether it be remorse for an act contrary to moral laws,—any one of these factors, either alone or associated, may be more or less predominant according to the individual.

Mysticism is another factor of these same manifestations. Without insisting too strongly upon it, we think that it is by means of mental restriction which it introduces into a physiological act that its intervention makes itself felt.

Masturbation may also be the starting-point in a woman of more or less permanent genital disturbances. Either on account of the uneasy conscience which it may cause in subjects who are inclined to be scrupulous, or by having introduced young persons too early to the sexual life to which they then yield themselves, it gives birth to a whole series of mental representations with the phenomena of association of ideas and comparisons which disturb normal sexual activity.

Sterility is responsible for a number of cases of sexual neurasthenia in women. Being sterile she considers herself to be abnormal and abased. Often she is reproached for her sterility by those around her, and she becomes obsessed on the subject. More often, to tell the truth, these patients become what we shall now study under the title of *false sexualism.*

Inversely, *the fear of pregnancy,* this great modern evil, may become the starting-point of sexual phobic manifestations. Its rôle is much the same in effect as that of incomplete coitus.

Frigidity on the part of the woman is at the same time a cause and an effect. From this point of view, we shall study it with the clinical forms of functional sexual manifestations in women.

All the mechanisms that we have just glanced at have an essentially restrictive action on the sexual life of the woman. She may, however, enter upon this form of nervous disease by a wholly different path. As a matter of fact, if the sexual instinct is susceptible of being inhibited by certain psychic phenomena, other mental representations are, on the contrary, capable of stimulating it.

In this sense sterility may come in again. It is, as a matter of fact, rather rare. More frequently the abstinence of the husband is the cause which deprives a woman of the satisfactions which she considers legitimate and concerning the absence of which she becomes obsessed.

Age may also have something to do with it, the much-talked-of critical age, when a woman, seeing the end of her sexual life approaching, tries to make the most of her last years.

Frigidity may also come in in this latter sense as well as in the restrictive sense, the woman wishing to prove to herself that she is not abnormal. We are not speaking now of sexual perverts, but of honorable, sometimes very austere, women who are the prey of obsessive ideas against which they struggle. Often their ideas do not take shape, but just as often, being depressed by these obsessions, they fall into very grave neurasthenic conditions of all kinds.

We have now reached the study of the clinical forms under which may be presented sexual functional manifestations, considered in themselves or in their consequences. We shall take up successively—

1. *Genital localizations properly so called (spasms, contractures, algias).*
2. *Feminine frigidity.*
3. *Neurasthenic states of sexual origin.*

1. *True Genital Localizations.*—These localizations may be of two kinds. One set corresponds to a mental representation of defence. Such are vaginismus and contraction of the adductors, which may occur either alone or associated. Others correspond to the externalization, or the projection of painful representations to the region of the genital organs. Such are genital pains.

These two kinds of genital manifestations may be complicated by the addition of urinary phenomena, increased micturition, pains in the bladder, etc.

Vaginismus consists of a painful spasm of the vaginal muscles, which takes place every time there is an attempt to penetrate into the vagina. Its result, we might almost say its aim, is to make all sexual approach impossible.

In the great majority of cases, the origin of vaginismus is of a sexual nature. It occurs as a consequence of clumsy defloration, or following an attempt at violation, or as a result of coitus which has been painful for some reason or other. It may be brought about by simple emotional fear of sexual approach. But sometimes the mental representation may be started by elements of a physical nature, and on the frequent existence of this has been based the theory of vaginismus or reflex spasm. It is certain, in fact, that in many cases,—and very naturally so, in view of the circumstances under which vaginismus occurs,—there exist traumatic or inflammatory lesions of the genital organs as a result of defloration. These lesions may be painful in themselves or on contact, and may enter into the genesis of the spasm.

It would thus be the initial production of pain that would determine the spasm at the moment of coitus. This perhaps may be the mechanism of certain forms of vaginismus,—superior vaginismus,—where a certain penetration is possible and where the vaginal contraction takes place only in the upper part. Finally, in certain cases it is not the vagina itself which is hyperæsthetic, but only the clitoris.

But, as a general rule, in all these cases the pain is due to a psychic mechanism and has nothing to do with any previous action exerted on the painful spot. It is, therefore, the fear of pain which comes into play. It is thus that we find vaginismus persisting in women who are morally distressed on account of their genital inferiority and who ask nothing more than to be relieved of it. One sees it even in prostitutes! It could not be otherwise when the mechanism of vaginismus, as a rule, causes a fear of the sexual act. This is the way in which the great majority of cases become established. It may be complicated or continued by one of the secondary mechanisms which we have just described, such as anxiety at the appearance of real pain due to lesions, or uneasiness caused by the possible memory of former pains.

Vaginismus may have still a different mechanism. The production of too strongly voluptuous sensations or a too intense psychic desire which is afraid of missing its satisfaction may also be the starting-point of it. This, however, is a very much rarer form of vaginismus, and in such cases the fixation is not generally lasting.

Confirmed vaginismus is a very painful affection; but on questioning patients they quickly reveal the preponderating mental nature of this pain, which often the mere approach of the male is sufficient to elicit, and sometimes the simple idea of the sexual act is sufficient to cause it. Sometimes it disappears suddenly without any apparent cause. Sometimes a change of partner will determine its disappearance. More often, and if it is not treated, it is a lasting affection. We have seen women who remained chaste through their whole life on account of vaginismus. It goes without saying that their conjugal happiness was peculiarly compromised in consequence.

A girl at eight years of age when playing with her brother received a violent blow on the labia majora. She told nobody about it, but believed that she had been seriously hurt. As she grew older there gradually grew in her mind the idea that this traumatism had deformed her genital organs. She was frightened at anything that had to do with the functions of that region. When she heard a confinement spoken of, she was seized with a feeling of terror. Believing herself malformed, she made up her mind to remain unmarried, but, being very unhappy at home, she did marry nevertheless when she was twenty-six years of age. When she was seen by one of us six years after her marriage, she had never yet been able to allow her husband to approach her, and no physician had ever been able to examine her on account of the foolish terror into which she was thrown at the moment of examination, a terror which manifested itself in extreme agony, which almost overcame her, as well as on account of the invincible defence of the adductors. This woman was all the more broken-hearted over her condition because she ardently desired to have a child. Isolation was the only thing that had any effect upon these symptoms, and when this patient was convinced that she was normally formed, and when she consented to dilate herself gradually by means of sounds which were increased in size by degrees, she became so qualified for her conjugal duties that ten months after her treatment, which had lasted two months, she became a mother. By the progressive dilatation of the hymen, practised by the patient herself, and by persuasion, the intense hyperæsthesia which she had experienced on the entrance of the vagina had completely disappeared.

Contracture of the adductors may exist in two different forms. It is sometimes produced in an intermittent fashion and is then frequently associated with vaginismus. This spasm of the adductors occurs under exactly the same circumstances as vaginismus, and is always determined by a sexual idea, which may be positive as well as negative. As a rule, this phenomenon is merged into the symptom-complex of vaginismus. This is not the same in permanent contracture of the adductors. The latter may be found in hysterics quite apart from any genital causation, as may be any other muscular contraction. It is none the less true, however, that in the large majority of cases, the contracture follows a sexual fixation. We have seen contracture occur after attempts at violation and after defloration. The fear alone of sexual approaches may also determine it. Sometimes this contracture is very violent. It is, as it were, the crystallization of the phenomenon of defence which is expressed in the contracture of the adductors,—custodes virginitatis. Sometimes a greater or less period of preparation is required to bring it about, as is the case in many hysterical manifestations.

When it takes place, the limbs of the patient are in extreme adduction, and the knees are tightly pressed one against the other. Sometimes one member overrides the other. If one tries to separate the limbs, the contracture grows worse, and one can feel the cord of the adductors, just as plainly as if it were a case of an organic affection of the hip. As a fact, there is no notable difference between this contracture of psychic origin and the contracture of organic origin which may lead to a coxalgia; in either case it is a question of phenomenon of defence. Here it is defence against the pain which movement causes. There it is a defence phenomenon against a sexual approach, which, although it may have become purely imaginary, is none the less capable of producing the same results. In both cases it is a reflex phenomenon, with a peripheral starting-point in the contracture of organic origin and a central starting-point in the neuropathic contracture. As a matter of fact, one instinctively defends oneself in the same way against a danger, whether it is supposed or real. This is a very interesting fact, because it opens up a vista of secondary theoretic considerations, which we shall examine a little later.

Contraction of the adductors thus created does not tend to improve spontaneously. It may last for a very long time, four years in one case observed by one of us. It may disappear under the influence of a strong emotion. It is susceptible of being dispelled by means of psychotherapy. Does it persist during sleep? This is a question that we shall take up when we study hysterical contractures as a separate subject. We might note, however, that its non-persistence during sleep would have no significance in modifying our conception of its origin. As a phenomenon of defence it is liable, as are all phenomena of defence, to disappear or to diminish during sleep. Contractures of organic origin—such, for example, as those of coxalgia—persist during natural sleep, because the pain, which gives rise to them, continues even during this state to be felt in a subconscious fashion. They disappear during chloroform anæsthesia, as do hysterical contractures, because in the chloroform slumber the painful sensation vanishes.

This contracture of the adductors is generally very marked. When it is not so severe, it may give rise to a group of symptoms creating hysterical coxalgia; but we shall meet all these questions elsewhere, so we will not dwell upon them now.

Genital algias, like the symptoms which we have just described, are generally of sexual origin, but, though they may be increased by the manifestations of the sexual life, their peculiar nature is that they are permanent manifestations which become in some way autonomous.

The thought of physical malformation, painful coitus, a rather profuse leucorrhœa, a real but temporary lesion, may be the origin of the psychic fixation of a painful symptom which, whatever its source, ends by being a pain of purely central causation.

In certain cases the pain, which is most frequently localized in the vagina, is in no way increased by contact or pressure. Under other conditions it would seem that there exists, by virtue of continued mental representation, a sort of educated sensibility, an erethism of painful sensibility, which causes vaginal sensibility to be perceived in a painful fashion. Sometimes simple contact then becomes extremely painful, and vaginal pain may develop or maintain the symptoms of vaginismus.

When once this algia is developed, it becomes an obsession. The patients are extremely preoccupied with it. By reason of its situation they may manage to hide it, and refrain from complaining about it. Sometimes they are perfect martyrs to it.

Very frequently vaginal algias are accompanied by urinary phenomena, pollakiuria, cystalgia, etc.

By the continued preoccupation which they set up, algias are apt to react upon the general health and to become the starting-point of serious neurasthenic symptoms.

2. *Female Frigidity.*—Female frigidity may include two classes of facts,—absence of sexual desire on the one hand, and on the other absence of voluptuous sensations. In reality these two orders of manifestations are closely allied, and we shall take up here only that frigidity which is due to the absence of voluptuous sensation, which may or may not eventually lead to the suppression of desire for coitus.

This is a rather frequent phenomenon, which is very little understood and is looked upon as of no importance, but which nevertheless is the origin of all kinds of troubles which react upon the conjugal life, and even upon the social life of the affected persons.

It may in certain cases be merely apparent. This is when the inadequacy of the partner is the cause. It is especially apt to be met with when the man is himself a sexual neurasthenic with extremely rapid ejaculations. We shall find cases like this further on. For the present we shall take up only the question of feminine frigidity in those cases where the husband for his part is equal to the occasion.

There are no voluptuous phenomena without corresponding mental representations, and as a matter of course there are none in the presence of contradictory mental representations. The whole mechanism of feminine frigidity lies in this proposition. Sometimes the cause of this suppression of a whole group of normal psychophysical reactions is found at the very beginning of the sexual life. And here again we see the overwhelming effect of clumsy defloration. The wife gets a feeling of disgust for the sexual act, and at the same time inhibits all potential possibilities of voluptuous sensations. Outside even of such conditions where there is a physical starting-point, there may be reasons of a moral nature. Perhaps she does not care enough for her husband, or has married him under protest, etc. At other times, and we have seen many examples of this, it is incomplete coitus practised from the start, either in marriage or in a less settled union, which is the cause of it. Then for one reason or another the relations become normal, but the frigidity persists.

Sometimes, finally, religious ideas are the cause of this, and there are women who, by virtue of their education, consider it shameful and degrading to entertain any sensual interpretations of the genital life.

Here is the case of a woman, the mother of six children, who is incapable of any voluptuous sensation. This is because at seven or eight years of age she handled herself. Her parents caught her at it and punished her severely. She was taught to abhor everything connected with her organs as shameful and wrong. When she was married, she submitted to her husband's approaches but would never permit herself to have any feeling. As the years passed she became gradually exhausted by these constant struggles against what she considered as immoral, and she succumbed to a very severe attack of neurasthenia at the age of thirty-three. When cured and equipped with more sensible ideas, after several months' isolation and psychotherapy, she still went two years—so strong had been her previous inhibition—without experiencing any pleasure in her conjugal relations, although, as she no longer felt any reproach on the subject, she greatly desired to enjoy such experience.

Under other circumstances it is the fear of pregnancy, or, inversely, the desire of maternity, in other cases, again, a too marked sexual altruism, anxiety that her companion should have his pleasure, which comes in as an intervening factor to inhibit all mental representations of a voluptuous nature.

A wholly different mechanism results, on the other hand, from an excessive desire for sensations of this kind. It is the fear of not experiencing them which engenders frigidity.

In fact the coldness or lack of passion maintains itself. In sexual phenomena all the psychological mechanisms of expectancy, memory, and association of ideas are developed to an extreme.

In the absence of all previous experience it is evident that the rôle which the imaginative faculties can play must be practically nil. This explains, moreover, why frigidity is such a common phenomenon at the beginning of the sexual life. But if the woman does not become obsessed by this frigidity, her education will go on rapidly. If she does become obsessed, or if one of the factors which we have described above should intervene, one can conceive how frigidity may sometimes become definitely established.

There are, as a matter of fact, wives who have passed their life without knowing any sensual pleasure. There are some who, being virtuous women, admit the fact, accept it as such, and pay no attention to it. During the sexual act they think of something else. Some of them in fact experience no pleasure until after several years of marriage. On the other hand, there are those who think of nothing else, and who go about looking for someone who can "transport them to the seventh heaven," and it is frequently for a reason of this nature that one sees women leaving their regular life, taking lovers, and becoming sexual perverts. One calls them seekers after sensations. There is an error in the last plural. They are not seeking sensations; they are seeking only one. They are more to be pitied than blamed, for they are the prey of a powerful and lasting obsession, which undermines their physical and moral life.

3. *Neurasthenic Conditions of Sexual Origin.*—Outside of the properly so-called genital disturbances, there exist in women a very large number of neurasthenic conditions which are of sexual origin, but purely psychic. A woman, much more commonly than a man, is apt to mingle her sentimental life and her sexual life. The phenomena of

the one react on the other, and *vice versa.* We shall try to show elsewhere that sentimental love is only a peculiar form of emotionalism, and that, on the other hand, the large majority of neurasthenic conditions have emotional phenomena as their basis. Everything that affects the domain of sentiment, or those spheres which are more or less closely dependent on it, is, therefore, by definition susceptible of becoming a basis of neurasthenic states. And this is the reason, we think, that we so often find, on questioning these patients, that the starting-point of their troubles has been in the sexual life.

These original troubles are of various natures. The rôle of sexual abstinence is considerable, whether it is a question of women who are more or less neglected by their husbands, or of widows, or of unmarried women who are obsessed in various degrees by their lack of sexual satisfaction or the wrong which their maternal instinct suffers. All the mechanisms which we have gone over at the beginning of this study may come in in the creation of intermittent emotional states. To these there are added more or less serious neurasthenic symptoms, whose origin one must know how to find, an origin which is often more difficult to discover because, when there are no positive sexual manifestations, it is very apt to be carefully dissimulated. It often happens that women have no idea themselves of the cause of their condition. There is thus established, as it were, a sort of compromise between the strength of the physical sexual life and the intensity of the sentimental life, unless the latter finds material for its development in the mental make-up.

It is, therefore, quite common to find in those who are chaste of necessity these conditions of excessive sentimentality, which are a source of continued emotional conditions, and which lead to the development of neurasthenic manifestations, even to extreme loss of weight and physical as well as moral asthenia.

These facts have an importance of their own, for they show how the phenomena of the physical life may react on the moral condition of people, and also because they offer explanation for a great number of conditions, which there is a very general tendency to consider as crypto-genetic and which are apt to be attributed to a series of organic causes.

Before leaving the study of pseudo-sexuals, we wish to devote a short paragraph to the conjugal reactions of sexual neurasthenics.

Conjugal neurasthenia of sexual origin is a very commonly observed phenomenon.

It sometimes happens that a husband presenting functional sexual manifestations holds his wife responsible and causes her to share his convictions. Under other circumstances this conviction springs up spontaneously in the mind of the wife, who, in view of her companion's impotence, imagines that it must be on account of some anomaly in her own constitution. Sometimes the wife is haunted by the fear of impotence on the part of her husband, and at the same time, while she is intensifying the source of his impotence by letting him see her state of anxiety, she is inhibiting herself and becomes cold, and finally ends by suffering on her own account for her frigidity. The inverse conditions may be presented, and the woman, being generally lacking in warmth at the beginning of her married life, may by her coldness cause her husband so much anxiety that he believes himself to be at fault. Hence there is excitement at the moment of sexual approach, with consequent impotence. In this way are born those conjugal neurasthenias which spoil the lives of married couples, and which become the starting-point of physical and moral depressions which are often extremely persistent, because rational therapy has not been applied to them or has not been called forth by confidences. Such patients, in fact, seem to have a peculiar feeling of shame in speaking to a physician about any such experiences. And we have seen people living together for ten or twenty years most unhappily, but always refusing to confess the true cause of the troubles which were disturbing them.

C. False Gynæcological Manifestations.—Apropos of this category of troubles we might repeat almost word for word what we have just said on the subject of false gastropathies. These are essentially progressive neuropathic disturbances created by medical suggestion. A slight leucorrhœa, an excessive or too long-continued flow at the menstrual period, if treated by local therapeutic measures, is often the beginning of weeks, months, sometimes years, of special treatment, during the course of which time there will be established by degrees all the subjective phenomena which the questions of the specialist have indicated,—heaviness of the lower abdomen, pains in the kidneys, rapid fatigue in walking or in standing. Other phenomena may become associated with the region of the urinary tracts or the digestive apparatus. The woman who is a false uterine will develop, by the gradual growth of suggested ideas, a false gastropathy or a false urinosis.

The starting-points of these various manifestations, however, are variable. Sometimes they are the slight quasi-physiological disturbances that we have already described. Sometimes it is a woman's great anxiety for maternity which has led her to consult a gynæcologist. Sometimes, again, it is the sexual manifestation which we have just studied which forms the starting-point of errors of interpretation, and turns the woman's mind toward the idea of some real affection of her genital apparatus.

And then the physician comes in, who often, instead of trying to turn the patient's attention away from her genital organs, believes it to be his right and duty to "try to do something." He inserts tampons, he draws up a special hygiene for her, and practises dilatations, when he does not resort to gynæcological massage, which, of all special therapeutics, is the one which is most apt to fix the patient's mind upon her genital regions.

We have happened to see a great number of women whose existence was absolutely centred on the idea of a metritis whose very existence was, to say the least, doubtful. In this way false uterines are started, and in this way are also set up pseudo-salpingitis and pseudo-ovaritis, because women who, after various suggestions, have felt more or less vague pains in those regions, have consulted physicians who have treated them for affections which they did not have.

And though the local phenomenon in itself may not be of much importance, its consequences may be extreme, by reason of the moral and material anxieties occasioned by the expense or the period of enforced rest, or the obsessions to which such treatment may lead. Very serious and intense neurasthenic states may follow, whose starting-point lies wholly in error of interpretation on the part of the patient, and also, we must add, on the part of the physician as well.

There is one more class for us to examine. It is of *nervous pregnancy* that I wish to speak. Here it is not usually a question of outside origin, but of auto-suggestion. There are some women who are haunted by the idea of maternity, because they either so greatly desire it or fear it. We then find developing in them a curious group of phenomena which simulate pregnancy, with the exception of uterine gravidity, even to its very last symptom. Suppression of the menses, or at least some irregularity, progressive enlargement of the abdomen, modifications of the breasts, and the so-called sympathetic disturbances, such as flushings, vomiting, etc., mark its stages.

Localized abdominal tympanism may be partially explained by more or less conscious modifications of the muscular tonicity of the walls —in their contractions and relaxings. If, on one hand, the sympathetic disturbances may unquestionably be of a suggestive nature, how can one conceive of suggestion as having any influence on amenorrhœa or modifications of the breasts? Is one not led to concede that organic modifications may be directly produced under the influence of a persistent mental representation?

In short, the signs of pregnancy, outside of the properly so-called physical signs, are sometimes so marked that they deceive even a physician. Certain cases have occurred in which a diagnosis could only be made by the prolongation of the signs far beyond the normal limits of gestation. But sometimes a false nervous pregnancy may be followed by false labor, the woman feeling all the pains, and parturition alone being lacking.

These observations on nervous pregnancy lead us to the study of a last phenomenon. We know that emotion may stop or suppress the courses. Therefore, may we not question whether amenorrhœa may, or may not, be a neuropathic manifestation? That it exists in a great many nervous conditions, in the course of mental anorexias and certain melancholic states, as well as in hysterics and even neurasthenics, is a fact of common observation of which there is no doubt. But how may it be interpreted? It seems to us very certain that in a large number of cases amenorrhœa is a result not of a neuropathic condition, but of a more or less marked cachectic state which has been brought about by insufficient food as a result of a primary neuropathic condition. Moreover, we see neuropathic conditions as a secondary development in chlorotic, anæmic, tuberculous, and genital patients in whom the suppression of the courses is a common phenomenon.

Outside of those cases of nervous pregnancy where amenorrhœa is a positive fact, and apparently of nervous origin, though rarely absolute, the question whether amenorrhœa may be considered as a neuropathic phenomenon still remains to be solved.

CHAPTER IV.

FUNCTIONAL MANIFESTATIONS IN THE RESPIRATORY APPARATUS.

NEUROPATHIC disturbances of the respiratory apparatus are evidently much less common than those which occur in the digestive or genito-urinary apparatus. They are, however, rather frequently observed.

We shall study successively nasal and laryngeal difficulties, then the respiratory troubles properly so called.

Nasal troubles are of diverse origins. Often in this case medical suggestion has come in. The patients really have a slight organic swelling, a slight congestion of the mucous membrane, an abnormal turbinated bone,—troubles which have no very great significance and which can be and should be treated in subjects who are not impressionable. If, on the other hand, one treats a neuropath in these conditions, far from improving him one will generally manage to fix in his mind the idea of a nasal affection, around which his psychism will become centred. Numerous troubles may then be set going.

The action of the ideas on the mucous secretion is a very common phenomenon. When has one greater need of a handkerchief than when one has forgotten it? In the same way we have seen nervous people imbued with the conviction that they have a nasal lesion, always going about with a handkerchief in their hands and using it twenty to fifty times an hour. Sometimes the mental representation leads to a repeated or constant snuffling. In this way there may be developed regular tics of nasal origin. Sometimes, again, the thing becomes complicated, and the patient, persuaded that he can no longer breathe through his nose, experiences a very marked inconvenience in his respiration, on which his attention afterwards becomes fixed.

Here, as in all other functional localizations, very serious neurasthenic conditions may follow by the usual mechanisms,—material anxiety, as a result of medical expenses, loss of interest in one's work, by reason of dissipated attention, etc. Although such cases are rather rare, we have nevertheless seen them.

Laryngeal disturbances are perhaps more frequent than those of nasal localization. We shall not take up here the subject of hysterical mutism, a complex manifestation which we shall meet elsewhere. We have before us three categories of patients: some are laryngeal phobias, others are attacked in varying degrees by aphonia, while still others present spasmodic phenomena.

Neuropathic manifestations, caused by the simple fixation of the psychism of the subjects on their larynx, are comparatively frequent, as may readily be explained by the multiplicity of functions which require the use of a good voice, as in the case of singers, actors, advocates, orators, and street criers of every kind. Let any slight laryngeal trouble which may happen accidentally last more than a day, or let even the unfounded idea of a possible laryngeal trouble disturb the patient's mind, and fixation may be produced.

Sometimes these patients go to consult specialists, who conscientiously assure them that there is nothing wrong; they go to see others, until at last they find a specialist who, perchance weary of arguing, will consent to treat them locally. The patients will henceforward and for a long time have false laryngitis. These are the patients whom one sees taking infinite care of themselves, swathing their throats in silk handkerchiefs, and sucking all the pastilles which are advertised in the daily press. A draft of air worries them; a change of temperature terrifies them.

Sometimes the phenomena do not remain purely psychic, and the situation is complicated. Such patients try their voices all day; they cough to clear their throats; thus a cough of purely nervous origin may be started, which though voluntary at first will a little later become purely automatic.

Things may go still further, and these same patients, by simple mental representation, however slightly they may respond to auto- or hetero-suggestion, may nevertheless develop more or less marked phenomena of aphonia or hoarseness.

Sometimes there is simple diminution of the volume of the voice, the patient hardly dares to speak, he whispers rather than speaks; sometimes there is hoarseness which is probably due to the muscular asynergias which the mental representation can create. Does not one often find, on the other hand, that under the stress of emotion the voice breaks and its tone is changed? This is what might be called a phantom voice.

These are the same symptoms that continued laryngeal preoccupation is liable to bring about. Here, as we have already shown elsewhere and as we shall continue to indicate many times again, when phenomena of preoccupation (or obsessions, if one prefers so to call them) become localized on an organ, there will finally be established in this organ the same symptoms which are apt to be suddenly or directly produced by an emotional shock.

Spasm of the vocal cord may also be met with in neuropaths. We have seen a case of this kind in the service of one of us, an old hysterical patient who was very peculiar and who had been examined by all the specialists without any one of them being able to attribute the phenomenon which she presented to any affected organ. It was a case of laryngeal spasm which occurred in a peculiarly intense degree when the patient was lying down, but which would continue when she was seated or standing, although it was then much less marked. It was accompanied by sounds of snorting and deep breathing. The snorting disappeared completely during sleep. The spasm had made its appearance after a violent emotion, and, once established, had at first been intermittent, but afterwards became permanent. Repeated examinations of the larynx showed a wide glottis, normal vocal cords, functioning easily and without paralysis or spasm. From the fact of her continued good state of health, the absence of cyanosis, and the total disappearance of the phenomena during sleep, and of their diminution during wakeful times in the night, and when the patient did not think that she was observed, and, finally, on account of the past neuropathic history of the patient, a diagnosis was made of hysterical functional spasm of the constrictor muscles. This diagnosis was further confirmed by the fact that on pretending to catheterize the larynx the spasm would disappear. This patient, who was under the observation of one of us for ten years, and in whom the affection dated back for fifteen years, has always been in the same condition.

Such intense manifestations are rare; but cases less marked, or only recurring at intervals, are frequently seen. These cases often have a particular genesis. Swallowing the wrong way has been known to give rise to them. A subject, having by a false attempt at swallowing introduced a little liquid or some solid particle into his respiratory tubes, is seized at the moment with a legitimate spasm. But after that he will live in dread, almost in expectancy, of this spasm, which may be produced by the slightest disturbance of deglutition, or even, without any trouble of that kind, by a simple mental representation, or on the occasion of any emotion, whether trifling or profound.

The respiratory troubles of neuropaths, properly so called, are extremely interesting to study, because they have a sufficiently distinct objectivity to enable one to detect them easily and analyze them, and to separate the different mechanisms which are liable to produce them. Here again we find ourselves in the presence of two classes of patients. The one comes under the head of phobics of diseases of the respiratory tracts. We shall take them up immediately. The others present effective functional disturbances.

Diminution of respiratory interchange is a common factor which is present in nearly all neuropaths when in a state of preoccupation or obsession. It is merely a normal phenomenon of which the continuity is abnormal. All phenomena of attention, expectation, or preoccupation, even in the most healthy individual, are accompanied by a diminution of the number and the depth of respirations. Watch a brain worker seeking for a solution of some difficult problem, watch a workman while performing some delicate and careful piece of work, look at a spiritually minded devotee while praying in church, notice the attitude of the listeners to an exciting story, and you will be able to verify the fact that in all these individuals their respiration is less frequent and less profound, and that, even without experiencing any emotional phenomena, they are obliged from time to time to draw a deep breath, on account of the organic need created by the insufficiency and infrequency of their inspirations and respirations during the period of attention.

Now, the nervous man while experiencing any symptoms is, as a matter of fact, in a state of *continued* attention, observation, expectation, and preoccupation, and he holds his thorax comparatively immovable, at least to such an extent that after a certain time he gets the habit of not breathing deeply enough.

We have systematically examined by means of a spirometer the volume of air expired by a great number of neuropaths afflicted with the most various symptoms. We have thus been able to ascertain the fact that all these patients show a diminution, which is sometimes considerable, in their vital capacity and in the amount of air they inhale.

As to the amount of respiratory interchange, we have obtained three hundred, two hundred, and even one hundred cubic centimetres, instead of the normal five hundred. As to the vital capacity, it rarely passes three litres, and the usual amounts vary between a litre and a half and two litres and a half in individuals who are otherwise normally constituted. We naturally in the course of examinations have guarded against any possibility of suggestion, contenting ourselves with merely showing the patient how the apparatus works, without telling him the object of our search and its probable result. In order that the patient shall have no knowledge of the results obtained, we always cover the dial of the apparatus on our first examination.

Here then we have established the first objective fact, and one which is fertile in consequences. On the one hand, it explains the rapidity of breathing while the patient is walking, speaking, or even standing still. On the other hand, it is quite certain that the insufficiency of respiratory interchange as a phenomenon of nervous origin may have consequences from the point of view of bodily reactions. And we should not be at all surprised if a certain number of the urinary modifications which have been pointed out in nervous patients might be attributed to phenomena of this kind, or the inverse, which may also be observed under special circumstances.

This very diminution of respiration may constitute an autonomous neuropathic manifestation, of which we have seen a very curious example.

Madame X., forty-two years of age and the mother of six children, was afflicted with a very peculiar respiratory trouble. At different times on one of her good days, and three or four times a minute on a bad day, the patient would draw long deep breaths exactly like what we commonly call a sigh of relief. The trouble went on for two years. It would appear coincident with all kinds of preoccupations. It was intensified by excitement. The fact of going to dine in town, or of receiving friends, etc., would make it considerably worse. Moreover, the patient noticed that several days before the appearance of her courses it increased spontaneously. In addition to this very peculiar phenomenon the patient showed signs of very marked astasia-abasia.

In examining the patient attentively when the phenomenon occurred,—and we might as well state at once that all that was necessary was to look for it and it would occur,—this is what one would find. The patient remained in an almost absolute state of apnœa for a certain number of seconds. We have counted these respiratory pauses with a stop-watch, and have found them to last from twenty to thirty seconds. The pause terminated by a long involuntary inspiration. It is evident that this long inspiration was directly dependent upon the apnœa; and when ordering the patient to breathe in a regular manner, at the rate of ten deep breaths in a minute, the phenomenon would not be repeated. The intensity and frequency of these deep breaths were in direct proportion to the attention which the patient brought to bear upon the phenomenon or the state of expectancy that she was in concerning it. Thus, fearing that it would occur while she was busy about her daily occupations, she always had with her an effective reason for producing it.

This patient had narrowed her life down to such an extent that she would no longer leave her home, and as a matter of course the neuropathic symptoms from which she was suffering, having become a veritable obsession, grew steadily worse.

Here, then, we have a first series of disturbances in which the mechanism of the attention is concerned as well as a more or less obsessive preoccupation, which disturbances may become singularly complicated when the attention is fastened on the respiratory tracts themselves.

Emotion very frequently has a strong effect upon the respirations, and under two different forms. Sometimes it has what we might describe as a sudden switching off of the respiratory function, which is cut short. The patients complain of their throats being contracted, they suffer from a sense of emotional restriction or oppression, and cannot breathe. When the emotion occurs again, it brings on the same phenomena, which may under certain circumstances have such an effect as to cause that diminution of respiratory interchange of which we were just speaking.

The usual effect of emotion in causing symptoms in the respiratory functions acts in quite the opposite way. A *nervous pseudo-asthma* forms the type of what we might call respiratory emotionalism.

Here are two examples which will help us more clearly to understand the genesis of this difficulty.

Mr. X., aged thirty-eight, had a small business in Paris. He wakened once in the middle of the night, thinking he heard a noise in his shop; he felt uneasy, and became quite disturbed, and then was taken with an intense polypnœa. He gasped for air, and was obliged to run to his window to get relief. This phenomenon lasted for several hours, then finally he gradually grew calm, but he could not go to sleep again that night. The next night he wakened again, this time without any cause of anxiety, but the same symptoms occurred. However, the duration of the attack was perhaps not quite so long. He went back to bed, and was able to get to sleep, but he awakened a second time and was seized with a second attack. In the weeks that followed this affection persisted, and our patient would be taken from one to four times in a night with symptoms of this nature. His attacks never came on in the daytime; so he never had a chance to let us see him in one of them, and we could not tell whether the period of polypnœa was preceded or not by a period of apnœa. According to the patient's description, it would seem that there was none, and that the polypnœa was produced at the moment of wakening.

What mechanism was brought into play in this particular case? It seems certain to us that the first attack had been brought about solely by anxiety and excitement. As to the following attacks, it was the memory of the previous manifestation which created them. As soon as the patient was reassured concerning his condition, he ceased to have any of these symptoms.

Another case, quite resembling this, was presented by a patient thirty years of age, a printer and political writer, very much interested in questions of the day, and who in the midst of an election campaign was suddenly awakened in the night. He thought he was called to his printing-office, and leaped suddenly out of bed, and was seized with an attack of oppression with polypnœa, which lasted about two hours, but finally passed off. The same phenomena reappeared on the following days, and when we saw the patient he had been suffering in this way for three months. In his case also we were not able to determine whether a period of apnœa occurred before the period of polypnœa.

It is unnecessary to add that these two patients believed that there was something very serious the matter with them, and that they were obsessed about their affection. They were convinced that they had uræmic and cardiac symptoms, or at least that they were asthmatic. Nevertheless, in each case their cure was only a matter of several days.

As to the pathological physiology of such symptoms, we possess no positive explanation in the absence of exact information concerning the way they act at the start. Are they patients who, under the influence of some emotion, have a period of "shortness of breath," with apnœa and a sensation of suffocation, followed by a period of a sort of compensatory polypnœa? Or, rather, is it not emotion which has been the immediate means of making them pant? The two explanations are equally plausible. It is possible also that both mechanisms may be combined in the same subject.

Such manifestations are comparatively easy to diagnose. In the absence of any cardiac or renal symptoms, one cannot help but think of true asthma. Such attacks, however, differ considerably from it, first by the absence of all secretory phenomena, and further by the very nature of the respiratory symptoms. If there are phenomena of oppression or anguish, these manifestations are accompanied by a polypnœa, and not a dyspnœa that is markedly expiratory as in asthma.

A third type of functional respiratory disturbances consists of a more or less extensive *immobilization* of the thorax.

Miss X., thirty-three years of age, was brought to us one day, as a general medical patient, to confirm a diagnosis of incipient pulmonary tuberculosis.

On examination, it was found that, as a fact, the vesicular murmur of the right apex was extremely diminished and almost absent. Percussion and auscultation while speaking or coughing, nevertheless, gave exactly the same results on both sides. On the second examination, which was a little more thorough, it was found that the diminution of the vesicular murmur was not confined to the apex only, but extended through the whole length of the right lung.

Now, this patient had never had a pleurisy or any respiratory affection of the lung whatever. What, then, could be the matter with her? In inquiring still further into the history of her disease, we learned that, six months before, she had had an extremely painful right scapulo-humeral arthritis. The respiratory movements had exaggerated the painful symptoms, and under these conditions the patient, in dread of the pain, had in a purely reflex way immobilized her right side. The pains had disappeared, but immobilization had remained. The habit was formed. As a matter of fact, the measurements showed less expansion of the thorax on the right side than on the left during the movements made by inspiration.

We have had the opportunity of seeing similar phenomena following a stitch in the side, an intercostal neuralgia, an eruption of shingles, or fractures of the ribs. Their origin is sometimes organic. Their persistence—which is indefinite, after therapeutic measures have succeeded in fixing the ideas in the patient's mind, and that long after the initial pain has disappeared—constitutes a neuropathic phenomenon, a more or less conscious phobic manifestation, through fear of a pain which no longer exists.

Finally, belonging to this same group, there is a functional trouble which is rather difficult to interpret. We mean that *sensation of continued oppression* of which certain neuropaths complain. It must be clearly understood that in this case we are not speaking of respiratory manifestations in the true sense of the word, but rather a cœnæsthetic phenomenon. As a matter of fact, this sensation of oppression is what goes to make up in part the feeling of anguish that melancholics experience. It is no less true that it is quite frequently experienced by simple neurasthenics. Bearing in mind what we said at the commencement of this study concerning the diminution of respiratory exchange in nearly all neuropaths, it may be that in it we shall find a mixed cause—an organic cause of neuropathic origin—of this sensation to which nervous people so often refer in telling their story.

We are speaking now only of a more or less continuous sense of oppression. Under the heading of transient phenomena, we have already seen that it plays an integral part in manifestations of emotional shock, and it may still be here again a question of cœnæsthetic phenomenon, or it may be caused by shortness of breath arising from some emotional disturbance.

To conclude, the study of these respiratory manifestations has enabled us to isolate three mechanisms. One is due to attention, a second is created by emotional states, and a third is formed in some way by the crystallization of bad habits. It has seemed to us that the troubles due to this last mechanism deserve to be included in the class of neuropathic manifestations. As a matter of fact, although the vicious attitude is in a general way an organic phenomenon, its indefinite persistence without any corresponding persistent organic change is seen only in neuropaths.

This threefold origin of symptoms, which the study of respiratory manifestations has permitted us to set forth, offers a general scheme for the interpretation of all functional symptoms. This is a question that we shall take up further on, but which we ought to indicate in passing.

We are now ready to take up the study of the *phobic manifestations* which have fastened upon the respiratory apparatus and their consequences.

Affections of the respiratory apparatus, and particularly pulmonary tuberculosis, are so frequent that there is nothing astonishing in the fact that psychic fixation should be located upon the lungs. What, on the contrary, is curious, is to see that they are, as a fact, comparatively few in number. False gastropaths, false urinaries, and false cardiacs are much more commonly met with than false pulmonaries. This is undoubtedly due to the fact that the imagination, except in characteristic hypochondriacal tendencies, is not apt to choose willingly such affections as are considered immediately dangerous. Neuropaths and patients with false organic diseases generally give them a wide margin, and, just the contrary to the case of hypochondriacs, they are not inclined to cultivate those affections which are looked upon as mortal.

Nevertheless, this group of false pulmonaries does exist; and the psychic genesis of their trouble is complex. Sometimes it occurs in individuals with tuberculous heredity. They have lost a father, a mother, a brother, or sometimes a child with pulmonary tuberculosis, and thus the idea of a possible or probable heredity haunts the patient, and becomes a starting-point of his psychic fixation.

Sometimes it is the fear of a possible contagion which gives rise to the orientation. There are innumerable examples of medical students, and even physicians, who at some time in their lives have believed themselves to be tuberculous, without having any real symptomatology.

Any real respiratory infection, such as the grippe, tracheitis, bronchitis, or a stitch in the side, is sometimes all that is necessary for patients to live for years under the impression that they are tuberculous.

Here again the physician is really often responsible for such an idea, which he has helped to fix by a too minute auscultation or too particular inquiry. How many people there are of this kind who have been worried by the persistent idea of the possibility of a latent tuberculosis, because they have been asked whether they have never spit blood, or whether they have never had a continual cough, or if there has never been any tuberculosis in their family.

But tuberculosis is not always the only subject for fear. Sometimes it may be asthma, sometimes emphysema, and sometimes chronic bronchitis. We have seen patients laboring under the false impression that they had pleural adhesions.

Once the psychic orientation is made, what phenomena may develop from them?

Of them all, a cough is by all means the most frequent. Haunted by the idea of a possible affection of the lung, the patients force themselves to cough to see whether there may not be some slight traces of blood in their bronchial secretions. This cough, which is at first voluntary, later becomes automatic. The patient feels a sense of irritation, a tickling in the throat, and he gets into the habit of keeping up more or less continuously this little dry, short, repeated hacking which is characterized by the name of a nervous cough.

Along the same lines *thoracic algias* are developed. The false pulmonic, by reason of being examined and palpated, gets to the point where he discovers some peculiarly sensitive region. The mental representation of this pain projects itself in the form of a localized pain in the chest, accompanied occasionally by a cutaneous hyperæsthesia of the region where the pain is felt.

Other manifestations may still be produced by a very different mechanism. Patients who believe themselves to be attacked in their respiratory tracts have an intense fear of catching cold. They get what has been called cold phobias. They load themselves with clothing, wearing two or three coats, which they take off and put on when going from one room to another. When they have their backs to the fireplace they will put something over their chests, so that two different parts of their body shall not experience any difference in temperature. If they get an idea that it is cold, they show very marked signs of anxiety. We have seen one person who under these circumstances would always break out into a profuse perspiration on his body. If he were not able to go in and change his linen immediately, he would be sick, and would have a bad cold for several days, during which he would coddle himself.

Finally, by the attention which these patients bring to bear upon their respiratory functions they are liable to have any of the real functional manifestations which we have just studied.

It goes without saying that such obsessive preoccupations seldom exist without finally reacting on the general moral and physical health of the subject. Whether by reason of their preoccupation they neglect to take sufficient food, or whether in accordance with medical advice they eat too much, they run the risk of becoming false or even true gastropaths. Worn and depressed, the false pulmonic may develop true tuberculosis; and finally, worried and distracted by his business and his preoccupations and having thus been made extremely emotional, he nearly always ends up with a severe attack of neurasthenia, if he has not been fortunate enough to have proper therapeutic help to stop the development of these things in time.

Let us repeat again, in connection with such patients, what we have already said about other phobic manifestations. They are not hypochondriacs. It is an error in interpretation which is at the bottom of their trouble. They can be perfectly and completely cured if one can convince them of their mistake. On the other hand, what physician can boast of ever having cured a hypochondriac or nosomaniac?

Before closing this chapter, there still remain a few words to say about two phenomena,—namely, hiccough and hysterical hæmoptysis. We have placed them here for definite reasons,—hiccough because it is not properly speaking a respiratory phenomenon, and hæmoptysis because it seems doubtful to us that it really exists.

We know that hiccough is caused by a sudden contraction of the diaphragm. This contraction is generally reflex. It may start from the peritoneum, or it may have a gastric, œsophageal, or respiratory origin. A purely neuropathic hiccough is hardly ever found except in hysterics. After examining very carefully everything that pertains to this phenomenon, of which we have seen a certain number of examples, we could not help but believe, that in these cases it was due to a more or less voluntary—or, if you prefer it, a quasi-simulated—contraction. Perhaps, however, the mental representation created by a real attack of hiccough occurring previously might have been sufficient to cause it. We would hardly dare either to affirm or deny it.

As for hysterical hæmoptysis, as in all the so-called vicarious hemorrhages,—that is to say, occurring instead of and in the same way as menstruation,—we are rather sceptical. That they have established hæmoptysis in hysterics there is no doubt, but that these hæmoptyses might not be due to an incipient tuberculosis is by no means sure. In any case, we cannot consider it a sufficiently well-established fact to be placed with any sense of surety among the classified functional manifestations.

CHAPTER V.

THE FUNCTIONAL MANIFESTATIONS OF THE CARDIOVASCULAR APPARATUS.

A. The Heart.—Of all the bodily functions the circulation is perhaps that which is least able to be modified by the will. Although one may stop one's respiration to a certain degree, and although a simple mental representation without the addition of any excitement or emotion is able, as we have seen, to hinder the process of digestion, there is no similar state of affairs in connection with the circulation. No voluntary action or mental representation is in itself able to modify the cardiac contraction, or alter the rhythm, or have any effect upon its strength.

It is true that the functional disturbances which bear directly upon the heart and the blood-vessels are all dependent on emotions. But, on the other hand, the same thing happens in the case of the heart that we have seen in the case of the various other parts of the body,—namely, there are phobic manifestations which may be followed by a certain number of disturbances. These fixations are themselves of two kinds. Sometimes the mental representation may modify the cardiac rhythm, but that is when excitement or emotion intervenes. Sometimes the real functional disturbances are connected with the heart when the latter shows no sign of any objective trouble. They have to do with manifestations which one might designate as peri- or para-cardiac. This outlines the plan of our study, and we shall take up successively—

1. *Action of emotion on the heart.*
2. *Phobias of the heart, and pericardiac phenomena;* remembering from now on this fact, that a phobic manifestation may be the starting-point of emotional phenomena and consecutive troubles.

1. *Action of Emotion on the Heart.*—The heart reacts to emotion or excitement in two opposite ways.

Sometimes, and usually under the stress of emotional shocks, the emotion slows down the heart-beats until *syncope* is almost produced.

Syncope, as a rule, is only a symptom. Nevertheless, there may be in some people a true specialization of the emotion which causes them to feel symptoms of syncope on every occasion when they are excited. This is one of the first functional manifestations which one is apt to meet in the realm of the cardiovascular apparatus. Repeated syncope, as a matter of fact, rarely occurs in connection with cardiac affections properly so called. It is much more commonly a neuropathic manifestation.

In the immense majority of cases the emotion is accompanied by a tachycardia. The latter may be extremely marked. The heart may reach 140 to 150 and even more pulsations a minute. The tachycardia may be accompanied by more or less severe cardiac distress. In such cases tachycardia is generally also the result of an emotional shock.

When less marked, it may be an habitual symptom of internal emotion. Sometimes the memory of an emotion or a more or less anxious waiting time or some continued anxiety will be enough to cause a tachycardia without any emotional shock. There are some patients who seem to be afflicted with an almost continuous tachycardia, which, however, is characterized by this fact, that it disappears during calm and dreamless sleep. A restless sleep or nightmare will bring it on, and it frequently happens that patients troubled in this way wake up with tachycardia.

Emotional disturbance of the heart is usually accompanied, on the one hand, by vasomotor phenomena, which we shall discuss further on, and, on the other hand, by respiratory troubles (*e.g.*, by polypnœa).

Rapid heart-beats, or *palpitations,* of which so many patients complain, are, as a fact, only the subjective impression of transient tachycardias, and from this point of view would deserve no special mention were they not often the starting-point of more or less intense phobic manifestations.

Tachycardiac phenomena and syncope may often be associated in this sense, that under the influence of an emotional shock a subject may first be taken with tachycardia and then more or less suddenly fall into a state of syncope. Arrhythmia may in some cases be associated with it, or follow tachycardia. In the nervous patients whom we have studied arrhythmia seems to us to be nothing more than tachycardia of very short duration. Bradycardia is associated with syncope. Occurring alone it does not seem to us to form a functional manifestation.

We shall not dwell upon the pathological physiology of these phenomena, nor on the mechanism of the action of the emotions on the medullary centres. We feel that the fact in itself is interesting which shows that under the influence of an emotional shock or an emotional idea the cardiac rhythm is susceptible of change. It permits us, in fact, to isolate one mechanism of the functional fixations which until now the various symptoms we have described have not brought out very clearly, because, as we have already said, in all the functions which we have hitherto studied the simple mental representation and voluntary activity might serve as a basis of an interpretation of the troubles which were detected.

2. *Phobic Manifestations and Pericardiac Fixations.*—Phobic symptoms centred on the heart are very frequently met with. This is very simply explained by the facility with which the heart—or, what comes to the same thing, its neural mechanism—reacts to all emotional manifestation. As there are no individuals who do not experience some emotions, there are none who have not, on some occasion, experienced emotional modification of the cardiac rhythm. The emotional state

being, on the other hand, as we shall see later, distinctly favorable to the establishment of all auto- and hetero-suggestions, it very frequently happens that some exciting disturbance accidentally affecting his cardiac apparatus makes a very great impression upon a patient, and he develops a phobia concerning his heart.

In other cases ideas of heredity come in. In the general opinion of the public, heart disease is hereditary. We have seen numerous patients who, because one of their ancestors had had some cardiac affection, believed that they must some day fall a prey to a disease of the same nature. The sudden death of one's ancestors is particularly apt to make such an impression. One such patient whom we have seen lived in the perpetual fear of sudden death, because her father, her maternal grandfather, and her paternal grandmother had died in this way. More definite information regarding these ancestors showed that they had quitted this life at ages varying between eighty-one and eighty-six years.

We must call attention to the fact, in passing, that there was a certain period when heart disease was very prevalent. In the melancholy poetry of the generation of 1830 it was considered quite the thing, if one were at all inclined to be sentimental, to believe that one's heart was a little weak. This has rather passed out of fashion. One nevertheless still finds examples of it in very emotional people whose hearts often beat a little faster because they feel too keenly. These subjects differ from those who have been impressed by some emotional shock, and who develop phobias on account of a fear of their heart, in that they nurse along their imaginary cardiapathy and make much of it, but it is seldom that that lasts very long. It is the kind of fad that passes away when they find something else to exercise their imagination upon.

In other cases, and these are much more frequent, medical suggestion has been called into play. There are young people, for instance, who for their whole life, or part of it at least, will carry about the impression that they have heart disease because, when they were growing up, they had some of the troubles which so frequently occur when one grows too fast. Such are anæmic young girls who have had some hæmic murmurs which their physician was ill advised enough to tell them about, and who, as a result, had become convinced that they were cardiacs. There are so many fine points that may be noted in a very careful auscultation, such as a slightly dull sound, or a hint of double beat, or an abnormal tone. It is really a question of extra-cardiac sounds. The patient is very carefully auscultated. This is repeated over and over, perhaps ten times, to discover finally that there is nothing the matter. There is, however, by this time, really something the matter, for the patient's imagination has been set going. He departs with the conviction that his heart is not absolutely normal, and begins to elaborate fancies which have a far-reaching effect on his after life.

Here, among a hundred others, we have a case of a chief of a battalion, who had chosen the soldier's life as his career and who loved his calling, but who for years had been haunted by the fear of sudden death. This was because, twenty years before, while at Saint Cyr he had had an attack of rapid heart-beats while performing some violent physical exercise. He went to consult one of the well-known specialists of the time, who, although assuring him that there were no lesions, was so unwise as to prolong his examination, and to mutter in a low voice remarks about the tone of one of the cardiac sounds. The man was convinced that his heart was in a much worse condition than the physician was willing to tell him, and his life was completely spoiled by it, for from that time on he always had a fear of sudden death, and on that account would not marry.

A postman at Halles, twenty-eight years of age and strongly built, came one day to the clinic of the Salpêtrière. He had had two attacks of syncope in the street the week before, and he was convinced that he had some disease of the heart, for, he said, that was the reason why he had been discharged on half pay from military service. Now, his heart was perfectly sound; but, haunted by the fear of his disease, he was always getting out of breath and was continually obsessed by the fear of dying suddenly. He was cured, after one conversation.

Here we have a patient in whom a physician has discerned a slightly dry mitral sound, here is another whose pulse has been found a trifle slow or slightly tense, and they have had their lives spoiled because a physician has mentioned before them the very unlikely possibility of mitral stenosis or an aortic aneurism. We have seen hundreds of such cases, which have always been brought about by ill-considered medical advice.

Under other circumstances, the heart is not the organ in question, but the patient's symptoms are such as might be attributed to cardiac affections, and these happening accidentally become the starting-point of a phobic fixation. Slightly swollen ankles in a patient with varicose veins, a sensation of vertigo, scanty urine during the hot weather,—such things will sometimes be enough. But in this class of ideas the one which most commonly plays the rôle of chief pathogenic factor is getting out of breath. The number of people who are concerned by rapid breathing is very great. At first it is purely an accidental phenomenon, connected with eating too much, or with not knowing how to breathe during any prolonged effort. Then, when the attention has become centred upon this habit of panting, the patient feels the functional respiratory fixations of which we have spoken, but he attributes the panting to his heart, and all the more when the panting is accompanied by a purely physiological tachycardia which is its necessary companion.

Under these various influences many patients are seized with a profound conviction that they have some heart lesion. Other mechanisms are liable to make the person believe that he has angina pectoris. All precordial pains and even those that are more remote are especially apt, by following the genetic mode that we have already studied, to serve as a starting-point of the psychic fixation. An intercostal neuralgia, a stitch in the side, or even a rheumatic pain in the left shoulder is sufficient for a foundation. These being the principal sources of phobic manifestations, how do the patients who are suffering from them react?

Sometimes these patients remain simple phobics. They do not develop any particular phenomenon of cardiac or pericardiac fixation. These are pure psychics, whose lives are practically spoiled by the conviction that they are in a very precarious condition on account of their hearts. This, in fact, is the most frequent expression of their trouble. We must repeat, in connection with these patients, what we have already said concerning our other phobics,—namely, that they are in no sense of the word hypochondriacs or nosomaniacs. Often, in fact, they are people who are of naturally a gay temperament, who would ask nothing more than to be able to enjoy all that there is in life, but who, either spontaneously or as the result of some medical suggestion, have misinterpreted an accidental phenomenon of their life, and have ever since dwelt shrouded in their error. But these latter always have a starting-point. When cured by persuasion, these patients become definitely well in contrast to the hypochondriacs or nosomaniacs. They are what we might call accidental, but not constitutional nosophobics.

Frequently, however, the phenomena are complicated. Two examples will enable us to grasp the way in which such complications occur.

Mr. X., fifty-five years of age, came to one of us on account of attacks of tachycardia, which would come on without any appreciable cause, and last for a time varying from a few minutes to several hours. These attacks would come on at any time whatever, as frequently in the day as in the night. They were accompanied by polypnœa, a sensation of smothering, and pains that were more or less sharp. The patient also complained, outside of his periods of attack, of sensations of vertigo, with the feeling that his legs were giving way beneath him.

There were no hereditary nor personal pathological antecedents. The objective examination was without results. The heart was perfectly healthy; the sounds were distinct and well-marked. There were no murmurs nor extraneous noises. Percussion showed no dilation nor displacement of the aorta. The urine was normal. The arterial tension was 170.

Here we have a case of real paroxysmal tachycardia or an imitation of the same. What really was the matter? The patient had been subjected to a very sharp rebuke from one of his employers. After the tirade was finished, on entering his office he had had an attack of vertigo and tachycardia, and association was immediately set up. The patient said to himself, "It is because I am ill that I have not been able to do my work as well as in the past.'' He went home. In the middle of the night he wakened with nightmare. He felt his pulse and found it very rapid. From that time on, in season and out of season, he was seized with these attacks of tachycardia. Soon there occurred the added phenomena of anxiety and of precordial pains. He believed that he had angina pectoris. His daily duties became impossible for him, and he was on the point of sending in his resignation. His condition became still worse. He could no longer go out without being seized with attacks of vertigo, with tachycardia and panting.

A few days of rest interspersed with several psychotherapeutic conversations were enough to control these troubles.

An emotional attack as the starting-point, consequent phobia of the heart, then the reproduction by emotional ideas of the same symptoms, to which were added, by mental representation, precordial pain and very pronounced vertigo,—such was the succession of phenomena in this patient.

Another patient, Madame X., thirty-eight years of age, was attacked by a combination of symptoms which were pronounced, by a physician of Paris, and not one of the least known, to be angina pectoris. Here we have the whole succession of facts as they occurred to this lady, whose case is quite like the preceding one.

Her husband, with whom she did not live happily, was an invalid and afflicted with a very repugnant disease, which created in our patient a series of emotional disturbances, under the influence of which she fell into a very marked hystero-neurasthenic state, with violent headache, loss of weight, and a state of general asthenia, etc. In addition to these latter symptoms she perceived that when she was upset her heart beat more rapidly. She was concerned about this and went to a physician, who asked her if she did not have painful symptoms, and a feeling of heaviness in the left arm, etc. It goes without saying that, under this suggestive influence, the phenomena he was looking for soon made their appearance. She then consulted a specialist in heart diseases, to whom she gave in recounting the history of her case the whole symptomatology to which she had attained. He made the diagnosis of angina pectoris—''possibly neuropathic,'' he added. The patient naturally was all the more impressed. The symptoms increased, and the attacks with tachycardia, pain, and angina continued.

On examining this lady, we found a slight left hysterical hemiplegia, which, in conjunction with the circumstances of the beginning of her trouble, threw some light on the diagnosis. It is quite probable that this hemiplegia was brought about under the influence of medical suggestion which we have just related. This influence in fact explains the heaviness felt in the patient's arm, but it does not integrally explain the other motor symptoms, for, as a matter of fact, the leg was included in the paralysis. The patient had never noticed it, nor had she complained of it, and it was only by the difference in the wearing out of her shoes that we were able to convince her of the reality of a trouble which was elsewhere shown objectively by diminution of muscular strength. A distinct hemianæsthesia was associated with the hemiplegia.

Here, then, is a case where, under the double influence of emotional phenomena and suggestion, we can see how a whole series of secondary disturbances may be built up around a cardiac phobia.

Under other circumstances we have seen a cardiac phobia creating by the same mechanisms conditions of astasia-abasia having as a starting-point a mental representation of vertigo. Elsewhere the symptoms of vertigo exist alone; in other cases it is a very rapid panting which produces them; in still others the patients complain of congestive pressure, etc.

If we now try to sum up what has gone before, we shall see that cardiac phobias may occur as the result of emotional accidents or morbid convictions from many sources. Then, under the influence of emotional ideas, the various effects that emotion may exercise on the heart are produced or reproduced. Finally, under the effect of mental representations which are auto- or hetero-suggestive in their nature, there will surge up numerous secondary pericardiac or paracardiac symptoms. The commonest of these are precordial pains or symptoms of vertigo. But, as in all manifestations of this kind, they may be extremely diverse, and give rise to the most unexpected associations.

B. Vascular Manifestations.—Here again the same division may be adopted, and we can describe the effect of emotion on the vascular phenomena, on the one hand, and, on the other, the phobic manifestations which may be associated with vascular affections.

Is it possible for emotion to have any effect upon the large vessels? The thing is possible, but has not been proved, and we feel that the arterial throbbings which many patients complain of when under excitement bear some relation to the modifications of cardiac contraction.

On the other hand, nothing is so common as vasomotor disturbances caused by excitement. The emotion or excitement acts upon the vasomotor, in two different ways,—either by vasodilatation or vasoconstriction. Vasodilatation is the more common, and is seen by the blood rushing to the face. It occurs only in slight emotions, more specially perhaps in connection with emotional ideas depending on purely internal emotion. Every one knows people who blush at everything and nothing. We have seen patients of this kind to whom it was a real infirmity, who blushed every time any one spoke a word to them, and whose social life was thereby peculiarly hampered. We have seen women who would plaster their faces with layers of paint to try to cover up this trouble. In their case the very fear of blushing would of itself bring it on. They were annoyed not only from the point of view of secondary interpretations to which their blushes might give rise, but from the æsthetic point of view. True erythrophobias arise in this way, mixed manifestations where the emotion plays a rôle, but where the mental representation is sure to come in also as a factor. Here is an important point from the doctrinal aspect,—namely, that a simple mental representation is enough to create vasomotor disturbances of this kind. It is wholly a question of vasomotor disturbance and hysterical œdemas which is to be solved in such cases.

The vasodilatation may not be confined to the face: it may spread, flushing the neck and extending down to the breast, like the blush of shame. It is very rarely observed anywhere else.

Vasoconstriction is a phenomenon which is observed in emotional shock. The pallor of the face, which may become absolutely bloodless, and general paleness of the skin are classic signs of great emotion. They may also play a rôle in the production of syncope by too great a flow of blood, or, by their action on the irrigation of the bulbar centres, etc., a rôle also in the production of tachycardia.

Is there such a thing as localized vasoconstriction? This is the same problem as that of the dilatations, but we shall take up these questions when we study the functional manifestations which affect the skin, and all that we shall do now is to retain these two facts,—namely, that under the influence of slight emotion or emotional representations, vasodilatations arise which are usually confined to the face, on the one hand, and, on the other hand, the existence of vasoconstriction which may or may not be confined to the face, as a result of emotions which are more often strong and sudden. We may add that there are individuals who, apropos of slight emotion, will pale while others blush; but the fact is rare, and, as a rule, there must be some emotion of external origin, or such a strong internal emotion as anger to cause such phenomena.

Phobic manifestations which have an effect upon the vascular apparatus constitute a group which is wholly modern in its creation. For this the great extension given to the conception of arteriosclerosis is responsible. To this extension the medical press as well as the daily papers, by spreading abroad communications of scientific societies, have assisted in impressing upon the minds of many laymen as well as of physicians extreme ideas concerning the importance of such a diathesis. To the multiplicity of therapeutic means must be attributed in some degree the multitude of patients, and the excessive advertisement of all kinds of medical or physical treatments for arteriosclerosis has called forth a remarkable growth in the number of devotees to this or that therapeutic method.

We have, for our own part, seen a great number of patients who, because their arterial tension was raised a millimetre too high, had had their minds directed by physicians to the idea of precocious arteriosclerosis, sometimes more or less generalized or more or less localized. It goes without saying that, from that time on, these patients are continually examining themselves, and end by really experiencing a whole series of difficulties of mental origin in their different organs.

We have seen a patient oriented in this way by his physician on the probable arteriosclerosis of the spinal cord, who experienced one after another all the phenomena of astasia-abasia.

Others listen, as it were, for their arterial pulsations. When their head is on the pillow they try to see if they can perceive the carotid pulsation. They finally get to the point where they can hear their pulse, and by that time they have developed insomnia. Others are continually feeling their pulse in order to note the supposed or real hypertension, etc.

Does this mean that we mistake the real and frequent existence of arteriosclerosis? Certainly not, but we think that the physician ought in his diagnosis to take into consideration the mentality of his patients and to realize that the word arteriosclerosis is a very dangerous one to speak at the present day, because the public at large is too much informed, and too badly informed, concerning this affection and its immediate or remote consequences. Under these conditions it is very sure that such a diagnosis will throw the patient into a state of excitement which will be apt to lead to a number of secondary manifestations.

Other neuropathic disturbances may arise from the idea of a possible aneurism, even from the greater uneasiness caused by superficial or deep-seated varicose veins, etc. We will not dwell further upon this, however.

This brings us to the end of the study of the functional manifestations which may act upon the cardiovascular apparatus. We have confined our description to those manifestations which we consider to be undoubtedly functional in their nature,—that is to say, connected with the phenomena of emotion or due to some external interpretation or mental conception.

But there is a whole series of other vascular disturbances which would lead to numerous discussions, and which we have purposely neglected. Without mentioning vasomotor troubles which we shall take up elsewhere, we have in this chapter passed by many phenomena which although neuropathic in their nature are none the less functional manifestations. We have not spoken of painful palpitations, properly so called, nor of arrhythmias, nor of neuropathic angina pectoris, which is sometimes very difficult to distinguish from real angina, nor of essentially paroxysmal tachycardia, nor visceral hæmorrhages of hysterics, nor cyanosis of the extremities. That violent or repeated or continuous emotion, and even mental representations when firmly fixed, may be able to influence such affections is most assuredly possible. But it seems to us rather far-fetched to place them in the list of facts which we have just been describing.

CHAPTER VI.

CUTANEOUS FUNCTIONAL SYMPTOMS.

THE functional symptoms localized in the skin are extremely complex. By their number and variability, as well as their pathogenic interpretations and the discussions to which they have given rise, they assume a rank of first importance, a rank which, however, is much more theoretic than practical.

For convenience in description we shall take up successively—

1. *Action of the emotions on the skin and the cutaneous functions.*
2. *Vasomotor symptoms,—lasting secretory or trophic, diffused or localized.*
3. *Phobic phenomena and their consequences.*

In a separate chapter we shall take up disturbances of general sensibility, mixed symptoms which are cutaneous in their localization and nervous in nature.

1. *Action of Emotion on the Skin and the Cutaneous Functions.*—The cutaneous symptoms which may be observed under the influence of emotion are numerous. Here, again, emotion may work in two different ways, according to whether it is a case of emotional shock from an external cause of some sort, or whether it is a case of emotional representations,—or internal emotion, if one so prefers to call it.

Of all these fixations, the commonest and the most classic, we might almost say the most literary, is the well-known symptom of horripilation, or goose-flesh. It is formed by the raising up of the pilary system. These are the individuals whose hairs rise on their heads, whose flesh creeps. This symptom always arises under the influence of fear, or, as its name indicates, of some horror. It may be a dramatic play, or the sight of an accident, or listening to the description of some scene of horror which causes it. It often has to do with circumstances quite apart from the individual, and which do not directly concern him. This phenomenon, reduced to its simplest expression, is nothing more than a sensation which amateur lovers of dramatic spectacles like to feel. When it is a case of intense emotional shock where the individual is personally and directly involved, horripilation rarely occurs alone, but is accompanied by many other manifestations.

Superficial vasoconstriction is a phenomenon which also frequently attends any great emotional shock. People express it by saying that they felt "their blood freeze in their veins." It is accompanied by general pallor of the skin. More often it is associated with a tendency to faint.

Superficial vasodilatation also has its colloquial expression. People say that they "turned hot" when speaking of an emotion or an emotional representation where this phenomenon occurred, which, however, really belongs to emotions of moderate intensity rather than to great emotional shocks.

Vasodilatation and vasoconstriction may or may not be accompanied by secretory disturbances of the sweat-glands. Generalized hyperidrosis as a result of emotion is one of the commonest occurrences. One may break out into hot perspiration or cold perspiration following vasodilatation or vasoconstriction associated with secretory disturbance.

Vasomotor and localized secretory symptoms may be transiently produced under the same kind of influence. We have already spoken of the flushing and paling of the face. This symptom is commonly expressed by saying "I turned red," "I turned as white as a sheet," etc. Perspiration of one part alone may also be observed. Here again it is usually the face alone which is affected. Under the influence of shame, or any other emotional cause, such as fear, for example, one will find that other surfaces are affected by localized hyperidrosis,—the palms of the hands, the armpits, the breast, the genital and perigenital regions, and sometimes the entire cutaneous surface. However it may be, we have seen that under the influence of emotional shock, or accidental emotional representation, the following phenomena may be produced: horripilation, vasomotor and secretory disturbances. These are facts to be remembered, for we shall have occasion frequently to refer to them in the following paragraphs.

2. *Lasting Vasomotor, Secretory, or Trophic Symptoms, both Diffused and Localized.*—In this field all the manifestations which emotion causes are transient as the emotion itself. But the time was, and it is only just beginning to slip into the past, when major hysteria was cultivated, when it was customary to describe a great number of lasting vasomotor, secretory, or trophic fixations which were considered as of a functional neuropathic nature. For some years now, the existence even of these troubles has been vigorously attacked. Babinski, in particular, has refused to admit them. According to this author, hysteria is no longer the great simulator, to use Charcot's expression, but it is the hysteric who is the great simulator. Trophic, secretory, and vasomotor disturbances are, according to Babinski, created by conscious suggestion, or in other terms by simulation. Under favorable conditions to observe them, and where there is no chance of subterfuge, they do not occur, no more than do the troubles of sensibility. This is in fact almost the same thing as the conception which was some time ago set forth by Bernheim, who limited hysteria to the crisis itself. In support of his doctrine, Babinski states that personally he has never been able to observe any-

thing analogous to the various troubles of this kind of which we are speaking.

Nevertheless, if we turn back to the old nomenclatures, these troubles would be extremely diverse and very frequent. Let us first of all enumerate them.

Those that belong to the disturbances of the sweat-glands are bromidrosis (perspiration with odor), chromidrosis (colored perspiration), hæmatidrosis (bloody perspiration), phosphorescent perspiration, generalized hyperidrosis, localized hyperidrosis, or ephidrosis, all of which have been in their turn described and studied.

The cutaneous trophic disturbances which form urticaria, white, blue, rose, or red œdema, pemphigus, hysterical eczema, gangrene of the skin, disturbances of pigmentation, vitiligo, lentigo, lichen, whitening of the hair, atrophy and falling of the hair, hypertrophy of the pilary system, and onychia have all been frequently mentioned and considered as hysterical in nature.

In the vasomotor disturbances we may place hæmatidroses, or bloody perspirations, hæmorrhages which occur without any lesion, ecchymoses, and finally, and above all, the classic hæmorrhages to which have been given the name stigmata (the production of marks of wounds recalling in their arrangement the wounds of Jesus Christ upon the cross), as in the case of St. Francis of Assisi and Louise Lateau.

Trophic and vasomotor disturbances may be associated and hæmorrhages may follow bulbous eruptions and œdemas, etc. The majority of these latter troubles occur after hysterical dreams, in which are presented to the patient's mind either the lesions themselves or causes which are likely to create these lesions.

On each one of these troubles, chapters and even volumes have been written, quite as many in France as in other countries. Charcot and the majority of his pupils have described them at great length and have considered them as having an unquestionable reality. Could all these careful observers, even men of genius, have been the playthings of deceivers, and taken in by suggestions of which they themselves and not their patients were the prey?

It is very certain that we are much more reserved to-day in expressing our opinion upon the existence of true trophic cutaneous disturbances in hysteria, and that one must be more suspicious than ever of simulation. We may frankly say, we must be systematically suspicious. In any case, these troubles, if they do exist, are by no means as common as they were thought to be not so very long ago. On one point, however, everybody is agreed, and that is that it is evident that the former intensive method of cultivating hysteria was of such a nature as to give peculiar encouragement to the art of simulation.

Other arguments may be brought to bear. First of all, the absolute proof of deception in a great many cases, and of such clever fraud that it sometimes required great subtlety to detect it, must in itself have a bearing on the subject. It is always the case in medicine, quite contrary to the exact sciences, that negative facts count for nothing and positive facts only have the value of proof. We note the relative frequency of troubles in the regions which the patients can readily reach,—the hand, the arm, the breasts, the thighs,—and, on the other hand, the rareness with which they occur in regions which are more difficult to reach, such as the back, for example. We also note that the troubles observed often bear a peculiar resemblance to lesions made by compression, by burns, or by blisters, which are the mechanisms most often employed by simulators.

In the same way, if one admits Babinski's conception, we find that the troubles in phenomena of this kind would not be confined to the periphery. What we ought to study is the mental condition which will engender a simulation which is sometimes wholly disinterested, sometimes even injurious and dangerous for the patient, such as was the case of a patient of Dieulafoy who, although a real auto-mutilator, allowed himself to have an amputation performed for the trophic disturbances which simulation had engendered.

There are always some facts of which simulation could not be the cause,—for example, muscular atrophy, which is not seldom found in hysterical contractures and paralytics, and which may sometimes be very pronounced.

The same thing occurs also for the fibromuscular retractions in the case of hysterical contractures which have lasted a long time. Such are the fibromuscular retractions of the adductors which are observed in the case of old contractures of these muscles, and which, as we have had personal opportunity to see, can only be broken up with great difficulty, under the influence of chloroform. Such, again, are the fibromuscular retractions of the sole of the foot which are seen in hysterical contractures of the lower limbs dating back a long time, and which are quite as intense as those which one finds in cases of peripheral neuritis (particularly in alcoholic cases), when they have neglected to move the joints of the foot every day. These fibromuscular retractions of the ball of the foot may persist—we have seen several examples of them—even after the contracture is cured, and sometimes hinder the patient so much in walking that surgical intervention may be necessary. In truth, it seems, from our way of looking at things, that hysteria, just like neurasthenia, consists rather in a peculiar antecedent mental state than in the accidents of any kind which seem to us essentially secondary. Nevertheless, if we withdraw from the ancient classical opinion, which admits the reality and the frequency of trophic vasomotor and secretory disturbances in hysteria, we are, however, not ready to adopt such an absolutely exclusive attitude as Babinski's.

We might on this point sum up our opinion in the following manner. All the phenomena which emotion or emotional representations are capable of creating in a transitory fashion are susceptible of existing in a lasting form in a psychoneurosis, whether they occur as hysterical phenomena, or neurasthenic phenomena, or associated phenomena.

Without entering, for the time, into a theoretic discussion of this proposition, let us confine ourselves simply to facts. Concerning cases of ecchymosis, or hysterical hæmorrhages, stigmata, and cases of œdema, we must, as a matter of truth, state that we have not sufficient positive knowledge concerning them.

On the other hand, we have been able to prove a certain number of cases where the vasomotor phenomena or the secretory phenomena were produced, without any possible chance of simulation, by simple mental impressions. We can only quote a few of them.

Mr. X., sixty years of age, was afflicted with a phobia of cold, of which we have already spoken in connection with respiratory manifestations. Very well. In the case of this patient we have been able to prove the objective existence of superficial vasoconstriction associated with abundant hyperidrosis: the skin would be cold where a few moments before it was of a normal temperature. The phenomenon was produced the moment a mental impression of the possibility of catching cold occurred. The mentality of this patient was, moreover, not that of an hysteric, but rather of a neurasthenic.

In the case of a patient in private practice, the mother of a family, thirty-eight years of age, and afflicted with absolute and flaccid hysterical paraplegia, one of us observed, over and over again, that, under the influence of an emotional condition of a very peculiar nature brought about by the fear of an intimate psychanalytic confession, there would arise vasomotor troubles of really extraordinary intensity. The skin of the entire body became cold, and the extremities of the limbs, the hands and feet, turned bluish black, as if they had been dipped in aniline ink, or as if the patient had taken an overdose of phenacetin. Then the whole surface of the skin would break out into an excessive cold perspiration.

In the case of another patient, sixteen years old, whom we saw in one of our services at the Salpêtrière, and who had been under treatment for hysterical paraplegia for months, but who was cured in a few weeks, the following facts occurred. When lying in bed, the lower limbs seemed normal; but when she was told to get up and try to walk, under the influence of the emotions caused by the idea of the effort she was to make, her limbs and her thighs immediately turned purple. A very marked vasodilatation had taken place, which grew still worse when the patient was standing. In this particular case there could be no question of simulation, or of compression by any constriction whatsoever about the thighs, for the phenomenon was developed and increased, as it were, under the very eyes of the observer.

In the three cases which we have just outlined, it was a question really of emotional recollections under the influence of a mental representation, and that, according to our way of thinking, is the usual mechanism in this whole category of disturbances. They have nothing to do with suggestion. These are what one might describe as specialized emotional phenomena, which always occur in identically the same way under the influence of the emotion. They disappear when, under treatment, the idea loses its emotional dependence.

These are, therefore, repeated disturbances rather than lasting disturbances, in the proper sense of the word.

It is very evident that, theoretically, the continuity of any emotional representation whatsoever is apt to lead to continuity of the emotional manifestation. Perhaps permanent disturbances are due to some mechanism of this kind; possibly, under the influence of the continued disturbance of an emotional origin, trophic phenomena may be made to appear. Theoretically this is possible, and in practice one of us has had the opportunity to see the bullæ of pemphigus develop without any possible intervention of simulation.

At all events, it is prudent to hold one's self in reserve concerning the setting up of trophic or vasomotor disturbances. They are certainly much less frequent than was formerly believed, but it would perhaps be extreme to deny absolutely the possibility of their existence.

But as a fact, and in addition to the three examples which we have quoted, we could narrate many others. There do exist vasomotor and secretory disturbances which if not permanent are at least repeated in the course of psychoneuroses, and this in an unquestionable manner, without any possibility of suggestion or simulation, but merely by the common mechanism of emotional action.

3. *Phobic Manifestations.*—We have already described in a preceding chapter a certain number of phobic symptoms which focus on the skin. We now wish to speak of that numerous class of patients who are afraid that they have contracted syphilis and who are almost uninterruptedly examining their skin. Usually these phobic symptoms spring up spontaneously in the subject's mind, without any emotional phenomena, as a result of some suspicious sexual relation. Sometimes the patient's mind becomes fixed on his skin as the result of some slight symptom, such as balanitis, herpes, or redness due to various causes. Sometimes it is a physician who is responsible. Having a very impressionable and suggestible patient to treat, and not taking into consideration this peculiar mental quality, he may have said to the patient, "Now keep a sharp lookout, examine yourself, and come to me at the slightest symptoms." At the first appearance of any redness, or a pimple, or a boil, the patient is greatly alarmed. The redness is, however, often caused by the patient himself, who has brought it about by continually pulling and pinching his skin while examining it. Sometimes the obsession lasts for a long time, and we have seen patients who for years after a dubious coitus were still examining themselves to detect possible tertiary symptoms, for they had been carefully warned that the secondary symptoms often passed unperceived.

Under other circumstances there is more ground for the obsession. There are patients who have really suffered from former attacks of syphilis, or who have been afflicted with psoriasis, or eczema, etc., and who live in the expectation of the appearance of some new symptoms or some new cutaneous growth. Hypochondriacs they certainly are not, phobics or obsessed if you will, but their phobias and obsessions are the accidents of extrinsic suggestion.

A whole series of other phenomena complicated with various suggestive disturbances may result from the psychic diffusion of symptoms which really exist. In these cases the patient is not obsessed about his lesion, but about his symptoms, and chiefly the symptom of itching.

One frequently sees patients who have a trifling itching sore, a slight chafing or eczema of the scrotum or armpits, etc., whose itching has continually spread further simply by psychic fixation.

Mr. P., thirty-eight years of age, had had a generalized itching for several months, which had become so intense that it was impossible for him to sleep. This itching obsession hindered the patient in all his affairs and he was obliged to give up his work. He ceased to take sufficient nourishment, and as a consequence developed a very serious neurasthenic condition. The starting-point of the psychic diffusion of this phenomenon consisted in a slight eczema of the scrotum. The interesting thing, but one frequently observed, is that before having this itching the patient had suffered from phobia of the heart for eight years as a result of a mistaken diagnosis, but from the day that his attention became directed to his skin he never gave his heart another thought.

Moreover, do we not often see the best-balanced people seized with a transitory attack of itching because they have been for a greater or less length of time with people who had the itch? The desire to scratch is contagious, and psychic impression is enough to start it going. Is not this a very typical example of an objective mental phenomenon? Although in the majority of people the symptom does not last, we have nevertheless seen people in whom the purely suggestive manifestation took such firm hold that they got to the point where they were convinced that they had an attack of the itch, or of pityriasis, and they would spend days, even weeks, seeking for objective symptoms. In view of the production of these purely subjective phenomena without any other cause than a mental representation, one can understand how easily a real localized pruritus may become diffused in neuropaths.

Under the influence of this itching, the patient feels the greatest desire to scratch, and the slight injuries to the skin caused by this scratching may become gradually spread over all the body, in parts that have nothing to do with the real lesion, and which may gradually establish one or other of these forms of real prurigo which are still so little known in dermatology, and which undoubtedly in a number of cases are caused by a purely psychic mechanism analogous to that which we have just described.

Phobic phenomena may also be established which have nothing to do with the skin, but are due to changes in the general health which may cause them through the medium of the skin,—the phobia of cold or of heat, or the fear of perspiring too freely, or—what is so frequently found among the working classes who are afraid of driving-in the sweat—of not perspiring enough. All this may be the starting-point of real education of the skin in thermic sensibility. Patients get to the point where they suffer at the slightest change of temperature, where they are always too hot or else too cold. One can easily picture the variety of troubles which may be created in this way. Under the influence of the emotional state into which the patient is thrown at any change of temperature which he must undergo, vasomotor symptoms may be produced, which would in a certain measure—but secondarily—justify the impressions felt by the patient and become the starting-point of the most pronounced fixation.

There is a whole class of neuropaths who are terribly afraid of even the slightest draught, and who feel one even when it does not exist. One of our clients who used to have this phobia,—which, however, was cured a long time ago,—tells the following story on himself: "I used to be so terribly afraid of the slightest draught that I would go into society as seldom as possible. One evening in a drawing-room I sat down before a closed door, and scarcely was I seated when I was aware of cold air on my back. I changed my place and established myself safely in a corner. At the end of the evening, I wanted before leaving to assure myself that the door before which I had seated myself at first was not tightly shut. I went up to it and looked at it, and then discovered that it was the door of a cabinet built into the wall."

We have seen very many such people with educated thermal sensibility and phobias concerning changes of temperature. Naturally the discomfort that they feel has generally been considered as of organic nature. They have been told that their circulation is not good, that arthritism was one of the pathogenic factors of it. All methods of treatment—massage, douches, and medicines—have naturally followed, which, when practised without any conception of re-education and without being associated with psychotherapeutic treatment, have only succeeded in orienting the patient's mentality more fixedly and increasing the intensity of the symptoms which he felt.

CHAPTER VII.

FUNCTIONAL SYMPTOMS IN THE NEURO-MUSCULAR APPARATUS.

WE SHALL study, in this chapter, all those dynamic or static muscular disturbances which may be observed in the course of the development of the psychoneuroses. Among these numerous and complex troubles, there are evidently a certain number in the production of which other factors than the neuro-muscular apparatus come into play. Their grouping is in fact merely symptomatic and purely schematic, all question of pathogeny and mechanism being set aside.

First of all, as the most important from the clinical as well as from the theoretical point of view, we shall study fatigue, fatiguability, and exhaustion, with their functional consequences, or, in other terms, physical asthenia.

In a later paragraph we shall take up disturbances of equilibrium and coördination. Then there will be another class of wholly dissociated facts—tremors, choreas, and choreiform movements—which will demand our attention.

Finally we shall pass in rapid review paralyses and contractures.

1. Fatigue, Fatiguability, Exhaustion, and their Functional Consequences.—In the sensations of fatigue, of which neurasthenics so often complain, two different kinds of facts must be studied. These patients have, very frequently if not constantly, the impression of being fatigued without having made any effort. This is a purely suggestive impression. On the other hand, they are truly fatiguable in this sense, that any real physical exertion exhausts them more or less rapidly.

We shall pass rapidly over the impression of fatigue itself. It may have several origins. In the emaciated neurasthenic who is already more or less exhausted, it is easily explained. At other times, and very frequently, it is a simple phenomenon of auto-suggestion, a memory of fatiguability which has already been experienced, but which is evoked more or less continually, if one might so put it. Under other circumstances, it is a question of a sensation which may be experienced by many people, quite apart from any neurasthenic condition, but which is reinforced in the case of neurasthenics by the elements of auto-suggestion.

The well-known fatigue on waking, in particular, which one finds in nearly all arthritics, only becomes a neurasthenic symptom when the person is obsessed concerning this sensation. It is the obsession and not the fatigue which is unhealthy, for this is in a way a constitutional phenomenon which most well-balanced individuals pay no attention to, because they know of how little importance it is, and that the fatigue which they feel will disappear under the influence of physical or mental exercise.

Fatiguability on making any effort is one of the commonest signs which is met with in neurasthenia. It belongs, one might almost say, peculiarly to this psychoneurosis. It explains the fact that the patient practically finds it impossible to make any physical effort without very quickly experiencing more or less intense fatigue and more or less complete exhaustion. It is a synonym for muscular asthenia, or amyasthenia, and, if we have employed the word fatiguability, it is because on the one hand it arouses no prejudice, and on the other it expresses the clinical fact itself. In fact, when one says asthenia, one seems to indicate by it a constant diminution of muscular energy. Now, although there is a great number—and, to tell the truth, too great a number—of neurasthenics who hold the theory of the impossibility of making an effort, there are others who are capable of effort and of considerable physical work, and who only complain of the impression of fatigue as coming not too quickly but being too strongly felt. How many times we have heard these patients say, "I do it, but it uses me up." Let us, therefore, preserve the old word fatiguability, and leave the term asthenia to those who maintain the organic and quasi-irreducible nature of the disturbances of physical energy in the neurasthenic.

Let us go on to the classic clinical characteristics of this order of symptoms. They may be very briefly summed up. We may say, as do all authors, that the neurasthenic tires more rapidly and that his tire lasts longer. Let us add that, according to a great number of observers, the neurasthenic is incapable of impulse and cannot be carried away by enthusiasm.

The neurasthenic tires very rapidly. This means that, given a certain constitution for an individual when he is in a normal condition of health, the work that he is capable of may be rated at 100, but when he is ill the work of which he is capable will not be equal to more than 50, 20, 10, or even less, and he will get to the point where the figure 1 would, in the case of certain patients to whom all effort is impossible, still be too high.

The tire of neurasthenics is very lasting. This explains that other fact that, while in normal condition the length of time equal to 1 would be enough for a patient to rest from work equal, for example, to 10, a neurasthenic would require rest equal to 10 in order to be able to start in again upon work which is equal to 1.

The rapidity and lasting quality of fatigue are two characteristics which have been demonstrated experimentally. Ballet and Philippe, by means of Mosso's ergograph, have shown that in a neurasthenic the power of muscular contraction is exhausted much more quickly than in a healthy man, and that in order to recover this power the time which would be sufficient for a normal individual, or even for a patient afflicted with muscular atrophy, would be too short for the neuropath.

Let us add at once that Ballet is none the less convinced of the psychic nature, in the greater number of cases at least, of such a phenomenon.

The neurasthenic is incapable of progressive endeavor. This has been said elsewhere, but it is Deschamps principally who has defended this conception. To describe this impossibility of progressive endeavor he uses the neologism "aphoria." To quote this author, "The asthenic, given a certain fixed quality of strength, is incapable of increasing his capital of energy by exercise;" and further, "If it takes a patient five or ten years to get to the point where he can walk five minutes more, one can hardly call that progressive endeavor;" and still further, "He [the asthenic] passes through successive degrees of strength; these are degrees of strength which endeavor is powerless to modify. An asthenic possesses to-day a definite capital of force; this capital is stable for the time being, and always yields the same revenue. To work beyond that makes him bankrupt,—that is to say, it brings on a state of intoxication or sharp attack. It is a capital which cannot be changed either by progressive endeavor or by medicines. It is necessary for the whole organism to be improved and transformed by the efforts of nature, aided by wise therapy, in order to place it on a little higher level. On this new level, he would possess a new capital of strength a little above that of the preceding, but which would remain the same for a certain length of time, and which cannot be modified by the impulse toward improvement." These short extracts help one to grasp Deschamps's conception. This author, who, moreover, is a good observer, is, according to our way of thinking, wrong in not pointing out with sufficient exactness to which special class of patients his doctrine applies. From his description, it would seem that asthenia—his asthenia, with permanence as its characteristic—forms an integral part of the symptomatology of neurasthenia, since he studies it side by side with headache, backache, etc. Under these conditions we are very far from sharing his opinion, which latter we even find peculiarly dangerous, because it is peculiarly discouraging. Any work treating of neurasthenia is almost sure to be read, and quite too often in any case, by neurasthenics, who—whether asthenic or not—always find for themselves sufficient strength to read such books, and to reread them. And we have seen subjects, imbued with the doctrines of Deschamps, who were only too ready to become crystallized, "imbedded" in their given position, because they were convinced that any rapid progress was impossible.

Let us add, however, that it is very true that one does meet, in the progressive improvement of neurasthenics, a certain number of difficulties which we must take into consideration. In this group of facts, as well as in those met with in the course of the psychoneuroses, we have to interpret the rapidity and tenacity of fatigue and the difficulties of progressive effort. These are the facts which are commonly expressed in comparing the neurasthenic to an electrical machine by saying that he has insufficient potentiality, and that his accumulators are charged slowly and discharged too quickly, etc.

It seems to us, first of all, necessary to study phenomena which are both physiological and psychological, and which underlie the production of fatigue in healthy individuals.

As a matter of fact, the human motor cannot in any way be compared to a mechanical motor. Here, for example, is a locomotive in good running order. Under all circumstances it would be able with a definite amount of coal to produce a certain amount of mechanical work, a work which may be translated into a mathematical formula. No matter what the circumstances might be, it could do neither more nor less.

Here, on the other hand, is a man in good physical health. Under these circumstances he would be capable of work whose value could be expressed by numbers running, for example, from one to twenty. The thing that limits physical work in a man is not lack of fuel, it is not even what might be called the wear and tear of his mechanism, neither is it the appearance of fatigue which limits his physical activity. He may, as a matter of fact, after he has felt his first sense of fatigue, do work of even a superior quantity to that which he produced in the period preceding his first sensations of tire. The thing that definitely stops his physical work, as also intellectual work, is an extremely complex phenomenon known as exhaustion. What we must first try to explain is how this exhaustion may be produced more or less rapidly, according to circumstances and to individuals.

All physical work from its start falls into four periods,—namely, getting started, automatic work, voluntary work, exhaustion.

First of all, what is automatic work? It only exists where there is an accustomed physical activity. An employé, for example, automatically and mechanically traverses the distance, whether it be long or short, which separates him from his office. A workman can ply his trade for many hours without, as it were, taking any notice of it: the work in this case will be in a sort of a way instinctive, and will obey to a certain degree purely mechanical laws. This automatic work reaches its limit at the first appearance of a feeling of tire. Apart from any external phenomena it may occur more or less rapidly according to the degree of enthusiasm which the individual feels. This enthusiasm is nothing more than the progressive adaptation of an individual to a definite piece of work. If such adaptation is perfect, it cannot help but increase the possible daily quantity of automatic work, and the latter is increased not only because the motor is in some way rendered more powerful by the enthusiasm, but also because the force produced is better utilized and is fully concentrated on the desired end. A man with this progressive sense of work possesses a better lever and he uses it better if, instinctively, without either will or reflection, he can use it automatically as well as intelligently. Let us repeat, then, that two elements enter into the expression of the enthusiastic human motor,—increase of production of force and also (we might almost say chiefly) a better adaptation, or, if one prefers it, a higher degree of harmony in the effort.

This amounts to saying that, apart from any question of enthusiasm, harmonious effort is always less fatiguing than badly applied effort, because in the latter case, for the same quantity of work produced, there must be a more or less considerable useless expenditure of strength. This is exactly what makes the difference between a good and a poor worker. The latter, because he does not know how to use his tools, will be much more apt than the other to feel the first sensation of tire.

This must necessarily be so, and largely because the first idea of weariness, even the accumulated impressions of fatigue, put a decided limit upon human work. One says of people, that they have energy, which means that, along with their margin of automatic physical work, they have a large margin of voluntary work. During this second period, and this is the classical expression, the man struggles against the animal in him; thus one sometimes sees frail people capable of miracles of energy. History furnishes numerous examples of this. It is none the less true that human energy has its limitations, and that there comes a moment when the will itself is incapable of undertaking any supplementary effort. The man is then exhausted.

Under other circumstances, it does not work in this way, and it seems that under certain given conditions the margin of automatic effort may increase almost indefinitely.

Under the influence of great emotions, or in the course of pathological conditions such as ambulatory automatism, or certain forms of cerebral excitement, a man does not struggle against fatigue, he no longer feels it nor perceives it, because his mentality is asleep, as it were, or because he has become monoideastic. All the physical and intellectual impressions other than those which have to do with the end he is interested in are, we might say, inhibited in him.

This fact is of great importance to us, because it shows how much distraction (the word distraction being taken in its etymological sense) facilitates effort, and because it also explains how, inversely, attention makes the effort difficult.

Here is where the manner of getting started counts. If one, as a matter of fact, begins any work with a feeling of disgust or anxiety or the conviction that it will not go on well, this work will soon become fatiguing, because a mental element has been added to it at the start, because the effort, instead of being automatic will be in some sense voluntary, and because being voluntary it must necessarily not be so perfectly adapted.

It is a common thing to say that one struggles against fatigue. This phrase expresses not only a phenomenon of the will, but also a physical fact. The gait of a tired man, if his fatigue has come from a walk less long than that for which he was prepared, is a stiff walk if useless effort is expended. It follows very clearly from this that under these conditions fatigue will be rapid. A few examples will make our idea clear. Here are troops on the march. At the end of the column are a certain number of laggards. Among them some are limping, but there are also a certain number of strong, hearty fellows, good country specimens, who are used to walking long distances and to hard work on the soil. These men have hundreds of times done much harder physical work than that which is demanded of them now. They have by no means come to the limit of their endurance. But to-day they have lost heart. They are disgusted with their calling. They have been homesick ever since they got up. During the whole time of their march they have been complaining about their hard lot; and here we see them lagging along, limping, dragging their feet, and all tired out, with the perspiration running off their faces. Let an officer come along who can brace up their courage, or let the music start up some air from home, and they will quicken their step, and later reach their halting place without a shadow of fatigue, without having felt the slightest need of putting forth any real energy. But, on the contrary, let them keep up their slow lagging walk for a few miles further, and they will drop by the way, overcome, used up, and exhausted.

Here are other examples. A runner and a bicyclist are in fine condition. A few days before one could have accomplished, without any sign of fatigue, eighteen to twenty-four and the other from ninety to one hundred and twenty miles. Let them, at the end of a few miles, however, begin to fear that they are not sure of the way, and they will find themselves exhausted long before they have accomplished the eighteen or the ninety miles. Why? Because their effort, instead of being automatic, will become conscious, and therefore less thoroughly adapted and more fatiguing. It is identically the same phenomenon which we have just seen in the case of the soldiers.

When an individual reaches his resting place after a long walk, he will feel more or less fatigued. The next day, on waking, he will find himself very stiff. If he stays in bed, he will feel the same fatigue for several days. If, on the other hand, he takes up his journey, he will often be able to finish it less fatigued, as far as his subjective impressions go, than he was at the start. The neurasthenic behaves in the same way, the question of degree and the moment that sensations appear being put aside. And if under the impression of fatigue he stops more or less absolutely, he will often retain this impression of fatigue for a much longer time than if he got back to work. It is by a mechanism of this kind that one explains in a purely subjective way the prolongation of impressions of fatigue in the neurasthenic. If his fatigue lasts, it is because he does not take up his work again.

In fine, the conclusion at which we wish to arrive, and which the facts seem to justify, is that exhaustion is only partially an organic phenomenon. Its rapidity is directly proportioned to the degree of consciousness in the effort. It is inversely proportioned to the degree of automatism in the effort put forth and to the energetic qualities of the person who is working.

All of this helps us very much to understand the peculiar nature of this rapid and easily acquired exhaustion of which so many neurasthenics complain. These patients really do not know what it is to feel that good healthy tire which is almost pleasant and comforting, because, from the moral point of view, it represents work accomplished. They only know that exhaustion which sometimes comes too soon and rapidly grows worse, and which, on the contrary, sometimes strikes them like a thunderbolt, but does not surprise them. These feelings are accompanied by various symptoms of anxiety, shortness of breath, emotional phenomena of every kind, accompanied or not by phobic symptoms. Such patients finally become very much limited in their physical activity; some cannot walk a hundred yards, others fancy that they cannot go down stairs. There are some who stay in their rooms, some even who never leave their beds; sometimes it is really true that the slightest effort plunges them into all those disagreeable sensations which we have just described. Sometimes, however, they are merely phobics in whom the fear of exhaustion inhibits all desire to make any effort.

This exhaustion does not, however, necessarily extend to all forms of physical activity. One person will be exhausted by standing, but can endure walking or long conversations. Another cannot walk for a greater or less length of time after his meals, because he holds that the work of walking combined with the work of digestion is too much for him. Still another finds that he is incapable of any effort whatsoever unless he has slept a given number of hours. "When I have spent ten hours in bed and slept nine of them," a patient said to us, "then I can do things. If I have only been in bed for nine hours and slept eight, I am incapable of doing anything." The most subtle distinctions, and the most varied associations in the domain of things possible and impossible, are likely to turn up in this connection.

One peculiar feature in the exhaustion of neurasthenics is the sudden appearance, without any warning, of intense fatigue which obliges the patient to stop at once. To phenomena of this kind there has been given the classic term, which is somewhat abused, of neurasthenical paraplegia.

Very often this phenomenon has a peculiar origin. It occurs in patients who, for one reason or another, have momentarily forgotten that they belong to the class who are so easily exhausted. Then, by the common association of some idea, they suddenly remember their condition, and experience, as it were psychically, the sum total of all the fatigue that they ought to have felt. Phobic symptoms then come into play. They are afraid that they are going to be used up. They are afraid that they cannot go any further, and they stop short without strength and without energy. These are the same patients who, when you try to explain the mechanism of their fatigue to them, will say to you, "But, doctor, you must see that my fatigue was real, because it overcame me when I was not thinking of it at all." Really they did not think of it before they experienced it, but they felt it because it was borne in upon them to think about it.

Here, if you like, is a typical example of such a case. One of us one day had occasion to examine a lady who was very neurasthenic and profoundly "asthenic." She said it was impossible for her to sit up for more than a few minutes, or to hold out her arm for the shortest time. When we examined her, her arm did as a fact fall weakly after it had been extended two or three seconds. The continuation of the examination revealed that hyperæsthesia of the scalp which is common among so many nervous people who are nevertheless not true neuropaths. This patient had a magnificent head of hair, very elaborately dressed. On remarking that on account of her hyperæsthesia she must find it very difficult to let anybody arrange her hair, "Oh, doctor," said she, "I would never allow anybody to touch my hair. I do it myself." This patient, who was not able to hold her arm stretched out for three seconds, could hold her two hands above her head an hour a day to arrange her hair and brush it at night. It is quite true that she had not given this matter a thought.

Furthermore, this physical asthenia of neurasthenics is essentially variable at different times. One such unfortunate was so profoundly afflicted that he believed that he could not walk for more than five minutes without being exhausted. But we were able while talking about his troubles to keep him walking up and down for an hour and a quarter, without his ever noticing it.

It is evident that this neurasthenic asthenia strongly resembles symptoms of the same kind which are met with in a convalescent. The latter, it is true, is capable of only such special effort as is suitable to his physical condition at the moment. In his case all his physical activities are simultaneously attacked. In the former, on the other hand, who is illogical, variable, and incoherent, asthenia is a symptom of purely psychic origin and of accessory physical origin.

We might add that its physical origin is mostly accessory, for two reasons: first, because in some slight degree there may come in some symptoms in the production of exhaustion in a neurasthenic which, although of psychic origin, nevertheless play the physical rôle to some degree; and, then, because true physical asthenias do exist in certain cases.

Sometimes, in fact, the neurasthenic is really tired. This is what we will call, if we wish to use the expression, a neurasthenic who has "arrived." Emaciated and weakened by lack of nourishment, because he has suffered from those disturbances of appetite and digestion which we have long since described, and because he does not eat enough, he cannot walk, because his motor apparatus is in such bad condition and because he is so poorly fed.

His asthenia is thus the most natural thing in the world. But it is nevertheless a superadded and purely secondary symptom which has nothing to do with the fatiguability which many authors hold to be essential.

What, then, is the mechanism of the phenomena of exhaustion which one finds in a neurasthenic? How, in other words, does it happen that his effort is cut short so quickly? This is the question which we have to solve. We shall explain at the same time the mechanism of non-inhibited expressions of fatigue concerning effort which one meets in certain patients.

Dubois, of Berne, attributes fatigue "to a conviction of helplessness, following a real sensation, and exaggerated by the pessimistic state of mind which the fatigue itself brings on, acting on our morale." "One ought not to call it fatigue when there has been no work performed," says this author; that is to say, in fact, that these fatigued patients belong to the list of "interposed symptoms" who, according to Dubois's theory, interpose a false idea into the reflex arc. This conception of Dubois's seems to me only permissible for patients who feel fatigued when in bed. And it is chiefly to them that his interpretation applies. Dubois, who elsewhere is such a strong upholder of the psychic nature of the symptoms experienced by neurasthenics, does not think but that the true neurasthenic may also suffer from true fatigue.

As a matter of fact, one sees neurasthenics who have been in bed for some weeks, who feel themselves incapable—on account of fatigue, so they say—of efforts which they do not even attempt. Such, from all evidence, are pure psychopaths, more or less abulic, whose mentality has become crystallized on the memory of some former fatigue that really did occur. Sometimes, also, they suffer from real fatigue by reason of insufficient nourishment. But such cases do not apply to our subject. We must say that neurasthenics are very rarely also abulic, as is apt to be said of them. There are some who, in struggling against their affliction and their sensations, waste a store of energy. If there are some who are incapable of any will power, there are also some who put forth all the will power that they once were able to exert. We have seen these patients to whom some physical task had been given. "If you wish it, doctor," they would say, "I will do it;" and these patients would make the effort that was asked of them, such as running a fixed distance. They would arrive at their destination, but wholly exhausted. Yet, nevertheless, the effort that was proposed was by no means excessive. What is the mechanism of this phenomenon? According to our feeling, if these patients willed well they did not know how to will; they willed badly. With the best intentions in the world they would never succeed in overcoming their difficulties. But this is what these patients attempt to do. It is true that they themselves have raised their own barriers. We must explain ourselves.

The first and by no means the least important fact comes from the mentality of the neurasthenic. He looks upon nothing with indifference. Every act of his physical life, as well as his intellectual life, is counted, meditated, observed, and preserved in a reminiscent condition which is more or less continually present. If, therefore, one asks such a patient to make a physical effort in which he may or may not at some previous time have had feelings of fatigue, instead of getting to work at it in a perfectly simple manner, as would a healthy individual, he is going to watch himself while he does it. Sometimes a memory of fatigue will come to him, and will appear again in the production of consecutive impressions. But this mechanism is neither constant nor necessary. The very attention which the patient brings to bear upon the effort that he is making is sufficient to disturb the action which he wishes to perform, because, from that time on, instead of being automatic, his effort becomes voluntary and insufficiently adapted.

One has only to watch these patients somewhat attentively in order to realize this fact. In walking, for example, there is nothing normal in the way in which they behave. Sometimes, anxious to know if they will be able to keep up till the end, they begin to walk as fast as possible without sparing their breath. Soon they begin to pant, and it is not physical fatigue, properly speaking, which is going to make them stop, but the difficulty which they will find in getting their breath. And very often, as a matter of fact, it is this extremely unpleasant sensation which such patients describe to us under the name of exhaustion.

Sometimes, on the other hand, they will begin to walk more slowly; they count their steps, as it were, asking themselves, at each step, if they will not fall exhausted before the next one. We have already seen how greatly the respiratory functions may be modified by attention, and how the attention to a certain degree inhibits the respiratory automatism. Just in the same way in the case of these patients, they may be obliged to stop on account of their respiration. Other phenomena are very apt to occur. In fact, in the normal condition in all the customary forms of physical activity the work that is willed follows automatic work. Our patient, attentive to his promenade, acts from the first as one who is greatly fatigued. He is continually causing an error of interpretation, and, by bringing his will into play, he has a psychological impression of blocking and is already fatigued. The application of his will, or of attention, which is only a form of will, is interpreted by a real return shock as a sensation of fatigue. Therefore, one of two things occurs: on the one hand, our patient, for reasons that we shall determine further on, is abulic, and he will almost immediately cease to make any effort, or, on the contrary, being very desirous to improve and to progress from the physical point of view, he will push himself, and then there will appear, as a result of his exhausted condition, or the feeling of stiffness which this patient will begin to experience, a whole new series of phenomena. Psychic tension has its physical and reciprocal reaction. This is a well-known fact. When one is striving toward an end, he puts forth every moral and physical effort of his whole being. One holds oneself tense while making any intellectual effort. Gesticulation and mimicry are only the classical expressions of this general law. Our patient, therefore, is going to stiffen up and draw himself together. His gait will consequently lose its freedom. Sooner or later he will be taken with pains in the back and cramps in the legs, and these sensations will be produced more quickly than formerly, or else a topalgia, probably lumbar, will soon occur. Our patient is from now on rather like an individual trying to walk with lumbago or an arthropathy. It is easy to see that under these conditions he will not go very far.

What we have said about walking we could repeat exactly for any manifestation of physical activity whatsoever when attempted by a neurasthenic, whether his general condition is affected or not.

On the other hand, one can see very easily how being convinced of a difficulty or one's own helplessness may inhibit effort. Here, for example, is an individual who, in a moment of enthusiasm, has leaped over a rather wide ditch. He comes back, computes the width of the ditch, and thinks he was very fortunate to have been able to jump across. Try to make him leap over this ditch once he knows how wide it is, and nine times out of ten he will fail in the attempt, or if he succeeds, in overcoming he will have had to put forth every effort, and when he reaches the other side he will sink down all out of breath.

Is this a case, properly speaking, of a moral phenomenon? It is simply a case of the intervention of psychic phenomena which are focussed upon an act which, to be performed under the most favorable conditions, ought to be in some degree automatic. It is no less true that it is in this way that the asthenia of a neurasthenic is encouraged and cultivated, an asthenia which serves to reinforce the memory of previous exhaustions. In the same way the automatic part which may exist, although it is more often very feeble, is still further reduced.

This, we think, explains very clearly why the neurasthenic cannot be worked up to further effort. He knows that he can walk without fatigue for five or ten minutes, or even an hour. During this time his effort will be normal, automatic, and unconscious. But the moment that he has passed what he considers to be the limit of his endeavor, the phenomena which we have just described will come into play. Unless he has had appropriate treatment, it is plain that the exhaustion will always come on at the same time. And this is why the neurasthenic cannot be incited to endeavor.

Here is a demonstration of this statement. Two patients came to us the same day; both were neurasthenics and incapable of long effort.

To each of them we ordered very progressive effort. During the first days their effort was without result. Our two patients, living at the same hotel, became acquainted with each other. They discovered, outside of the pale of their diseases, mutual sympathies and the same interests and tastes. They decided to go into training together. From that time on, it began to come of itself, and in a few days the progress made was considerable, enough to convince the patients that they were gaining. What had happened? Following the advice which had been given them, they had been careful not to speak about their illness, but, talking of various things which offered them distraction, they were enabled to make constantly increasing efforts without any difficulty.

As to the relapses, under the influence of training, of which Deschamps speaks, we have never seen any. The whole reason lies in the fact that the patient, in the course of his exercises, is never allowed to get to the point of exhaustion. This, as we shall see later, is a simple matter of supervision.

To sum up, we will say that there are two forms of asthenia in the neurasthenic. One has to do only with the symptoms of fatiguability. It is that of the abulic neurasthenic, who stops the first moment that he feels the slightest sensation of fatigue. The other may continue to the point of exhaustion; he is the neurasthenic who is still endowed with energy. In one case as in the other the automatic work is very largely suppressed. In the second case alone there come in what we might call disharmonies, which rapidly create a peculiar fatigue.

It goes without saying that these disharmonies do not necessarily and inevitably lead to exhaustion. This is the case with patients—generally, however, those who are mildly affected—who may go beyond their first feeling of fatigue without being exhausted by doing so. These are those to whom we alluded above who say, "I do it, but it uses me up." In their case, we must add, the psychologic factors of distraction come into play. These are they who, not being strongly obsessed, still have a taste for their work, during which they forget from one time to another that they are sick. This is the reason why complete exhaustion may be indefinitely put off. But that is not enough to prevent their feeling fatigue which is much greater than under normal conditions and which is also very effective.

Does this mean that we consider that, outside of the psychophysical mechanism which we have just set forth, the neurasthenic may always be capable of the same effort which he could make when he was well? Certainly not, and we do not attempt to deny that in certain patients there is a very real fatigue. But to what does it respond? Not certainly to a real physical inferiority, but rather to the mental condition of the subject. The human organism, from the point of view of fatigue, cannot be dissected into parts. There is not one physical being, another moral being, and another intellectual being separated by impassable barriers. We all know the physical fatigue which comes from emotion, preoccupation, or intellectual work. We come away from a long discussion, or some slightly arduous task, worn out in body. The regular quantity of daily work that one can dispose of represents the sum of physical, intellectual, or moral effort. And what happens in the case of the neurasthenic? The things that can create and do create in him the effect of legitimate fatigue are all those obsessive preoccupations of which the mentality is the seat. These are the facts which we shall take up later, when we shall attempt, by the aid of the data furnished us by psychoanalysis, to make up the synthesis of the neurasthenic.

However this may be, and as far as the true primary asthenias are concerned, frankly speaking we have never met them, except under very special circumstances, and in patients who in other ways show signs of constitutional mental degeneracy,—*i.e.*, the phenomena of psychasthenia of Janet, which, according to many psychiatrists, bears a close relation to a periodic psychosis. In the latter, certainly we find associated with mental and moral deficiencies physical deficiencies which are almost as difficult to remedy as it is to change their psychic defects. Therefore, we must say again that even in these latter the asthenic manifestations are variable.

There are also (it is a question of diagnosis) individuals who have become prematurely aged, who are, if you will, asthenic, but in whom it is a question, taking it all in all, of a process of senile involution which is only abnormal from the point of view of the time at which it has occurred.

As in the neurasthenic, he may show signs of false fatigue, due to error in mental representation, premature fatigue, by reason of having entirely suppressed the automatic period of his effort, and true fatigue resulting from the lack of nutrition caused not only by his obsessions and preoccupations, but brought on more often by disharmony of effort. In the neurasthenic who is under careful direction this fatigue is the commonest of his symptoms; it is also, according to our opinion, the one which yields most easily to appropriate therapy. This idea seems to us of the utmost importance, for it is very much more encouraging to patients than that which takes it for granted that for a very long time, or always, they will remain in that state of definite lack of strength.

We have now glanced over the general fatiguability of neurasthenics and the mechanism of their exhaustion. We must next speak of phenomena of the same order but whose lack of logic is much more apparent. We allude to the localized amyasthenias.

We have spoken here of certain patients who are exhausted by all kinds of efforts but who are nevertheless able to do some one thing without fatigue. Here we have to do with individuals whose incapacity for work only extends to a given group of muscles, which contract under definite conditions.

We meet with the most varied types of such fatigue fixations. The inability to remain standing for any length of time is a symptom of this kind, and by no means the least frequent. It is needless to say that this difficulty in standing is found in association with other symptoms of general fatiguability. But one may also find it alone. These are the patients who can walk for a long time, can lift weights, and swing dumb-bells, etc., and yet who insist that they are exhausted at the end of a few minutes or even after a few seconds of standing on their feet. There are some who, in order not to use up their strength, get to the point where they are obliged to make their toilet in instalments.

The mechanism of this phenomenon is varied. Very often it is connected with a lumbar topalgia. In other cases it is the memory of some previous exhaustion, caused by having been obliged to stand for a long time, which causes it. We know that standing is the usual attitude of conversation. Now, while he is conversing, the neurasthenic throws himself entirely into his conversation, and it is not rare to find it resolving itself into a monologue rather than a dialogue. What fatigues him then is not so much the standing as the conversation, during which he sometimes expends much strength without paying any attention to managing or saving his breath. After a little time of such exercise, he is out of breath, distressed, and exhausted. There is an error in interpretation which makes him attribute the symptoms of a wholly different origin to the fact of standing.

These are the initial phenomena, but whether it is a topalgia or a previous memory which is present at the beginning of the symptoms the results are the same.

It must, in fact, be remembered that the act of standing is not an indifferent phenomenon. It is apt to cause a feeling of muscular fatigue in the strongest people, and one cannot remain standing for any very great length of time without a change of position, by letting the weight rest first on the right leg and then on the left for example, in order to allow the muscular groups which are in a state of tonic contraction time to rest. But even under these conditions one finds oneself obliged, at the end of a certain length of time, to sit down.

How would this affect the neuropath who is troubled by a lumbago or who recalls the exhaustion he felt as the result of standing upright at some former time? In two very different ways. Sometimes he does not hold himself erect. He is continually changing his position, and therefore performs what is a much more rapidly fatiguing work, according as the sensation of fatigue is reinforced by former mental representations of the same kind. Sometimes, on the other hand, he stiffens himself, holds himself perfectly still, and holds his breath, and the time during which he remains standing will be marked to some degree by the limit of the possible duration of continued voluntary contraction. This duration naturally varies according to the energy of the subject, following the intervention or not of respiratory troubles analogous to those which we have already described, and according also to the psychic reinforcement of the mental impression which is felt. In both ways this duration will not be very long, and it is chiefly under these conditions that such patients, standing as stiff as pickets, are apt to declare themselves exhausted at the end of a very short time, sometimes not more than a few seconds.

Here it is a question of an amyasthenia attacking the muscles whose tonic contraction is necessary to the erect position. Other muscular groups may be attacked in a still more specialized way. We refer to false professional cramps. Here is a most characteristic example.

Miss N., thirty-two years of age, is a talented pianist, in love with her profession. When we saw her in 1908, she had been obliged to give up her professional work almost completely for nearly eighteen months. Each time that she tried to play the piano she would invariably be taken by feelings of very painful lassitude, located principally in the right arm, but in the left arm also, though in a less marked degree. In spite of all her efforts, she would very soon be overcome by the pain and obliged to stop.

Having been obliged to give up many things in her life, and seeing the possibility of being forced to abandon her art, which constituted her only moral resource, it is needless to say that she was very profoundly depressed.

The origin of these symptoms went back to a slight rheumatic pain of the right shoulder, which had for several days occasioned rather painful sensations, and on account of which she was obliged to give up her daily musical exercises. Then progressively, at the same time that the articular pain grew dull, before disappearing entirely, the phenomena which we have just described appeared. The patient had consulted many physicians, and the most remarkable diagnoses had been made,—myositis, neuritis, etc. There were some who spoke of pianist's cramp, and who hinted to our patient that she would probably be obliged to give up her career. The greatest variety of treatments were tried,—hydrotherapy, mechanotherapy, electrotherapy, hypnotism, local applications of every kind, etc. In short, the patient, being more and more persuaded that her trouble was chronic, suffered more and more and grew more and more hopeless. The objective examination showed nothing: the articulations of the shoulder, the elbow, the wrists, and the fingers were free. The muscles were supple, there was no painful point anywhere along the line of the nerves, and sensibility was intact. This patient was cured in a few weeks: she was able to take up her former occupations in their entirety when the mechanism of her condition, both in its present and past history, had been made clear to us and to her.

It was, in fact, very simple. The patient, being attacked at first by real rheumatic symptoms, was overcome with dismay at the possibility of being obliged to give up her career. She insisted on working in spite of her pain. She insisted upon playing in spite of everything. The result was that she at once stiffened herself to the task in order to play. She thus lost all her suppleness, and the fatigue against which she was struggling by steeling herself to still further effort only appeared more quickly, more insistently, and more painfully.

The method by which the facts of this phenomenon were brought out deserves to be described. All movements, particularly those of writing, were accomplished with the greatest ease. There was something in that which convinced us of the functional nature of the phenomena experienced. But is not the same thing true of professional cramp? What made the proof clear was the fact that writing also became fatiguing to our patient, and gave her the same painful impression as in playing the piano, when the things which she wrote, instead of being a simple copy, had to do with very interesting facts. She would then hold herself tense; her pen would scratch the paper; her handwriting would change and become cramped. In a case of this kind, could the immediate facts be explained by the intervention of any mental representation or by a direct auto-suggestion? No, we do not think so. We hold that it is chiefly a phenomenon of disharmony, very similar to those which we have previously described. The specialized, localized lassitude of our patient was a real fatigue legitimately felt. It was such as any woman might experience if, instead of playing in a manner which was to some degree automatic, she should play while holding herself stiff and tense. In fact, these patients are at the start in the condition that others are in after several hours of practice. These are not patients who do not want to do anything, and who are of the tired abulic type and inhibited by a wrong mental representation. They are patients who, because they are only too anxious to do things, inhibit what in their particular cases might be called their mechanism. Although they are old professionals, they behave like débutantes.

We have also seen another patient whose symptomatology in some points was almost identical. We have also in like manner seen employees helpless with writer's cramp, which was due to phenomena of the very same nature as those that we have just described.

This only serves to show how necessary it is, in cases like these, for the diagnostician to be careful and minute in his examination, for a careless diagnosis may lead to veritable disaster, careers ruined, and lives spoiled. One appreciates also how baneful an influence a physician may exert by making the conviction sink deeper into the patient's mind that he may have some definite loss of power. It is this conviction which, as a matter of fact, is at the base of the whole procession of symptoms. And if in the intermediary mechanisms we find disharmonious facts coming in, which have hitherto been considered of little value in what concerns the initial principle of things, we agree with Dubois. The important psychological fact, however, from the point of view of the moral treatment of these patients, consists in this: in their case the will is not absent—quite the contrary—but it is badly applied.

Phenomena of the same order seem to us to be able to account for certain clumsy movements of which the patients complain. Some will say, for example, that "they can hold nothing in their hands." In many cases, it is true, this is due to "nervous movements;" but in some circumstances, nevertheless, it has seemed to us that our patients, being cognizant of their awkwardness, or believing themselves clumsy in some incident that has accidentally happened, only loosen their hold upon objects because they were holding them too tightly. At the end of a short time their quasi-spasmodic contraction is relaxed and the object falls. It is true of nervous people more than of others that trying to do one's best is fatal to doing well.

2. **Disturbances of Equilibrium.**—In order thoroughly to understand the mechanism of disturbances of equilibrium which one observes in the course of the psychoneuroses, we are obliged to refer to clinical observation. We might add that it seems useless to call attention to the fact that the observations to which we refer are of recent date. We are not wholly convinced, in fact, but that many troubles which might have been described at one time, when hysteria was a more or less consciously cultivated disease, were nothing more than troubles due to education, for which simulation and suggestion were both partly responsible.

We shall, therefore, first turn back to some observations in which all the cases which we have been able to study are almost identical one with the other.

Here is the first history, already published by one of us, which furnishes an example of an hysterical symptom following immediately and bearing a direct relation to an emotional shock. It was the case of a young girl who, on seeing her dog, to which she was very much attached, run over by a train on a railway crossing, felt her limbs give way beneath her, so that she sank down on the ground. She had to be carried home. Thenceforth she could no longer walk or stand up. If she tried to get up, she would immediately fall. Nevertheless, when she was examined in bed, there was no disturbance of general sensibility nor of the muscular sense, nor any motor incoördination. Her muscular force was intact, she could draw up and stretch out her thighs, legs, and feet; she could resist passive movements when pressure was brought to bear on any part. It was not a case of paralysis, but of disturbance of equilibrium. This patient was cured in eight days by isolation with psychotherapy.

For the last twenty-seven years a lady, fifty-two years of age, had been confined to her room and could not walk without hanging on somebody's arm. Hers was a case of great emotional fear, whose symptoms had a very curious and definite origin.

When she was twenty-six years old and had been married two years, she was dining one day in town with her husband. In going down the stairway of her hostess's house, either because she was affected by the cold or perhaps because the dishes which had been served at dinner had disagreed with her, she was taken with vertigo and giddiness, and finally with vomiting. She was taken home in a carriage. The next day she found that she was not able to get up. The moment that she stood upon her feet, it seemed to her that everything was turning around her and that she was going to fall. A physician was called in, but, instead of attributing her trouble to the results of indigestion, he made the diagnosis of hæmorrhage of the brain. He told her husband that it would be impossible for his wife to live in Paris; that it would inevitably follow, when she went out again, that her equilibrium would never be perfect, and she would be exposed to the danger of accidents in the traffic of a great city. The husband was convinced. He made a home for his wife in the suburbs of Paris, but, as his business took him to the city, he was obliged to leave every morning and not return till evening. His wife, left alone all day, did not dare go out of her room, where she lived like a prisoner. Things went on in this way indefinitely. Every attempt that she made to get up or to walk or go out being followed immediately by the same symptoms of loss of equilibrium, she finally, after a certain time, gave up trying to make any effort, and thereafter she never walked unless there was some one to hold her up.

On examination, it was found that in bed this lady had preserved the muscular strength of her lower limbs, but the moment that she wanted to get up she would sink down, either all at once or very quickly. She could sometimes take a few uncertain wavering steps before she wholly lost her equilibrium.

At the end of a month's treatment these symptoms, which were purely functional in their nature and which for twenty-seven years had spoiled the best part of her life, had completely disappeared.

A third example is furnished us by a lady of thirty-two, who was very emotional. She had been sick three years when we saw her for the first time. The physicians who had treated her made a diagnosis of a disease of the spinal cord. They had made several applications of hot irons and had put blisters upon her. They had given her mercurial injections and large doses of iodides, etc. In short, she, as well as everybody around her, was convinced of the organic nature of her disease, and that it was probably incurable. She came to us hobbling painfully on two canes, only putting one leg forward when she had so placed one of her canes that she was sure that she could lean firmly and securely upon it. When her supports were taken away from her and we tried to make her walk, she held out her arms as if to balance herself, then put one foot forward. It would then often happen that her limbs would suddenly give way, and she would try to recover herself by drawing herself up quickly. In the course of these two movements,—the one involuntary and passive, and the other sudden and voluntary, but incoördinated,—she would always lose her balance, and her faith in the gravity of her disease would only be the stronger.

Objectively the patient showed no sign of organic affection. But we discovered very easily the existence of a left hysterical hemiplegia, which was very slight, and which had passed wholly unnoticed by the patient herself and by the physician.

The origin or cause of the affection was more difficult to discover, and it was only after some time that we succeeded in obtaining a complete confession from our patient. She was living with her husband and mother-in-law. The latter made her life anything but happy. She was the regular mother-in-law of the melodrama and continually aggravated her daughter-in-law, who, always trembling lest her household peace should be upset, got to the point where she could not even see her mother-in-law without having a serious emotional disturbance. "Each time that I saw her," she told us, "I felt as though I were ready to fall. My limbs gave way under me." These impressions, which at first were produced only when in the presence of the one who caused them, ended by being felt continuously as the young woman lived in the constant recollection of a scene that had just passed or in the anticipation of one to come.

A few weeks of calm with appropriate treatment were sufficient to cause these symptoms to disappear.

In the three observations which we have just given we have to deal with objective disturbances of equilibrium. In a very great number of cases the patients complained of purely subjective troubles. We shall come across these patients again when we study vertigo and sensations of dizziness. For the time being, these are the only objective disturbances without vertigo that we shall interpret.

Stasobasophobia, which is confused with what is called paralytic astasia-abasia, is a very peculiar phenomenon, but one whose purely mental mechanism is easy to grasp.

In a normal state, when we are standing still or when we walk, our static or kinetic equilibrium is assured by a series of tonic muscular contractions which, though they have an organic centre of reinforcement in the cerebellum correspond none the less to special mental representations, and which act so that in a given situation the tonic contractions are instinctively and automatically increased or diminished.

A comparison with the phenomena of speech will perhaps better explain our idea. When a child learns to speak he registers what have been called motor images of articulation. When he learns to hold himself upright, or to walk, he registers motor images of static or kinetic equilibrium. When he knows how to talk, the functioning of the motor images of articulation become automatic and unconscious. When he knows how to walk and to stand up straight, the corresponding motor representations have also become absolutely instinctive.

But let there be a lesion which destroys the base of the third left frontal convolution, and the idea, though persisting, cannot be expressed by a spoken word. How natural that the subject should be greatly upset on not finding the words he wants and that he should hesitate and stutter.

The same thing is true for walking and standing; and, if one can conceive the existence of disturbances of equilibrium from cerebellar lesions, with localized or generalized affections of the muscular tonus, one can also conceive of the existence of disturbances of the equilibrium dependent upon the loss of the mental representations corresponding to the necessary contractions to insure equilibrium. The patient no longer knows how to stand upright or to walk. He has forgotten how he ought to begin, just as we have seen how, under the influence of a lesion or an emotion, our subject either could not or did not know how to find the words he wanted.

As to the various influences capable of inducing these peculiar manifestations, they are of two kinds, which, moreover, are apt to be confused. Sometimes it is a question of emotional shock, and sometimes phenomena of a phobic nature are the cause.

Let us suppose that it is the question of an emotion. Here again we find the rôle of specialized emotion which we have already had to point out so many times. The giving way of the limbs is an emotional form of reaction that is well known and classic. It seems that among certain subjects when the emotional current is once directed it will always follow the same channel, and that, whatever may be the nature or the intensity of the emotion experienced, it will always be translated in the same way. A young woman, afflicted with hysterical paraplegia, remembered that it was always usual for any emotion to "take her in her limbs." All that was necessary in her case was a more intense emotion than usual for the purely classic symptoms to become continuous. One can conceive, therefore, from this that by an analogous mechanism stasobasophobias may be produced by emotional shock, or rather by the crystallization in some way of a specialized emotional action.

Under other circumstances it is a question of phobic phenomena. Here things may be interpreted in a double sense. Sometimes the patients are so convinced of their helplessness that they do not even make enough effort to enable them to stand up on their feet or to take a single step. They just let themselves go, and sink down helpless. Our second patient would be a good example of this mechanism. Elsewhere the phobic action is exercised by the intermediation of the emotional action. The patients are so afraid of falling that they are always in a more or less intense state of excitement, which is accompanied by a more or less perpetual forgetfulness of the coördinate efforts which they must make in order to stand on their feet or walk. The rather frequent association of agoraphobia with stasobasophobia brings this mechanism into evidence. These patients, who, being agoraphobics, are seized with a feeling of dread the moment that they see an open space before them, are under these conditions often subject to feeling their limbs give way beneath them, and display every evidence of the emotional pathogeny which we have just been trying to explain.

In fact, basostasophobia is a pure phobic manifestation or one associated with an emotion or else an exclusively emotional manifestation. Let us add that the symptomatic *ensemble* is not always complete,—that there are patients who are only basophobic and who still find it possible to stand with varying degrees of ease.

We now come to astasia-abasia. The phenomenon which constitutes it has been defined by Charcot and Richer as motor helplessness of the lower limbs, through lack of relative coördination in walking (abasia) and in standing upright (astasia). It is a functional ataxic symptom involving walking and standing. The patients whom we have just now been studying had lost all ideas of mental representations corresponding to the tonic contractions necessary to maintain equilibrium, but here it is quite another matter. There is no suppression, but there is anomaly due to incoördination. The muscular contractions may be present, but they are not adaptive, and only produce an unstable equilibrium.

On the other hand, we are not wholly convinced from the facts but that there is a possibility of considering astasia-abasia only as a syndrome wide enough to take in the most diverse cases which unite the objective disturbances of walking and standing.

In the first place, there is no true clinical type of astasia-abasia. There are as many different aspects as there are patients. Then that form of astasia-abasia of the so-called paralytic type, that in which the patient cannot leave his bed, seems to us likely to be confused with stasobasophobia. To consider this form as a maximum of incoördination does not seem to us to conform to clinical reality.

As for the other clinical types of astasia-abasia, they also, we feel, should be considered with some reservation.

We have seen hysterical choreas whose walking was disturbed by the incoördinated movements. We have seen people afflicted with a general tic taken with a falling attack during which their limbs would give way sideways or vertically. We have seen the association of stasobasophobia with hysterical hemiplegia giving rise to supplementary disturbances. Our third observation was of a typical case, and we have seen other similar cases. One of us had the opportunity of seeing at a former time a certain number of patients afflicted with so-called choreiform or shaking or leaping astasia-abasia. Since the cultivation of hysteria has been given up he has not met with a single example, and he is inclined to think that what he saw were symptoms which were more or less directly suggested.

In fact paralytic astasia-abasia is confused with stasobasophobia without any possible differentiation. It seems to us that what has been designated under the name astasia-abasia apart from stasobasophobia, which has already been analyzed, consists, on the one hand, of the symptoms which hysterics have learned to show, and on the other, of essentially morbid associations to which, in a more or less marked phobic condition, are superadded the phenomena resulting from choreas, tics, paralytic and paretic conditions.

Does that mean that incoördinated motor states of a neuropathic origin cannot exist? A wider view must be taken, and, if one confines oneself to looking upon incoördination as a non-adaptation of movements intended for a definite end, it is very certain that phenomena of this order are met with and very frequently among neuropaths. But this is not a question of ataxia properly so called. It is neither a central ataxia nor a peripheral ataxia. The movements made are coördinated. The error lies in the judgment which the subject brings to bear upon his movements in order to accomplish them. The movements which follow are perhaps not adapted to the end in view, but they are adapted to the ideomotor representation. These phenomena enter, in fact, into the class of disharmonies of psychic origin of which we have already spoken. A healthy subject is on the point of losing his equilibrium, in a certain sense, as a consequence of a false step. In order to save himself, he will go through a series of movements which will throw him to the other side. Can one then say that he lacks coördination? The adaptation has been insufficient on account of an error of judgment. But, having once made this error, the rest of his movements have been coördinated and the end accomplished.

It is the same thing with neuropaths, with this difference, that, in certain subjects, it does not require any abnormal phenomenon or anything outside of themselves to produce it. All that is necessary and sufficient is for them to have an error in the mental representation, which is sometimes primitive, and disharmonic movements will be produced, creating a real incoördination, which, physiologically and pathologically speaking, is nevertheless not a true ataxia.

Here, for example, are basophobics who try to walk because they have been convinced of the necessity of re-educating themselves. At first they do not dare to put one foot before the other. Then they plunge forward and all at once take such a stride that they lose their balance. It is practically the same thing as stepping off into the air, which will throw the best-balanced person to the ground. More timid than ever, they will at first try to widen the base of support and will straddle their legs in such a way that they will resemble the lines of an arrow-head. Then they try to make a forward movement. It goes without saying that the very position which they have taken disturbs their centre of gravity so that they cannot perform this movement without losing their balance. Other patients begin by stiffening all their muscles, which they relax on one side in order to advance. It is plain that they will be overcome by the contraction of the opposite side.

One could without difficulty go on enumerating such disharmonic phenomena. May it not be possible that troubles of this kind which have been considered as astasic-abasic are developed more often in the basostasophobics? But may they not also exist in individuals who, for one reason or another, are not sure of their static or kinetic equilibrium? One can see, according to this conception which we hold concerning them, that they have nothing to do with the real disturbances of motor coördination.

On the other hand, phenomena of the same order exist elsewhere than in the lower limbs. We have already pointed out that the localized amyasthenias and awkwardness of neuropaths were often due to manifestations of this kind. We do not insist upon it, and shall content ourselves with drawing attention to the fact that the common characteristic of this kind of motor disturbance is overshooting the mark. We are far from believing, as may be seen, the conception that the majority of neuropathic manifestations, and particularly those in neurasthenics, are disturbances due to lack of will power. Other disturbances of equilibrium, of almost exactly the same mechanism, have to do with the vertigoes which are so frequent in neuropaths. We shall take them up when we study vertigo itself. The latter, inasmuch as it constitutes a disturbance of equilibrium, should be studied with the mental manifestations properly so called, for reasons which we shall develop later.

3. **Choreas, Choreiform Movements, and Tremors.**—We would like to glance, in this paragraph, at the general group of *involuntary movements* which may be observed in the course of the psychoneuroses. We shall not study the more or less hereditary tics or tremors of degenerates. These latter are symptoms associated with special mental conditions, and which on this account do not come within the scope of our work.

Three types of involuntary movements may be observed in neuropaths. There are *choreas,* which are the exclusive property of hysteria so far as the neuropathic manifestation is concerned. In neurasthenics as well as in hysterics, we may find *tremors.* Finally, there are in certain subjects, and particularly among children or adolescents, little involuntary movements which in some measure resemble *tics* if one considers them alone and thinks only of the movement produced. These are false tics.

Hysterical chorea is a well-known phenomenon. Like all the choreas it consists in the appearance, in those subjects who are affected by it, of involuntary irregular and incoördinate movements. It seems to us that the classical descriptions of hysterical chorea include two very different kinds of facts. It seems to us that the whole class of choreas with rhythmic movements which are no longer incoördinated, but recur at irregular intervals to reproduce movements made in ordinary life, such as leaping, dancing, etc., should be eliminated at the start from the list of the symptoms of the psychoneuroses such as we understand them. As a matter of fact, all these types of chorea have almost wholly disappeared from view in recent years. It seems to us that here, as is the case with so many other hysterical manifestations, they were the direct results of cultivation and of more or less direct suggestions, which required essentially, but to a varying degree, the willing coöperation of the patient.

Major hysterical chorea is not very frequently seen. Here the wild movements go to their furthest limit. This major chorea may be unilateral—hemichorea—and be accompanied or not by hemianæsthesia. One of us has seen a case in which the incoördinated movements were extremely marked in both upper and lower limbs. On the other hand, the minor hysterical choreas appearing more frequently in children, and particularly in girls of from thirteen to seventeen, after puberty, are very frequent manifestations. There is not a clinic at the Salpêtrière where one does not see two or three during a consultation. In the service of one of us at the Salpêtrière there have been from ten to twenty of these patients a year under treatment by isolation.

More often these are merely slight symptoms, little convulsive movements of the hand with awkwardness in taking hold of things, slight shakings in the arms or in the shoulders, and slight contractions of the muscles of the face. It is very rare to find any serious affections of the lower limbs. There may be slight trembling at different times during the day, which incidentally affects the gait, but that is about all.

Hysterical chorea may exist on one side alone. This is true for perhaps twenty-five out of a hundred cases. More often it is bilateral. Taking it all in all, it is a neuropathic phenomenon which is generally mild, and rapidly recovers under appropriate treatment.

What is the origin of these troubles? Very often they appear coincident with an emotional disturbance. But it is rather rare to find them established with their full intensity at the start. They are progressive troubles, starting, in the majority of cases, either in the hand or in the shoulder, and radiating from that point, while the attacks increase in frequency and intensity. We do not believe that they are due to a purely emotional disturbance, for different factors, it seems to us, enter into play. Suggestion by imitation explains a certain number of cases. Sometimes there are epidemics in a school where chorea—by suggestive action—becomes contagious. Sometimes the patients are children living with neuropathic parents who have some form of tic. We have seen one case of this kind in a child who was taken with progressive chorea following an attack of nerves on the part of her mother. She had seen her throwing herself around, and the movements which the child made were nothing more than attempts to imitate the mother.

At other times, and the case is very frequent, they occur in children who have been amusing themselves by making faces or some more or less extravagant movements, and who end up by making automatic pseudo-tics. One of us has seen several examples of this kind, among others that of a little girl nine years of age, who for two years had been sent away from every school because she would incessantly turn her head so that she could tuck her chin under her right arm. She was cured after eight days of isolation.

Under other circumstances they occur in children who hold themselves badly or who are awkward. They are told to stand up straight, and are reproached because they "can hold nothing in their hands." Following this, choreic movements may develop as a sort of objective excuse. Again, chorea may be a sign of constitutional psychomotor mental instability, but it then occurs in psychopathic children, who are not included in our present study. Here the movements are always much more apt to be incoördinated voluntary movements than true choreic movements.

What, then, in these manifestations is the part played by emotion, which clinically is active in establishing them as well as bringing about their occasional intercurrent modifications?

It seems to us that emotion must act by favoring the initial suggestion. On the other hand, all involuntary movements and all incoördinations, even of organic origin, are always increased by emotion. It would seem that even in subjects afflicted by these troubles there exists a certain more or less conscious power of regulation which emotion causes to disappear, while at the same time increasing the intensity of the objective phenomena.

This is all evidently hypothetical; but, while we fully admit the rôle of emotion in the genesis of hysterical choreas, we nevertheless think that direct or indirect suggestion is often cause for them.

Tremor occurs in neurasthenic patients as well as in hysterics. Neurasthenics are sometimes seized in their upper limbs with small, quick, irregular tremors. Sometimes one can see in these patients a real intention tremor, which is exaggerated in proportion to the will brought to bear upon the voluntary movement.

This tremor frequently appears under the stress of emotion, but after this has passed the tremor disappears more or less quickly, to reappear under the influence of the same causes which created it. Under all circumstances rest causes it to disappear.

The tremor of hysterics is essentially polymorphous. Appearing after any moral or physical shock it may have any rhythm. As a matter of fact, one finds in hysterics a vibratory tremor with short, rapid oscillations, which may be either localized or general, and may last only for a few hours after an hysterical attack or may in some cases become permanent. It persists in spite of rest and only disappears during sleep. Movement and emotions exaggerate it.

Slight rhythmic tremor is the most frequent. There are several forms of it.

Intention tremor of the Rendu type disappears, at least for a few moments, during absolute rest. It is exaggerated by movement, and its oscillations increase in extent in proportion to the movement which is made. When the patient stands up, if he tries to walk, or even if he remains seated for a certain time, the whole body is, as it were, shaken by tremor.

Localized in the lower limbs this form of tremor constitutes the paraplegic type, and simulates the tremor of spasmodic paraplegia; but suddenly straightening the foot will stop the trembling instead of increasing it.

Purely intention tremor exists only during movement and disappears wholly during rest.

It is in the group of slight rhythmic tremors that hysterotoxic tremors belong, like those which are met with in mercurial poisoning (Letulle).

The slow tremors of hysterics have rather a wide swing. They may be generalized or localized. All these kinds of tremor may be combined or succeed one another in the same subject, becoming complicated by choreiform movements and incoördinations of all kinds, which give them an essentially polymorphous aspect.

At the present moment we have only very uncertain data concerning the pathophysiological physiognomy of tremor in general. Our reluctance to express ourselves concerning the mechanism of their appearance will, therefore, naturally be understood.

It is perfectly evident that emotion is able directly to cause tremor. In popular parlance any one speaking of the effect of emotion will say that he "trembled from head to foot." It is quite possible that we still have to deal with that specialized action of emotion which we have already spoken of so many times. A person who has once trembled under the influence of an emotion will be seized with trembling the next time he is overcome by emotion.

And yet, is it not possible to conceive that the tremor may be encouraged by itself? The fear of trembling and the discomfort which it causes the subject who experiences it become factors of the emotion which make the trembling lasting. It is possible in this way to explain that tremor of neurasthenics which disappears during rest and calm, but reappears with every emotion. The fact that the tremor may be exaggerated during any volitional act is also explained in this way. For the nearer a person approaches to the desired end the more his emotional condition is increased by the fear that he may not attain it.

There seems to us no shadow of doubt but that formerly a great number of cases of hysterical tremors were largely due to more or less voluntary suggestion and imitation. But this interpretation nevertheless does not seem to be applicable to all the clinical facts.

It appears to us that to a certain degree tremor may be considered as a phobic manifestation. If, in fact, one admits that the theories of Debove and Boudet explain the pathogeny of this trouble, which theories apply chiefly to intention tremor, and make the phenomenon depend upon contraction of antagonistic muscles, one can conceive that any more or less subconscious movement of arrest may create a tremor during any voluntary movement, for the essential characteristic of phobic manifestations consists in phenomena of arrest or recoil.

On the other hand, all that it is necessary for a healthy person to do to make a limb tremble is to stiffen it. One sees, therefore, that certain tremors may persist by reason of the very state of contraction into which the subject puts himself when he becomes concerned about his tremors and tries to stop them.

Finally, there exist a whole series of nervous movements, which, however, are only secondarily neuropathic, to which we might give the name "perfection movements." An illustration will explain better what we mean by this term.

We were called to treat a young man, sixteen years of age, for "nervous movements." These were located in the left shoulder and the right side of his face. Sometimes our patient would be seized two or three times during the day, and sometimes twenty times in an hour, with a sudden contraction of the left shoulder, which he would raise. He would also experience contractions of the side of his face in the same irregular way, but as a whole less frequently than in the shoulder. These would draw the line of the mouth out of place and to the right.

There were no other appreciable involuntary or incoördinated movements. This young man was skilful with his hands and showed no lack of strength. He was psychically normal in his character. He came from nervous but not neuropathic stock, and in trying to find any nervous symptoms in the family we had to go back to a great-aunt who had been afflicted with tics. It was just this possible heredity which had disturbed his family, and which had led them to dwell upon the subject and to allow our patient to become disturbed more than there was any reason for, considering how slight the difficulty was.

As a matter of fact, this young man had just passed two years in bed for a coxalgia. He had been almost continually in a recumbent position on the right side, with his head leaning on that arm. In this position he was able to read. As it was very difficult for him to make any movement (for he was wearing a plaster cast) when he wished to speak to the attendant who was always with him, he would not move, but would twist his face a little to the right. The result was that after a time there was a slight muscular predominance on the side in question, and, when he was examined in repose, it was found that the right labial commissure was slightly turned upward. For the same reasons the right shoulder was found to be a little lower than the other, as could easily be seen when he was undressed.

From that time on, the movements made by this young man were movements of rectification or of adjustment, which tried to raise up the fallen shoulder and to bring back the twisted axis of his lips. But his family, being unduly disturbed by the symptoms, kept continually speaking to the young fellow about it; the movements consequently became more frequent, and increased daily, even hourly, according to the degree of attention which was brought to bear upon them. The young man, being noticed so much, began to brood over his trouble, and, feeling annoyed by the discomfort arising from his trifling deformity, he instinctively made the necessary movements to overcome it.

It seems to us that a great many of these nervous movements so frequently seen in youth are due to some mechanism of this kind. They are the instinctive correction of vicious attitudes. It goes without saying that to call attention to them only makes them worse.

Perhaps a certain number of hysterical choreas might be placed with symptoms of this kind, which become more or less diffused according to the degree of attention and auto-suggestion which is brought to bear upon them.

We shall not dwell any longer on these manifestations, which are important only in so far as they are considered so. They often disappear spontaneously without any treatment. Their real interest lies chiefly in the mistaken diagnoses which are frequently based upon them. It is often possible, without a thorough examination, to take them for the starting-point of tics or hysterical chorea, and, if a physician does not take their exact nature into account, he may commit some such therapeutic error.

4. **Contractures and Paralyses.**—A contracture is a persistent tonic and involuntary contraction of one or several muscles of the body. Paralysis consists of the more or less complete abolition of the voluntary motor power (the striated muscles) and of reflex motor activity (smooth muscles).

Functional paralyses and contractures—that is to say, those that have no relation to any organic lesion—are met with chiefly in hysterics.

We shall pass rapidly over the clinical characteristics of hysterical paralyses and contractures. The paralysis may take the form of a hemiplegia, monoplegia, or paraplegia. It is frequently associated with superimposed disturbances of sensibility. The symptoms which permit the differentiation of these paralyses from organic paralyses are very well known, and we shall not dwell upon them. One point only seems to us of interest to remember (we shall see why in a moment), and that is that so far as the face is concerned one much more frequently observes a glossolabial spasm than a facial paralysis properly so called.

The contracture may be monomuscular, may affect a group of muscles, a segment of a limb, one limb, or several limbs. The rigidity may be extreme and unyielding. It brings about deformities which are sometimes very marked and which are rarely met with in other contractures.

The condition of the reflexes in contractures and in hysterical paralyses is a subject still under discussion, and we shall take up the problem further on, when we study the possible modifications of the reflexes in the course of a psychoneurosis.

Although from the semiological point of view these troubles are well classified, and have definite characteristics which everybody admits, the same is by no means true as far as their nature and pathogeny are concerned. We shall find in studying the contractures and paralyses the very same difficulties in their interpretation as those which we met when we were studying the disturbances of sensibility.

The solution which Babinski offers is extremely simple, and is in consequence not considered so attractive. According to this author, it is as necessary to have an act of the will to relax a muscle as it is to contract it. In the hysteric this voluntary action is suspended, the result being a paralysis if there is a permanent relaxation, or a contracture if a persistent contraction.

This is the hypothesis, but do the facts bear it out? First of all, parenthetically, we would like to throw some light on the connection which is often found (we do not say that it is always the case) between contractures and paralyses. How is contracture brought about in organic paralyses? In the great majority of cases it is caused by a predominance of the extensor muscle activity in the lower limbs and of the flexors in the arms. We do not, as a matter of fact, believe—and one of us has already, in 1900, made this point clear—that organic contractures may be explained by the existence of paralyses of certain muscles with a hypertonia of others. Here, as a matter of fact, the position of the limbs is the same as that seen in tetanus or in strychnine poisoning—namely, flexion in the upper limbs and extension in the lower. In other words, in hemiplegic contractures of organic origin the limbs take the position which is imposed upon them by the "resultant of the antagonistic forces of the muscles in a state of hypertonicity" (Dejerine). But in hysterical contractures the position of the limb in the majority of cases is the same as in organic contractures. In other words, in the hysterical hemiplegic or paraplegic all the muscles share in the contracture, as in the case of organic lesions. This is, however, not always the case and in hysterics one may observe contractures which fix the limbs in a position other than that resulting from muscular predominance, and this occurs under certain special conditions, as we shall see immediately.

With this parenthesis, the first question which we should ask ourselves is the following. On what occasion did the hysterical paralyses and contractures appear? The predominant etiological circumstance is undoubtedly emotion. The latter (and it is an important fact) may act very suddenly, leaving the patient paralyzed or contracted all at once, without his even having had time to know it. In a recent discussion of the Neurological Society,—December, 1909,—several facts of this kind were reported. One of us, in particular, reported several. The most convincing perhaps concerned a woman of the people, who was without education or instruction, having always lived in her own environment and being wholly ignorant that any such thing as hysterical contracture existed. Up to the time of her accident she had never shown the slightest neuropathic phenomenon. One day while she was very carefully preparing a meal, this calm and placid woman fell into a violent rage with her husband. She worked herself up into an intense state of emotion. Her husband sneered at her, and she tried to box his ears. But at that very instant the upper part of her right arm was seized with a contracture. We could mention several cases of paralysis which have been produced under like circumstances. One fact, therefore, is certain,—that an emotion, of itself, and without any suggestive intervention or any voluntary participation on the part of the patient, may suddenly create contractures and paralyses.

A second question, whose solution would be rich in theoretical results, has to do with the persistence of hysterical paralyses and contractures during sleep. The discussion of the Paris Neurological Society, in May, 1908, on hysteria, considered this question of contractures during sleep alone. It would be interesting to know whether hysterical hemiplegics settle themselves down comfortably to sleep, and whether they are able to modify their positions during sleep. So far as the contractures are concerned, very contrary opinions were held. Babinski denied the persistence of contractures, while Raymond affirmed them. As a matter of fact, it is extremely difficult to learn the facts about such things. Hysterical individuals are apt to sleep "with one eye open," and one can hardly examine them without waking them. One fact, however, seems to be of value. If an hysterical contracture is relaxed during sleep, how can one explain the existence in certain of these patients of fibrous adhesions which sometimes cannot be overcome even with the use of chloroform? We have seen one patient of this kind who had had contractures in three limbs for some years, and in whom there was every evidence of periarticular fibrous adhesions, which still persist, even though all signs of contracture have long since disappeared. If, in the case of this woman, the contractures had disappeared during sleep for, say, eight to ten hours out of the twenty-four, it is not very likely that these anatomical changes would have taken place. We have seen a similar case of a double contracture of the adductors, dating back for four years, as a result of an attempted violation, in which there existed fibromuscular adhesions which were very difficult to break up under the influence of chloroform.

Hysterical contractures and paralyses, Babinski said, are made and unmade at will under the influence of suggestion. We feel that some distinction should be made in the cases. There are two forms of hysteria. There is cultivated hysteria such as was formerly seen at the Salpêtrière, and there is real non-educated hysteria. Without any possible question, Babinski's ideas apply to patients of the first group. In those cases, as a matter of fact, with the more or less conscious connivance of the patients, one can get almost anything out of them that one wants. It was an hysteric, you may remember, one of the stand-bys of the hospital frequenting the general medical wards, who, when they wanted to make him sign his dismissal card, said to one of us, "But, sir, I can have a hemiplegia, or a hemianæsthesia, or a contracture, whatever you will. Am I not an interesting patient?" The mythomania of this class of patients, their dramatic instinct, and often their practical interest as well, make them lend themselves very readily to the most diverse suggestions. This applies to professional hysteria which understands its duties, its advantages, and also its slight inconveniences. This discussion has nothing to do with these patients. The case is not the same with accidental hysterics, who are very often honest people, and who are quite properly disgusted when on being seized with a paralysis or a contracture they find themselves considered to be more or less simulators. With these patients it is much more difficult to make the symptoms appear or disappear rapidly. One sees hemiplegias and contractures persisting sometimes for a very long time in spite of all suggestions. As far as the production of paralyses or contractures in hysterics by direct suggestion goes, we ought in truth to say that, as that is contrary to our therapeutic method, we have personally never made any attempts along this line. We are, therefore, obliged to refer to authors who, like P. Janet, have stated that it was very difficult and generally quite impossible to produce lasting paralyses or contractures by suggestion.

Babinski draws another argument from the actually far greater infrequency of hysterical paralyses and contractures in comparison with what one used to see formerly. As a matter of fact, it is very evident, after what he has just said, that all the manifestations of cultivated hysteria have disappeared, reducing the frequency of such manifestations to its just proportions. It is none the less true that, speaking only of hospital practice, one of us still treats each year in the Salpêtrière service a rather large number of paralyses and contractures of hysterical origin. This, however, is a purely negative argument, and cannot be considered as favoring one conception more than another.

Our personal conviction is, therefore, that there exist hysterical contractures which are true contractures, coming within the definition that we have just given,—that is to say, which are at the same time permanent and involuntary. We also believe that there exist troubles by non-intentional suppression of the voluntary motor powers, and which are hysterical paralyses. The same phenomena which an emotion may call forth transiently may be rendered lasting by an hysteria. For we frequently see emotion leading up to pseudoparalytic manifestations, such as the giving way of the legs, the impression of being about to sink to the ground, etc. "Emotion takes one by the arms and legs."

But here, as for hemianæsthesia, we will very willingly admit the secondary intervention of mental representation. It is the very nature of hysteria to fix, in the individual, sensations or conditions which would normally be transient, and it is quite probable that, secondarily to the emotional phenomena, the hysteric is psychically convinced of his helplessness, and cannot get hold of himself physically. This is how the systematization of the paralyses or hysterical contractures comes about, as a result of the fixing of some set of mental representations upon a functional muscular group or a segment of a limb or a part of the body.

Other contractures seem to us to have a wholly different origin. They are what might be called contractures of defence. Here, for example, is a woman on whom rape has been attempted, or one who is attacked by vaginismus, which has brought on a contracture of the adductors. Here is an individual who has added an hysterical contracture to a more or less painful joint. It would seem to us that we have here a case of immobilization in the position of defence against the rape or against the pain. These patients, on the other hand, although they may have often shown themselves indifferent to the symptoms, are very far from being indifferent to its cause. They think about it the whole time. They are sometimes literally obsessed by what they have had to go through, or by the painful symptoms of which they are the prey. The persistence of their contractures is, in fact, merely the objective manifestation of the persistence in their psychism of the creative cause itself. These are in a certain sense phobic manifestations. When we call an act to mind we visualize the movements which produced it. Contractures, in fact, persist because the patients continue to defend themselves in thought. On the other hand, treatment shows the reality of such a conception, for the patients are only cured when they cease to be afraid, when they are no longer in the slightest degree influenced by the impression which gave rise to the symptoms. It is quite possible that the contracture may be variable in such cases and that it may cease during sleep, but these patients sleep very little. Again, we must add that not all such contractures are due to hysteria, and that even in those patients who have true hysterical contractures they do not try to manufacture their symptoms nor are they aware that these are due to hysteria.

We have now finished with the functional fixations which affect the muscular apparatus. This chapter, although containing so many ramifications, is nevertheless only too incomplete, and during the course of our later descriptions we shall meet with a whole series of disturbances which we have omitted here because the neuro-muscular apparatus is not the only one that comes into play and because they are better classified elsewhere.

CHAPTER VIII.

DIFFUSE OR LOCALIZED DISTURBANCES OF SENSIBILITY.

FIRST of all, how does general sensibility behave under an emotion? Two distinct classes of facts and of wholly different mechanism may be observed.

If it is a question of intense and prolonged emotion, without mental representations or without the anxious waiting for some painful phenomenon to appear, general sensibility may be completely deadened. The subject is totally anæsthetic. This may occur equally under the effect of emotions which are called sthenic as well as under those which are depressive.

A soldier on the field of battle, a man rushing to a rescue in a fire, may be wounded without even perceiving it. In the same way in a railroad accident, or in an earthquake, sensibility may completely disappear, and individuals who are seriously hurt may be seen wandering distractedly over the scene of disaster without taking any notice of the injuries which they have suffered. Such facts are classic; history furnishes many examples of them.

The mystic uplift of the mind, or religious emotion, if one so prefers to call it, is able to bring about the same effect. The history of the martyrs is full of stories of individuals who have undergone the direst suffering without showing any signs of pain. It is a very different matter, on the other hand, when people are expecting something which will give them pain. In these cases the phenomena of sensibility receive, on the contrary, a psychic reinforcement. It even happens that individuals will have the impression of pain before the thing which will give them pain has touched them. This is the case with the patient who screams before she is touched; and, although this cry is often called forth by fear, yet it is also often true that a mental representation alone will be enough to make her feel a painful sensation which she believes to be distinctly localized.

Moreover, under these conditions real pain is peculiarly reinforced. A simple touch may become extremely painful, which without this emotional expectancy of pain would scarcely be perceived.

These hyperæsthesias may be diffused or localized according as the subject is uncertain of the point where he ought to feel the painful sensation or as he is forewarned and has fixed his mind upon the probable region of the pain. Under these last conditions localized hyperæsthesia may be accompanied by a total or relative anæsthesia of other regions. This is a fact that is well known to operators, especially to dentists, who fix the attention of their patients on one point while they are operating without pain, or with very little, on some other point.

Under these circumstances it is not a question of a pure and simple emotion. The pain is not caused by an emotional shock, nor is it due to a more or less continuous emotional condition. The emotion here is complicated with expectancy, which is a psychic phenomenon, and we are quite ready to believe that hyperæsthesias are often really phenomena of suggestion, the emotion coming in as a factor of suggestibility.

But, acting directly and without the intervention of anything that would cause pain, continued emotion may bring about a state which, if not that of hyperæsthesia, is at least one of hyperexcitability, in the course of which all contacts are painful and accompanied by sharp reactions, a state of hyperexcitability which in certain cases may very distinctly demonstrate the exaggeration of the reflexes.

It is very evident that all these phenomena concerning general sensibility are, properly speaking, purely central phenomena. The skin only comes into question as being the part that is touched. It has seemed to us, nevertheless, that these troubles, like those that we have already described, ought to be studied according to their subjective localization. It is none the less true that general sensibility is not confined to the skin alone. Certain mucous membranes share in it. The connective tissue, muscles, and bones are subject to it, and what we have just said of disturbances of sensibility which are emotional in origin may be very naturally applied not only to the cutaneous sensibility, but also to all the points of the body on which any traumatic action whatsoever is liable to cause a mental representation of pain.

One objection might be raised resulting from the fact that under certain conditions we have considered expectation as an emotional phenomenon. It is very certain that at the first glance expectation would appear, on the contrary, to be a phenomenon of reason. Then, too, expectation alone is not enough to create those phenomena of psychic reinforcement of pain of which we have spoken. When expectation is reflective, cold as it were, it does not increase pain; it even enables one by the intervention of the will to suppress any outer sign of it. But let the attention in an impressionable subject be mixed with emotional elements or phobic elements, and the pain will be reinforced. This is exactly where the interesting theoretical point comes in. It lies in the rôle that emotion will play,—viz., the rôle of emotional mental representation of which we have already spoken, and which we shall come across again and shall develop at length, when, after finishing the analytic part, we shall reach the synthetic study of functional localizations.

The rôle which emotion plays is no less distinct in the production of subjective disturbances of sensibility. We know that emotion very frequently produces phenomena of cœnæsthesia. Sensations of thoracic tension, impressions of painful contractions of the abdomen, painful genital or perigenital sensations, may, however, be produced just as well by an emotional shock as by a subcontinuous emotional preoccupation. Our very decided impression, which is drawn from a great number of clinical facts, is that many of the profound persistent pains which are met with in neurasthenics, and which are described by the name of algias, have no other origin.

As a matter of fact, disturbances of cutaneous sensibility in the course of the psychoneuroses are of two kinds. They may consist of purely subjective disturbances or of disturbances which are easily proved to be objective. The latter themselves include two varieties. Sometimes they have to do with phenomena of anæsthesia, sometimes it is a question of hyperæsthesia.

We must, therefore, take up successively:

A. *Objective disturbances of cutaneous sensibility: (a) Anæsthesia, (b) hyperæsthesia.*

B. *Subjective disturbances of sensibility.*

A. Objective Disturbances of Cutaneous Sensibility.—*(a) Anæsthesia.*—The anæsthetic disturbances which we have been able to observe in the course of the psychoneuroses are numerous. In a general way they include at one and the same time all forms of sensibility,—tactile, thermal, pain, and even deep sensibility. Also, as a general thing, they are classified among the hysterical symptoms, and it is very rare that anæsthetic objective disturbances of sensibility are met with in neurasthenics. The topography of this class of disturbances rests on classic findings. Its essential characteristic is what we might call its geometric limitations. These hysterical anæsthesias appear band-like, as a pair of cuffs, or occupying a region covered by the trousers or the socks. Their name indicates that they attack a limb or a portion of a limb, and that their upper and lower boundaries are distinctly determined by a circle. On the trunk they may appear as anæsthetic spots, or limited areas of anæsthesia.

But of all the anæsthetic manifestations which hysteria may create, the one which is considered the commonest is undoubtedly hemianæsthesia. This hemianæsthesia—which fetters not only general sensibility but still further special sensibilities, which is often, to employ the classic expression, sensorially sensitive—strikes exactly one half of the body and leaves the other half strictly alone. As a rule, it attacks the left side. As is the case with all hysterical troubles, it is much more frequent in women than in men.

The very existence of this hemianæsthesia, as far as hysterical stigmata are concerned, has been called into question by some authors, Bernheim first of all, and then Babinski, who is the chief one to stand out against it, as well as against the segmentary anæsthesias.

According to this author, the hemianæsthesia would be due either to a medical suggestion or to an auto-suggestion by imitation. Patients who have seen other subjects examined for this hemianæsthesia, and its existence established, are persuaded that they ought to show the same symptom. From that time on, if they do not feel, it is because they do not wish to feel. But here we must explain ourselves, for the question is singularly complex.

If we could but find a subject in whom suggestion had suddenly produced a hemianæsthesia, everybody would be convinced. It would unquestionably be an hysterical symptom. Babinski would call it "a pithiatic symptom"; but the word has nothing to do with the thing, and this author would be the first to recognize the fact that such symptoms are found only in those individuals who were formerly called and who, except by Babinski and those who follow him, are still called hysterics.

There is consequently no doubt that, whatever may be their origin, hemianæsthesiæ as well as segmentary anæsthesiæ are hysterical stigmata. But this is not the question under discussion.

The important thing is to know whether, in certain individuals, under the influence of emotions or of emotional representations, or some other mechanism, and outside of the conscious intervention of the will of the subject, disturbances of sensibility with definite topographical limitations are liable to be created. The question, in other words, is whether the subject who cannot feel anything simulates his anæsthesia or really does not experience any painful impression. For, if we admit that under the influence of even a direct suggestion sensibility may really disappear, the whole theory falls to the ground. As a matter of fact, it would really be strange if a rather vivid emotion or a personal direction of the mentality of the subject could not produce the same effect as that brought about by a suggestion, which is after all an indifferent element, and one would be led to conceive that the disturbance of sensibility in hysterical individuals might in truth be brought out by suggestions, but with very much more reason by any psychic traumatism whatever that was able to create them.

Hence the prejudicial questions which it seems to be our duty to solve are the following: Can the hysterical individual who is in a state of apparent anæsthesia really feel anything? Is the anæsthesia always a phenomenon of suggestion? Where does the break come in that causes the non-transmission of the peripheral stimulus to the superior centres?

Can the hysteric who is in a state of apparent anæsthesia really feel anything? It is quite evident that as far as tactile sensibility is concerned the problem can never be solved. A simulator can always say that he does not feel what he touches, even though the stimulus may have been transmitted and recognized. As far as this mode of sensibility is concerned, one could fall back upon the fact of non-attention. In order to feel impressions as slight as those produced by simple contact, it is evident that the subject must try to pay attention as to whether he feels them or not, and, if voluntarily he turns his attention away and fixes it upon something else, it is possible that the slight tactile impression may not be felt, by a simulation which is unconscious in a way, but which would none the less enter into Babinski's conceptions. We must also add that in reality the subject will, on the contrary, almost always have his attention drawn to this sensibility by the very circumstances of the examination. He will consequently be in that condition which would lead a normal subject to perceive contacts which he would not feel in daily life, psychically speaking. And, on the other hand, in the clinic it generally appears that disturbances of sensibility in an hysteric are in direct proportion to the attention which the subject brings to bear upon them, and that they diminish when the attention is turned away.

There is, however, one mode of contact which is apt to produce very decided impressions. We refer to tickling, which in certain individuals provokes extremely violent reactions which the will is wholly incapable of stopping. How, then, can it be possible for one to tickle the sole of the left foot, for example, of an hysteric, with impunity, without calling forth the slightest reaction, when the same thing on the right foot will bring about an extreme reaction which the will is powerless to inhibit? This is a disturbing fact, and one which would suppose a very peculiar strength in the will of the simulator. We shall come back, however, to this point when we study the cutaneous reflexes in hysteria.

However it may be, we must not admit that the problem, as far as tactile sensibility is concerned, cannot be solved. But as regards thermal sensibility and sensibility to pain the case is not the same. The fact is that one may lay very hot bodies upon the skin of hemianæsthesic hysterics, and that one may pinch them violently and even stick pins in them, without their showing that they feel the slightest sensation. In certain cases of hemianæsthesia in men, one of us has been able to apply excessive pressure on the testicle of the anæsthesic side without the patient giving any sign of noticing it. Of course the simple statement of a patient is not enough to convince one. It is true that one can by the will suppress part of the customary reactions to pain. One can keep from crying out. One can in a certain measure involuntarily inhibit a part of the reactions of defence which pain usually brings about. But can one inhibit all of them? Can one prevent that instinctive shrinking which so generally occurs? Above all, can one prevent those vasomotor phenomena—the flushing or paling of the skin, for example, the contraction of the brow, the narrowing of the palpebral fissure, etc.—which follow states of sharp pain? This seems to us doubtful at the least. Nevertheless, these phenomena are not produced in hysterical individuals, and, further, there has been seen, in a certain number of cases, the absence of local reactions, such as a flow of blood after a prick or ecchymosis after pinching.

The great argument in favor of the theory of simulation lies in the fact that hysterical individuals are rarely afflicted with involuntary traumatisms. In anæsthesias due to some organic cause, in syringomyelia, hæmatomyelia, and anæsthetic leprosy among others, it very frequently occurs, and it often happens that the anæsthesia is noticed for the first time when the patients burn themselves without perceiving it. But this peculiarity is rather rare in these affections, for in hemianæsthesiæ by cerebral lesions and in the anæsthesiæ of tabetics it is only occasionally found.

Among hysterical individuals the phenomenon is very rare, because, it is said, these patients know very well how to guard themselves from contact with anything that is too hot, which means that they are warned by the heat of a body,—in other words, they can feel. The argument has its value, but does not seem to us final.

In the first place, as a matter of fact, although it is rare for an hysterical individual to be burned without feeling it, it is nevertheless not an absolutely exceptional fact, and we have had examples of it in patients to whom the thing really happened. But, on the other hand, as hysterical hemianæsthesia occurs on the left side in the greater number of cases, it is evident that accidents of this kind would not be apt to happen as often as in the cases where it is bilateral or when the right side was affected. Finally, it is very certain that from the point of view of pathophysiology psychic anæsthesia does not perhaps act in quite the same way as organic anæsthesia. This is a question which we shall take up again very soon.

However it may be in the presence of a case where the pain leads to no reaction, and in the presence of the actual facts of involuntary traumatisms, we cannot help but admit that hysterical anæsthesiæ seem to behave very much like real anæsthesiæ. It is very certain that the partisans of simulation could always uphold their opinion, and one would never be able absolutely to prove to them that a subject was not simulating; but it would be necessary in such cases for the simulators to be very strong and very much on their guard. Nevertheless, there exist cases of anæsthesia which have developed from the start in patients so young or so slightly educated as to make such a knowledge of simulation seem truly extraordinary to us. Still another argument of the same psychological order seems to us to have some value. This is the fact that it is extremely rare for hysterical individuals to complain of their anæsthesia. They are much more apt to tell one that their arm or their leg has a feeling of heaviness in it. They do not make the slightest mention of their analgesia or their thermoanæsthesia. How under these conditions could they even get the idea of simulation?

These last considerations bring us to the second question: Is hysterical anæsthesia always a phenomenon of suggestion? In this theory it is claimed that hysterical anæsthesiæ are simulated under the influence of divers suggestions. We have just seen why we do not believe that they are either always or even very often simulated. We do not believe either that they are always due to suggestion, at least—and of this we are very positive—as far as their first manifestation is concerned.

Medical suggestion, or suggestion by imitation, is what the holders of this theory call it: As far as suggestion by imitation is concerned, it appears, if one refers to the discussions which took place in 1909 at the Neurological Society of Paris, that a certain number of neurologists, including one of us, were in a position to affirm that they had had experience with hemianæsthesiæ occurring in patients who had never had anything to do with hysterics. On the other hand, the very special topography of these anæsthesiæ, whether they were segmentary anæsthesiæ or hemianæsthesiæ, eliminated all idea of extra-medical suggestion. As a matter of fact, one knows that the limits of hysterical anæsthesiæ are absolutely regular, particularly in hemianæsthesiæ. Therefore, we defy anyone whomsoever to be tested in those regions where the circles of Weber are rather large and to indicate exactly, within one or two centimetres at least, the superior and inferior boundaries, or to tell exactly, we repeat, where the pincers or the pin which is used in exploring the sensibility crosses the median line. As one cannot voluntarily exactly locate the median line, no matter how keenly one pays attention, how can phenomena of auto-suggestion by imitation, while at the same time creating anæsthesia, endow these patients with such a specialized sensibility that they are able to have more precise ideas of their cutaneous topography than in a normal condition?

On the other hand, suggestion by imitation is, properly speaking, only a form of simulation. Suggestion, by its very definition, means the involuntary introduction into the mentality of the subject of phenomena which were previously strangers to him, and whose acquisition has no reasonable cause.

If, therefore, the phenomena of hysterical anæsthesia were always phenomena of suggestion, there would always be also phenomena of medical suggestion. One would then have to start examinations of the course by which a veritable education of the sensibilities is produced which could give rise to the precise topography of these disturbances.

That medical suggestion is exercised in a great number of cases, and particularly in those hysterical individuals who have had some little training, is a fact that cannot be doubted. But it seems to us to be going too far to generalize and think that all the examinations of sensibility which have been made up to the present have been vitiated by suggestive elements acting as much on the subject as on the observer.

To show the rôle which medical suggestion can play, a rôle which in certain cases we do not try to deny, different arguments have been brought to bear. First of all, it has been claimed that the frequency of anæsthesia on the left is due to the fact that, the observer examining with the right hand, and proceeding naturally in his researches on thoracic sensibility of the patient from right to left, the latest impressions perceived by the patient were on the left, and that consequently suggestion had considerably greater chances of being made on the left-hand side.

This argument hardly deserves discussion, for it implies that one always studies sensibility beginning on the right-hand side of the body. To us the criticisms which are made concerning the methods of examination of sensibility are much more important. It is evident that any process of examination which draws the attention of the subject to his sensibility contains in that very fact an element of suggestion. It is certain that, if one asks the patient, "Can you feel better on the right than on the left?" or says, "Tell me as soon as you feel this less distinctly," etc., one directly suggests his anæsthesia to him, just as, in other cases, when one puts the question to him, "Where am I touching you?" one suggests to him that he must be able to feel. There are, however, many methods employed which, in the majority of cases, even when practised by physicians who are not on their guard in this matter, contain no element of suggestion. They are such as are used when testing for thermoanæsthesia. In the majority of cases they lay a hot or a cold body on the skin of the patient and ask him, "What do you feel? is it hot or cold?" This is the natural question which we have heard asked almost spontaneously even by very young students.

Now, under these conditions, where the patient is not asked if he feels anything, but where he is asked to define the nature of his sensations, if there be a suggestion it will only be a negative one. Nevertheless, among nearly all hysterical individuals afflicted with disturbances of the sensibility, there is a superposition of anæsthesia and thermo-anæsthesia.

We shall not dwell upon this, and, though we are persuaded that one is justified in doubting the rôle which suggestion may play in hysterical anæsthesiæ, we nevertheless think, for all the reasons that we have given, that, in its creation at least, hysterical anæsthesia is not always due to immediate or even to remote suggestion. We have, as a matter of fact, during the last year, observed several cases of hysterical anæsthesia—hemianæsthesia, anæsthesia of a leg, cuff-like bands—in subjects who had never had any previous medical examination. Finally, we conclude this criticism of the theory which holds that sensory disturbances of hysterical individuals are always the outcome of some medical suggestion by asking how it is possible that this suggestion never produces hyperæsthesia, but always and only anæsthesia? On the other hand, for those very cases where suggestion might have come in, it will have to be explained why this suggestion, which is impossible for the great majority of people, can be realized in certain subjects only, and precisely in those who are called hysterics. The solution of the problem of hysteria would be set back rather than advanced.

Where does the break take place in the non-transmission of a peripheral stimulus to the cortical centres?

This is a third question to which it seems necessary to try to make some reply. As a matter of fact, anæsthesia may be produced by very different mechanisms. One may theoretically conceive of the existence of an anæsthesia due to a lack of stimulation of the peripheral nerves even under the influence of a normal stimulus, to lack of transmission, or lack of reception of the stimulation produced, and finally to a lack of perception. This last form of anæsthesia supposes simply the suppression of mental images which lead to a knowledge of and judgment concerning the peripheral stimulation. It is, properly speaking, psychic anæsthesia. In the immense majority of cases hysterical anæsthesia belongs to this latter group, as may be clearly seen in studying the clinical characteristics of this anæsthesia. If, as a matter of fact, conscious sensibility has disappeared, there persists a subconscious sensibility which expresses itself by the dilatation of the pupils following the unfelt painful stimulation, which shows itself also when the subject is distracted, and which at all events allows instinctive phenomena to persist, whence the rarity of unperceived traumatisms in hysterics as well as the persistence of cutaneous reflexes in them, due to the complete integrity of the primary and secondary reflex arcs.

But we have seen that this immunity of hysterics to unconscious traumatisms is not as complete as we have been led to believe. On the other hand, there are cases where the cutaneous reflexes are abolished on the side of the hemianæsthesia while they persist on the sensitive side, which wholly eliminates the hypothesis of the congenital absence of the missing reflex. One of us has been able lately to establish in three patients suffering from hemianæsthesia the unilateral suppression of the plantar cutaneous reflex and of the fascia lata reflex. He was able in another patient to establish in the same way the suppression of the cremasteric reflex. Now, these facts are evidently difficult to interpret if one persists in considering hysterical anæsthesia as a purely psychic anæsthesia, so much so that one is led to ask oneself if under some circumstances the anæsthetic trouble does not arise from another mechanism, and if the interruption in sensibility may not occur at some lower plane.

In short, if we sum up the conclusions which have been developed by this discussion, we must admit that they are all of a negative nature, and that, to our way of thinking, hysterical anæsthesiæ are neither always phenomena of simulation nor always phenomena of suggestion nor always purely psychic anæsthesiæ.

We now come to our personal conception of these phenomena. In our opinion, there exist three classes of hysterical anæsthesiæ. In the first series of facts one may place the cases due to simulation. In the second group of cases we shall range the patients in whom the disturbances of sensibility are directly due to suggestion. Finally there remains a third class of patients in whom the disturbances of sensibility seem to us to be residual emotional phenomena.

Like all the other conceptions, our way of looking at this is evidently only an hypothesis, but it is an hypothesis to which the facts seem to point with peculiar directness. We showed, first of all, at the beginning of this study, that emotion was able to suppress sensibility completely by producing absolute side-tracking, and that under such circumstances it was really a question of total anæsthesia, and not purely psychic anæsthesia, such as we had seen in accidents happening to people who were psychotic or in a state of great mental excitement which they did not even try to avoid. The subjects under such circumstances paid attention to nothing and felt nothing. When the state has passed and the emotional cause has disappeared, the sensibility may return; but the anæsthesia may also persist, either by auto-suggestion which is preserved in an individual who remarks that he has felt none of the various injuries which he has experienced, or it is a question of a simple residual phenomenon independent of all suggestion. In the one case as in the other, the topography of the residual disturbances—the anæsthesia being psychic originally, but with inhibitions and multiple irradiations and added complex phenomena—will always appear in accordance with the usual mental representations of the sensibility,—that is to say, according to regional representations. Hence the segmentary anæsthesia, and hence the hemianæsthesia.

This theory will explain the numerous cases where one sees disturbances of sensibility directly following some emotion, and chiefly an "emotional shock," of which we have also been able to observe several examples, and without which there would have been that cumulative period which usually precedes hysterical attacks.

In other words, we admit that the phenomena which emotion can create are the phenomena which the hysterical individual is able to preserve.

The emotion, at the same time that it modifies the function, inhibits the corresponding mental representations, and what remains after the emotion naturally bears some relation to the antecedent representations. The latter are evidently subordinated to questions of education, reasoning, and all sorts of acquisitions. We do not feel any pain or anæsthesia in the territory of a nerve; we feel it in the arm, in the wrist, or the hand; we feel it on the right or on the left side; and this is why hysterical anæsthesiæ are hemianæsthesiæ or segmentary anæsthesiæ, superimposing themselves, so to speak, on the antecedent mental representations. These broad mental representations, which are in some degree primary, command the whole series of final representations. If we feel a pain, the psychic localizing is made in a progressive fashion; one has a pain in such a finger, or such a joint, or at a certain part of the hand. The secondary manifestations are subordinated to the primary representation which includes them all. And in the emotional residue, in the phenomena of auto-suggestion, which, as we shall see further on, cannot be separated from the emotion, the localizations take place according to the primary mental representations. It is the whole half of the body, the whole limb, or a segment of a limb from which sensibility disappears.

The question which remains to be solved would be to find out if the mental representation corresponds to anatomical facts; if the mode of psychic localization of impressions corresponds to the regional cortical distribution of sensibility, just as the hysterical paralyses may correspond to a regional distribution of motor images. It is very certain that our intellectual acquisitions ought to comply to cerebral anatomical conditions, and be superimposed upon them. And under these conditions there would be nothing extraordinary if, as regards territory, the hysteric hemianæsthesia should be identical to the organic hemianæsthesia. Thus we may conceive that emotion may act almost anatomically, and its effects become secondarily localized.

This long digression outside of the realm of clinical facts, and evidently purely hypothetical, has nevertheless appeared to us justifiable. Further along, in our general study of the psychoneuroses, the full theoretical importance of this interpretation of facts will appear more clearly.

Outside of these limited anæsthesias one may observe, as a result of great emotions, a general anæsthesia, extending over the whole tegumentary surface. During hysterical crises it is a common occurrence, but it may linger after the attack. Usually it resolves itself into a hemianæsthesia, or a residual segmentary anæsthesia, which fact also helps to prove the truth of our idea.

Finally, disturbances of sensibility may be less marked and appear as a simple hypæsthesia. As this slight disturbance is very difficult to determine without bringing in the element of suggestion, we would be quite inclined to believe that there is often opportunity for more or less conscious simulation. The patient who pretends not to be able to feel as distinctly, but who feels all the same, who hesitates about the exact limitations of his sensations, is, by the very nature of things, directly susceptible to suggestion by the examination, and one should at least be very reserved in making any statements concerning the objective reality of such manifestations. We shall not dwell upon the clinical characteristics of these various anæsthetic disturbances. We have pointed out the majority of them in our theoretical discussion. Nevertheless they are quite classic. The equal affection of all kinds of sensibility, association with sensory disturbances, involvement of deep sensibilities, the equality of the degree of anæsthesia at all points, at the base as well as the extremity of the limbs, their ready disappearance under psychotherapeutic influences, are each and all the peculiar attributes of this kind of manifestations.

(*b*) *The Hyperæsthesiæ.*—The hyperæsthesiæ—or, what is the same thing, the hyperalgesiæ—consist in the objective increase of painful sensibility. When they are very marked, tactile sensibility becomes in a certain way sensibility to pain; sometimes a very light touch, simply brushing over the hyperæsthesic region, is enough to produce very marked impressions of pain.

When arising in this way, a hyperæsthesia localized in any one area of the skin is an hysterical phenomenon. The hysterical zones, the ovary and the breasts, etc., which have in their day had a certain celebrity, are in reality hyperæsthetic zones.

The mechanism by which these zones are developed is variable. More often—not always, however—they are the result of pure hetero-suggestion. Sometimes auto-suggestion may come in, and the cutaneous zone in which the objective hyperæsthesia has been established becomes either subjectively or actually painful, without, however, in the cases in which we have been interested, our being able to detect any real nervous lesion. We have seen neurasthenics suffering from vertebral topalgia,—that is to say, from a purely subjective disturbance of sensibility—who, by establishing an hysterical association, have developed a distinctly exaggerated sensibility in the theoretically painful zone. As for the hyperæsthetic localizations, they defy all description. Like all suggested manifestations, and quite the reverse from anæsthetic troubles, they are not fixed, and have no definite limits and no permanence without a repetition of the suggestive actions which created them.

We cannot say as much of generalized hyperæsthesia due to emotion, of which we have already spoken at the beginning of this chapter. It is a frequent phenomenon not only among hysterics, but also among neurasthenics. It is even a common phenomenon in daily life. Every person who is at all neuropathic has undoubtedly had moments when, to use a popular expression, he has felt his nerves all "on edge," where the idea of being touched seemed insupportable to him, or where the slightest jar would throw him into an emotional state with sometimes considerable exaggeration of feeling. These conditions, which may be found among nervous people—neuropathic candidates, but not yet real neuropaths—when they are suffering from more or less continued care or worry, are not lasting. Among neurasthenics who are suffering emotionally from some continuous cause, this condition is often found in a persistent form, and particularly in those forms of neurasthenia that are predominantly psychic, where the patient is in a tense, excited state rather than depressed.

Here it is evidently a case of hyperexcitability or psychic irritability rather than hyperæsthesia properly so called. This hyperexcitability is not limited to the domain of general sensibility, but it can extend still further, to the domain of special sensibility, and even to the general *ensemble* of all vital manifestations having a psychic tinge.

If only as an aid to diagnosis these facts ought to be pointed out. It is no less true, however, that such phenomena, really belonging to the emotional state, are of a nature which suggestion may develop but cannot create. This is a fact which is also of importance, and to which we shall return.

B. Subjective Disturbances of Sensibility.—All the spontaneous sensations which are produced apart from any stimulus, and whose general *ensemble* represent subjective disturbances of sensibility, are excluded from the program of our study. In order to consider subjective disturbance of sensibility as a functional manifestation we should have to admit that there are some organic phenomena that are not susceptible to explanation. This is the same as saying that we cannot consider any disturbance of the sensibility due to vascular or nervous actions, either direct or indirect, as a functional phenomenon.

Topalgias, or central psychic algias, constitute practically the great majority of the subjective disturbances of general sensibility, which have been described in the course of the psychoneuroses.

These topalgias willingly abandon the domain of superficial sensibility in order to attack the region of visceral sensibilities. A number of painful phenomena, which graft themselves on the many phobic states which we have already seen, and which we shall have to analyze, are in reality only manifestations of this kind. As a matter of fact, these are very often regional manifestations: pains in the kidneys,—neurasthenic backache,—vertebral pains, pains in the nape of the neck, the famous neurasthenic helmet. Sometimes the painful sensations are by the patient more definitely localized in the face, the forehead, the head, the back of the eyeballs, or on some point of the vertebral column, such as the coccyx or the region of the neck.

These pains are of varying intensity. Movement increases certain of them, particularly the coccygodynia. When they are very sharp and generalized, they constitute akinesia algera, characterized by absolute impossibility of the patient's making a movement without feeling painful impressions, from which he gets into the habit of such a complete immobilization that, like a paralytic, he cannot leave his bed. In a less marked degree this phenomenon is common among neurasthenics. It enters as an essential factor in the so-called physical asthenia with which these patients are afflicted.

These painful impressions almost always belong to neurasthenia. They are essentially phenomena of a suggestive nature, and later we shall find this fact,—namely, that, in anything that concerns subjective disturbances as well as those of sensibility, the neurasthenic is even more suggestible than the hysteric.

The majority of these phenomena come about through the psychic fixation on the part of the patient of some pain that had once been experienced or some emotional sensation which had once been felt.

The following case is in this respect most interesting. It is the case of a man, fifty-six years old, who for fifteen years had suffered from a localized pain at the pit of his stomach, coming on, without any relation whatever to the time of eating, in the form of attacks so intense that he could neither sleep nor suppress his groans. The pain was not clearly defined by the sufferer, and none of the classic diagnoses seemed to fit it. It was not a burning sensation, neither was it a boring or tearing or stabbing pain. In fact he could not compare it to anything. The only definite idea that he had about it was of its intensity, which he stated to be very distressing, as was likewise the calamity which it brought into his life, which he considered as hopelessly spoiled by it.

Now, upon analysis this pain proved to be nothing but the fixation of an impression of pain.

As a matter of fact, its onset coincided with a whole series of emotional traumatisms, caused by the loss of his money and losing of his position, to which anxieties were added family cares and troubles of all kinds. During a period of eighteen months, while the patient's affairs seemed to be going better, these painful phenomena disappeared almost completely, but only to reappear without further interruption when his temporal and emotional affairs were again upset. On examination no objective sign whatever could be found, but palpation of the epigastric region, which was easy and which did not bring on muscular contractions of the wall, nevertheless always started a subjective pain in the patient.

He had naturally seen a great many physicians, who had all ordered local medications, whose therapeutic effects were nil, but which had had the result of fixing more profoundly than ever in his mind the conviction of his incurability.

By the simple means of appropriate psychotherapy, this patient was completely cured in a fortnight. This was partly due to the fact that it was a question of a typical pain, and also to the fact that our patient was sufficiently strong minded to allow himself to be treated by *shaming him out of it*, which constitutes the only therapy for such an affection.

Sometimes there seems to be no starting-point and the pain is created wholly by suggestion. To appreciate this fact it is only necessary to question, on the one hand, educated neurasthenics who know by heart the classic symptomatology of the affection of which they complain, and, on the other hand, neurasthenics belonging to the poorer and badly educated classes of society. Then one can see that the helmet headache, the pain in the nape of the neck, and pain in the spine are extremely frequent among cultivated people, but much rarer among the others.

On the contrary, pains with a complex mechanism, connected with the psychic fixation which has come about in connection with some real thing, pains in the kidneys, that whole class of visceral pains, and simple headaches without the classic stamp, are met with equal frequency in the two classes of patients which we have just designated.

Another element comes in, which is the education of the sensibilities as the result of the attention, whether emotional or not, being focussed on some one point or other of the organism. There is no question that one may succeed by focussing the attention, even though it be more or less complicated by phenomena of emotion and suggestion, in educating a visceral or peripheral sensibility in just the same way as a blind man or a clever artisan educates his tactile sensibilities. But these facts ought to be put in the group of hyperæsthesiæ rather than in the list of purely objective disturbances of sensibility. They are in reality phenomena of localized hyperirritability, which may be compared in their own particular domain to the diffuse hyperexcitabilities which we have already studied.

As a rule, a central pain begins by being intermittent. It is a pain that is felt once, then forgotten, then felt again at the end of several days, and whose reproduction strengthens the memory. Then by progressive stages the suffering becomes continuous. It is a pain which is dull and heavy, not sharp and poignant. When the patient is left to himself it is persistent, allowing him very little rest, but nevertheless it is rarely a factor of insomnia. As is the case with all psychic pains, as well as all organic pains with psychic reinforcement, distraction—this word being taken in its etymological sense—causes it to diminish or disappear. This, from the point of view of their treatment, is a most important fact.

These localized pains are extremely interesting from every point of view, first on account of their mechanism, and also on account of the various difficulties in diagnosis which their presence involves. The errors in diagnosis to which they lead are made in two ways,—either one mistakes a symptom connected with an organic disease for a central pain, or, on the other hand, one does not recognize the functional nature of the sensations perceived by the patient. We shall come back, however, to this question of diagnosis.

In addition to central pains, there are other subjective disturbances of sensibility which may be observed in the course of the psychoneuroses. These are abnormal sensations, but neither severe nor painful, which belong to the group of what in France are termed the dysæsthesiæ. Restlessness in the limbs, vague feelings of heat or cold, without any associated vasomotor disturbances, prickings, creeping, tickling sensations, etc., are all distinct impressions which may be found in patients exclusive of any organic phenomena, occurring either accidentally or more or less permanently. They may coexist with phenomena of hypæsthesia or anæsthesia, and also be found as isolated phenomena.

They are observed in hysterical individuals in the periods immediately following attacks, but they may just as well be objective manifestations in the domain of sensibility due to slight paralytic disturbances. One meets with them also in neurasthenics, but more often they are merely a suggestive association in connection with some phobic manifestation, which presents itself in the region whose sensibility is disturbed.

We are now, as far as we are able, done with the disturbances of general sensibility. We are far from having enumerated them all. We have in particular neglected what are called paræsthetic manifestations,—that is to say, disturbances of objective sensibility which are neither hyperæsthesiæ nor anæsthesiæ. These disturbances (polyæsthesia, fusion or summation of sensation, exhaustion of sensation, impossibility of localization, etc.) are but very rarely met with in the course of the psychoneuroses, and only in hysteria. If we repeat, on the other hand, that, in the domain of objective sensibility in hysterics and in the domain of algias and suggestive sensibility in neurasthenics, every trouble must be studied individually, it will make it sufficiently clear why and how and in what measure our study is incomplete. Volumes might be written and have been written on this subject. We must be satisfied for the time being with having related the commonest of these disturbances and having shown how they may become established under the triple influence of emotion, suggestion, and education, and by those phenomena which are directly connected with them, such as memory, attention, etc.

CHAPTER IX.

FUNCTIONAL MANIFESTATIONS OF THE SENSE ORGANS.

In this chapter, as in the majority of the succeeding chapters, we have two kinds of troubles to describe. There are, on the one hand, a whole series of phobic manifestations which may act upon the sense organs as on any other part of the body, while, on the other hand, there are functional fixations, properly so called, translating themselves into phenomena which, although they are subjective in origin, have none the less an objective appearance. So far as these latter manifestations are concerned, it is often very difficult to differentiate them from purely psychic fixations. The sense organs are, in fact, only anatomical projections of the brain, projections by which the latter comes in direct contact with the external world. The functions of the sense organs being essentially functions of knowledge, and knowledge being a psychological fact, it happens that many of the troubles which are experienced are in reality psychic disturbances which we must study elsewhere.

One is, nevertheless, in the right in describing functional manifestations of the sense organs when it is a question of the difficulty being localized in a single one. It is of course understood that some psychic disturbance is the cause in such cases, as in all functional manifestations, but the specialization of these disturbances allows them to be considered as having a certain autonomy.

We shall take up successively the functional disturbances of sight, hearing, smell, and taste.

The functional disturbances of *vision* which have been spoken of in hysteria are extremely numerous. More often they are unilateral, or at least in most cases predominant on one side. They are usually, therefore, associated with hemianæsthesia, and form a constitutional part of what is called sensitive-sensorial hemianæsthesia.

Of all the functional disturbances of vision narrowing of the visual field is assuredly the most classic. Bilateral, with considerable predominance on the anæsthetic side, it is chiefly characterized by this fact, that it becomes continuously more marked during the course of the perimetric examination, so much so that during a prolonged examination the successive fields of vision grow progressively narrower until under certain circumstances the visual field may become a mere point.

The hysteric is quite unconscious of the diminution of his field of vision. It in no wise hinders him in any of his daily duties which demand good eyesight. And he never in any way loses his sense of orientation.

The perception of colors may be modified in the hysteric. In his case the narrowing of the visual field for colors is just the opposite of what one observes in lesions of the optic nerve. Instead of the fields for green and red being the first to disappear, leaving the fields for yellow and blue intact for a longer time, in the hysteric it is red which persists longest in the vision. In hysterical achromatopsia red may be the only color that remains.

Other ocular phenomena observed among hysterics are sufficiently defined by the words dyschromatopsia, total achromatopsia, micropsia, megalopsia, monocular polyopia, kopiopia, and painful accommodation. These phenomena naturally are only specific when one has seen that there is absolute integrity of the fundus and ocular structures and that there are no coexistent errors of refraction.

Pupillary symptoms, such as myosis, bilateral or unilateral mydriasis, pupillary inequality, slow pupils, modification of the condition of the pupils during the course of an attack, etc., have been described in hysteria.

Other symptoms have also been pointed out which involve the extrinsic eye muscles and those of the eyelids, such as blepharospasm in clonic, tonic, or pseudoparalytic form, blepharoptosis, ophthalmoplegia, with conservation of all the intrinsic movements, strabismus from muscular spasms, loss of muscular sense of the eye muscles, etc. Finally a certain number of cases of unilateral amblyopia or of hysterical bilateral amaurosis have been established. We shall attempt in a little while to interpret these various troubles.

What is more interesting, to our way of thinking, is a whole series of manifestations of a phobic nature which may be met with in neurasthenics. The commonest of all consists in rapid fatigue of vision. For one reason or another, these patients afflict themselves by bringing auto-suggestion to bear upon their sight. Sometimes it is because under the influence of an ophthalmic migraine they have had scintillating scotomata, or else under some influence of a similar nature they have suffered from photophobia. Sometimes it is a medical consultation which has directed the patient's ideas. One finds him then providing himself with glasses of different colors, which he changes according to the atmospheric condition. The rapid consequence of this mental state is that such patients imagine themselves to be continually with a veil before their eyes, and think that they are unable to read anything that is a little difficult, or to continue for any length of time without experiencing intense ocular fatigue. There are some who every two or three minutes close their eyelids to rest a theoretically fatigued vision, there are even some who abandon part of their occupations, and there are still others who go so far as to shut themselves up in a semi-darkened room.

What is the nature of these troubles? Is it true, as has been said, that it is a real asthenia of vision which attacks these patients, corresponding to a general asthenia, and considered by many authors as organic? According to our way of thinking, the mechanism of this visual fatiguability is in fact of the same order as that of amyasthenia, but, like the latter, has nothing to do with organic phenomena. That the fatigue felt by these patients is real is very doubtful, but from what does it come? It appears to us that it is generally due to disharmonic phenomena which come into play. The patients grow tired quickly because they hold themselves too tensely, because their vision, instead of acting in an almost unconscious manner, is voluntarily made to act and is strained and overattentive. We are only speaking now, it must be understood, of the function itself, for we do not have to take up the modifications in relation to the trouble of perception, these latter being in fact pure psychic manifestations. The patients, in short, tire themselves just as any healthy subject would tire himself if he fixed his gaze in a very determined fashion upon a given point. Other phobic manifestations which are due to the prolonged preservation of a passing impression may also exist. One sees patients of this kind who will complain for weeks of a foreign body which has long since been removed from the eye, and who, by reason of making movements of their eyelids, pressing the eye with their handkerchiefs, and bathing it with all sorts of liquids, end up by having a true conjunctival irritation, accompanied by a more or less continual lachrymation.

It is by this mechanism that we see a certain number of neurasthenics creating for themselves what they call "a peculiar sensitiveness" of their eyes, and reacting by objective manifestations to impressions of cold, or to irritations caused by too strong a light, etc. As a matter of fact, these are phenomena of auto-suggestion and of unconscious simulation.

Concerning the true nature of the ocular troubles in hysterics of which we have just spoken, it seems to us that a certain number of distinctions ought to be made.

Of all the ocular or periocular phenomena which hysterics may present, and which have been subjectively verified by a number of good observers, the most classic—namely, the narrowing of the visual field—is perhaps still the one which carries with it the least conviction. It is quite possible that this supposed stigma of hysteria might have been in many cases directly suggested by the medical examination. The narrowing, as a matter of fact, is exaggerated with the observers, and varies in the course of the same observation. The fact that these patients have no difficulty in anything that has to do with directing their walk, their orientation, the nature of obstacles to be stepped over or avoided, etc., offers still further arguments in favor of the purely suggestive—and apparently hetero-suggestive—nature of this phenomenon. It is very evident that in a perimeter examination the subject whose attention has been fixed upon a given point will have a tendency, to a greater or less degree, to see nothing but this isolated point. This is, moreover, very much in accordance with the mental condition of hysterics, in whom the whole field of consciousness may, as has been said, be concentrated on a single perception. Although persisting in the instinctive or automatic mentality, none of the other sensations raise themselves up to the higher plane of perception. What under these conditions would be narrowed in the hysteric is not his visual field, properly speaking: it is his field of visual consciousness. We then have to do with an essentially subjective phenomenon, wholly different from other neuropathic ocular manifestations.

Pupillary disturbances, such as myosis or mydriasis, are generally attributed to a spasmodic action affecting the constrictors or dilators of the pupil. How shall we understand the mechanism of this spasm? The interpretation which may seem the more plausible, although it is none the less wholly hypothetical, consists in supposing that it is a question of the fixation of the pupil in a state of accommodation determined for sight at a distance (mydriasis), or for sight near to (myosis). This, therefore, would be at bottom nothing more than an exaggeration in intensity and duration of a normal phenomenon. When a subject is in a condition of concentrated attention,—or, on the contrary, when he is lost in revery, and his eyes "look into space, seeing nothing,"—there is produced a contraction or dilatation of the pupil. It is, therefore, a question of function indirectly submitted to the will, and one can very well understand that the hysteric whose eyes are "lost in space," or have a fixed stare, may have a permanent dilatation or constriction of his pupil.

So far as bilateral amaurosis is concerned, it is thought that there exists a true blindness of psychic origin, where the patients can no longer see, because they really do not look. In such cases there is only an exaggeration of the narrowing of the visual field, and a suppression not of sensation, but rather of visual perception. Here again the action of suggestion preponderates, but it must be understood that manifestations of this kind may be self-created by the inhibition, as it were, of all visual mental representations. It is not unusual to see people who under the influence of strong emotions almost completely lose all visual idea, so that they no longer distinguish obstacles or recognize a person right before them. It is very evident that in cases of this kind automatic elementary visual perception persists even when conscious perception has disappeared.

Paralyses and contractures of the extrinsic ocular muscles—which are, however, very rare—seem to us to be pathologically identical with those of paralysis or contractures of other muscles of the body: contractures of defence, so to speak, by the voluntary turning of the eye in a given direction; paralysis or contracture by paralyses of the opposing muscles, by loss of ideomotor representations of direction of sight, in a given sense.

As far as the phenomena of achromatopsia and of dyschromatopsia are concerned, they seem to us to share the same direct suggestive action as narrowing of the visual fields.

Neuropaths may present a certain number of fixations of the *auditory apparatus.*

In the same manner that we have just seen, that a psychic blindness may occur in certain hysterics, so in this same class of patients cases of psychic deafness may be found. This, to tell the truth, is a very rare manifestation, and in the cases in which it has been observed one must make a good many reservations. As a matter of fact, it has not been proved that simulation cannot come into play in these cases. Theoretically, however, one can conceive of the existence of psychic deafness with a pathogeny quite similar to that of the blindness of hysterics.

Other troubles which are much more apt to be met with in hysterics seem to us to be far more important. Hysterics often complain of their auditory functions. They say they hear poorly, cannot follow the conversation when several people are talking together, and are obliged to have the same words or phrases repeated several times. These are, in reality, phobic manifestations. They happen on the occasion of some incident connected with hearing, and have two different mechanisms. It is always a question of what one might call deafness of attention. Sometimes, however, it is due to lack of attention, and sometimes to excess. Here, for example, is a patient more or less preoccupied, concentrated upon his own condition, and experiencing all kinds of feelings of depression. It is quite evident that under these conditions he would be likely to hear only in part or inaccurately whatever might be said to him. This is deafness due to distraction. It may happen that the patient has noticed this, and that he is disturbed by having heard badly, and, if it so happens that medical intervention has further fixed his mind on the subject, he may have auditory disturbances due to excess of attention. The excess of attention paid to the hearing of one word hinders the hearing of the following word. Here again is a phenomenon of the disharmonic order attacking the normal automatism of the function of hearing.

Another manifestation consists in irritability to noises. Neurasthenics will very frequently tell you that they cannot bear the slightest noise, and that certain noises in particular are extremely irritating to them. Is this one of those signs of irritable weakness in neurasthenics which, according to a number of authors, forms the essential characteristic symptoms of this affection, or is it a special susceptibility of audition? This point must be made clear.

In all kinds of emotional states, and states of concentration, in which the subject absorbed in himself loses, so to speak, contact with the external world, it is very certain that all sensory stimuli are felt more vividly. It is the same phenomenon as that which makes a normal individual start on hearing some noise which he was not expecting.

One might say that the sensation is reinforced by the surprise which it occasions. In the neurasthenic the same thing is true, and the best proof of it is that he is insensible to sounds which he himself voluntarily makes. His irritability to noise is, as a matter of fact, only an outward expression of his concentration on himself.

On the other hand, this same irritability to noise is found in all subjects who are psychically depressed, in whom under these circumstances there exists a very real condition of irritable weakness. The condition of the nervous system in these cases is only an expression of the general condition. It may happen, in a certain number of neurasthenics who are emaciated and more or less cachectic, that factors of this nature intervene in causing the phenomenon.

Finally,—we might almost say, above all,—phobic phenomena may play their rôle in the genesis of this very special irritability. The patient who is exasperated by noise—whether he regards it as an external sign of the slight attention which his family pays to his condition, or whether he has interpreted his lack of sleep as due to the disturbances or lack of quiet around him—adds a psychic factor to his auditory perceptions. The irritability in this particular case is purely mental, and has nothing to do with any auditory trouble. Other mechanisms intervene by association of ideas, with the result that when a noise has once been the cause of a disagreeable sensation the same noise always reproduces the same impression.

Other patients complain of buzzings and thumping in the ear. There are people who attribute persistent insomnia to manifestations of this kind. Sometimes this is due to memories which are continually recalled. There are patients who by reason of the presence of a little wax in the ear, or for some other reason, have accidentally had buzzings in the ear. When the cause itself has disappeared they continue to experience the same phenomenon. In reality it is nothing but a pure psychic recall. Sometimes medical treatment has intervened,—catheterization of the eustachian tube, massage of the tympanum, etc., have been practised when the trouble was purely subjective,—with the prompt result of turning the patient's mind and fixing it on his ear, thus transforming sensations which should have been merely passing into a veritable obsession, which the patient externalizes in various degrees. Under other circumstances, these would be patients who, as a result of some emotional experience, might have felt sensations of dizziness, and who were told that they had "auricular vertigo." Still other circumstances may be the cause of establishing the phenomenon.

As for the drumming and whistling and buzzing sounds which patients notice in their ears, they are facts which are very easy to explain. They are due simply to the fact that the subjects whose attention has been brought to bear upon them have succeeded in being able to hear their arterial beating, a thing which any one may learn to do with a little attention. But, although the phenomenon is common, the consequences which the patients draw from it are not so. Sometimes very strong obsessions arise, so much so that the subjects who are afflicted by them spend their nights in watching for and experiencing these sensations, which are perfectly natural, but are magnified out of all proportion.

Finally, there are no effective localizations in the auditory organs which in neurasthenics, if the physician is not careful to understand his patient's moral condition, but may become the starting-point of an intensive diffusion of symptoms with phobic manifestations of all kinds.

The *olfactory apparatus* is not spared in the course of the psychoneuroses. Under the name of anosmia we shall consider the loss of olfactory sensations as found in a certain number of hysterics, either isolated or associated with psychosensory hemianæsthesia.

We shall come back very soon to sensory hemianæsthesia associated with psychic hemianæsthesia. As far as bilateral anosmia is concerned, it seems to us to develop from a mechanism which is comparable to that of psychic blindness or deafness. In this instance also there is no suppression of sensation, but suppression of perception, and the very patients who pretend that they do not smell the odor of a strong perfume will make good their escape, for example, from an environment filled with odors of gas. The automatism persists in such cases even when the conscious and voluntary idea has disappeared.

There are also secretory and vasomotor modifications of the olfactory mucous membrane which may be of a purely neuropathic nature. It has been thought that epistaxis in certain hysterics might be considered as a supplementary flux occurring instead of and taking the place of absent menses. This is, however, far from being the fact. In the first place, amenorrhœa in the hysteric is much less frequent than one is led to believe, and under these same conditions epistaxis is not frequent. It is really only a question of coincidence in such cases, and the relation of causality between these phenomena is probably due to the mental vagaries current at some period rather than to any real pathological association.

We cannot say as much for nasal hydrorrhœa. This is a phenomenon which may be observed not only in hysterics, but also, much more frequently, under certain special circumstances, in the neurasthenic. The nasal secretion is, as a matter of fact, liable to be directly influenced by the psychism. And the latter, on the other hand, is capable of directly creating sensations identical to those which result from a real nasal secretion. It is so true, that, in an individual with the least tendency toward any neuropathic traits, it is only necessary for him to notice that he has forgotten his handkerchief in order to have this simple idea cause him the most intense and legitimate desire to use one. It is the same mechanism of this supposed susceptibility of the mucous membranes which one finds in a certain number of neurasthenics. There are some who pretend that they are so extremely delicate that they cannot stand any change of air or environment without catching cold. As a matter of fact, it is simply a question of psychic fixation on the mucous membrane. It is possible for a more or less abundant nasal secretion to be produced by psychic mechanism; but even if this phenomenon does not take place, the patient wants to use his handkerchief, and does so. He spends several hours in this way, until his eyes have become swollen and filled with tears, and his nose slightly congested, when he has the great satisfaction of displaying to himself as well as to others the effect of a violent cold. As a rule, it does not last. These are the colds which linger for two or three hours, which caught in the morning have passed away by lunch time. Unfortunately, however, it does not always happen in this way, and often the idea may become fixed and diffused into a veritable obsession which spoils the patient's whole life. We do not wish to slander the specialist on this point; it has happened many times, however, that we have seen such a psychic fixation which has had a most disastrous effect upon the patient's life and which was almost wholly due to medical suggestion.

People who have made themselves ill along the lines analogous with that which we have just described and find themselves excessively prone to coryzas go to consult a specialist. It is very rare that they are not upheld in the necessity for this consultation by receiving some prescription,—nasal douches, slight cauterizations, powders, or ointment to snuff up. More often the specialist, who has perceived how mild the trouble is or that it really does not exist, has not, however, given due consideration to the mental condition of the subject who is afflicted. He may have said to the patient, "It is a very trifling affair. Do thus and so." This would seem to be a very unimportant statement, but often it is too much. It is enough in any case to make the patient believe that he was justified in being uneasy and to make him henceforth give himself up to a series of physical and mental gymnastics in the matter of autoöbservation. An obsession quickly follows, which is serious not so far as its object is concerned, but in itself, and by the disturbance which it brings to normal life by throwing a whole symptomatology which had hitherto been subjective, into objective form. This obsession will progress more rapidly and become more tenacious if the patient is put through a course of surgical treatment, such as removal of the turbinated bones, cauterizations, galvanocauterizations, etc., legitimate perhaps in themselves, but which the moral condition of the patient should interdict, just as in serious cardiac conditions the use of chloroform would be interdicted.

We have seen subjects—and they were not hypochondriacs—who had led a most miserable life for months, even years, because it had been shown and proved to them that they were not able to breathe as well through one nostril as through the other. In fact, we might repeat for these patients all that we have said for our false gastropaths.

Finally, there is one last fact bearing upon *smell* which concerns the manner in which odors are borne by neuropaths. It is understood that hysterical individuals in general, and in greater degree those afflicted with anosmia among them, are wholly indifferent to odors. The same is not true for any great number of neurasthenics. These latter may experience in the presence of odors in general, and of certain odors in particular, a very special irritability, going so far as to form a real phobic manifestation. It must be understood that we are not speaking now of obsessions in regard to odors, a mental manifestation which may be met with in certain neurasthenics who are perfectly aware of the obsessive nature of the phenomenon experienced by them. Here the question is not at all the same; the neurasthenics make a phobia of odors just as they do a phobia of noise, because the odor disturbs them in their meditations, and because, having once been annoyed in this way, they are more or less continuously calling up the sensation which they once experienced by the fear of its repetition.

It is possible for matters to go still a little further and for certain patients to be haunted by odors. This is a case of a more marked mental phenomenon, but one which never has the intensity, the tenacity, or the autonomy of the manifestations of the same kind which are met with in the well-defined psychoses.

Taste may also present a certain number of derangements in the course of the psychoneuroses. Unilateral diminution of taste is found along with psychosensory hemianæsthesia, associated with the disturbances of all the other modes of sensibility. The phenomenon may be so marked that patients are incapable of differentiating sugar from salt on one side of the tongue, which difference they can determine immediately if the object is placed on the other side. We shall discuss the interpretation of this phenomenon a little further on.

Total ageusia, as an isolated symptom, has been observed in certain patients with hysteria. As an independent fixation it is a rare phenomenon. What is very commonly found in many patients is disturbance of taste of all kinds, associated with digestive troubles. Take, for example, a mental anorexic or a neurasthenic suffering from a false gastropathy; it is very common to hear these patients complain of the lack of taste in all their food. Inversely, one can find subjects in whom the gustatory sensations are exaggerated. They find their dishes too well done or underdone, with too much or too little seasoning, etc. Finally, it is customary to find olfactory irritability associated with gustatory irritability.

In reality there is no perversion of taste. If the gustatory sensibility is tested it is found to be normal. There are only purely subjective symptoms attending the anorexia of these patients, and this is so true that from one day to another, depending upon the mental orientation of these patients, their excessive sensibility in the matter of taste may suddenly pass over into a characteristic lack of taste. In one hotel they may find the cooking insipid, and in another they will find the seasoning quite too high. In this case there is nothing but an exterioration or projection upon the given organs of a psychic digestive systematization.

Under other circumstances the disturbance of gustatory sensibility is only a disturbance of character, a particular expression of the patient's general pessimism. But in any case it does not appear to us that gustatory irritability—like all the other irritabilities—should be exalted into the position of an autonomous symptom.

In concluding this chapter there now remains for us to give a general view of the mechanism of psychic hemianæsthesia associated with hemianæsthesia of general sensibility. One knows that in these patients this psychic hemianæsthesia is constituted by the presence of a peripheral anæsthesia in addition to a narrowing of the visual fields, with or without other associated ocular disturbances, and by a diminution or complete suppression of auditory, olfactory, and gustatory acuteness.

Although it is possible, in a certain way, to get an idea of the mechanism of sensory hemianæsthesia, which has, as a matter of fact, a cerebral topography, and at the same time what we might almost call a mental topography, the same thing is not true for psychic anæsthesia. Here, as a matter of fact, the disturbances are more wide-spread, and still further—anatomically speaking—their peripheral distribution does not correspond in any way to any cerebral topography. But, do they correspond to any mental topography? In other words, as all sensory stimuli lead up by anatomical paths to bilateral cerebral stimulation, and as the cerebral topography is, as a matter of fact, bilateral, is the mental topography unilateral? Or, if one so prefers to put it, are there fields of consciousness which respond to unilateral psychic stimuli? This seems evident when one recalls that all psychic impressions are accompanied by a constant idea of the localization or the position of the objects which have caused the psychic impression. There are, moreover, ideas and judgments which in a more or less automatic manner largely determine our equilibrium, our sense of direction, and all our relations with the external world. Therefore, it is very certain that all our localizations are made in relation to the median line. All sensorial stimuli which are susceptible of localization are situated either on the right or on the left. This is the same thing as saying that conscious perceptions correspond to a certain extent to a unilateral distribution of sensorial sensibility. In these conditions, one can see that the inhibition of a certain number of mental representations may lead to the creation of sensorial hemianæsthesia. But one can also see how preponderant must be the action of auto-suggestion and hetero-suggestion, as it is a question here of mental processes which are already complex. Emotion, which in a great majority of cases is the chief factor in the production of hysterical disturbances, acts as a whole. Outside of the physical phenomena which it may bring about, it deprives an individual of his judgment, of his will, of his mental equilibrium; but it does not attack mental phenomena as complex as those which we must admit are attacked in order to be able properly to interpret psychic hemi-anæsthesia.

One may, however, conceive of another interpretation. It might be possible, psychologically speaking, for the functions of sensibility and of localization to be so closely united that they might be confused. What the hysteric would lose under these conditions would not be the sensibility of the right half, or more usually the left half of his body, but rather visual, acoustic, olfactory, and gustatory hemi-sensibility. What would be lacking to him would be the whole apparatus of localization, or, if one so prefer to call it, of exterior consciousness of the right or left side, with all the general and sensorial sensibilities which belong to it. One would thus understand the curious association, which is entirely anti-anatomical, if one might so call it, which hysterics make when they superimpose upon an anæsthesia of general sensibility the psychic disturbances that one recognizes.

All this evidently is pure hypothesis, whose only merit as an hypothesis is that it enables one to take a rational conception of things, and may, in consequence, have some chance of being right.

CHAPTER X.

NERVOUS AND PSYCHIC MANIFESTATIONS PROPERLY SO CALLED.

ALTHOUGH all functional manifestations spring directly or indirectly from the psyche, it does not follow on that account that the nervous apparatus itself has nothing to do with them.

We have already seen that neuro-muscular disturbances and disturbance of the sensibility which we have studied constitute the nervous manifestations properly so called. Nevertheless, a certain number of points remain for us to study, and we shall take up successively in this chapter—

A. *Disturbances of sleep;*
B. *Headache;*
C. *Disturbances of the reflexes;*
D. *Disturbances of speech;*
E. *Acquired disturbances of psychological functions;*
F. *Phobic manifestations fixed upon the cerebrospinal axis.*

A. Disturbances of Sleep.—These are extremely numerous and infinitely varied in neurasthenics. They occupy a preponderant place in the symptomatology. They are the source of a whole series of secondary disturbances. Thus we ought to study them in some detail.

It is far from easy to really understand these troubles, for, at the present time, there is no theory concerning sleep,—or, rather, there are too many, of too contradictory a nature.

One does not know what sleep is, but there is no author who does not believe that he has the right to define insomnia. One takes it for granted that it has a pathological physiology, while ignorant of its normal physiology. Hence, the pathogeny of sleep disturbances becomes, to a certain degree, individual. This man—we speak, of course, only of purely neuropathic conditions—does not sleep because he is under too great tension, and that man because he is too much relaxed, another has too much or too little acidity in his urine, a fourth is so feeble that he cannot tire himself sufficiently, etc.

It seems to us that, if one wants to get a little more definite idea concerning the mechanism of sleep disturbances in the neurasthenic, it ought to be enough to acquaint oneself with what occurs in the healthy man. The study of conditions which permit sleep to be regular, the search for causes which may occasionally disturb it, may be able, it seems to us, to furnish sufficiently exact ideas to explain the great majority of irregularities which sleep may undergo in the course of the psychoneuroses.

First of all, there is no doubt that sleep is a natural function of the body, and that a series of waking and sleeping states forms as necessary a rhythm, for example, as the contraction and relaxation of a muscle. Sleep is a general function of all organized beings. According to some naturalists, it exists even among plants, and there is perfectly rhythmic. Among animals, psychic life seems to be limited to their bodily life, sleep appears with the disappearance of all peripheral stimuli and all demands of organic life. As far as the animal is concerned, the psychological doctrine of sleep of Claparede is quite exact. According to him, sleep constitutes a true "reaction of disinterestedness." The dog that has eaten a full meal, having no interest in any action outside of himself other than the needs of his body, sleeps. It is the same way with a very young child. In the case of the latter one might almost say that sleep is the natural condition, out of which he emerges when he is hungry or when some peripheral stimulus awakens him. But, in proportion as the child's age increases, things are modified. Instead of sleeping eighteen or twenty hours a day, he does not sleep more than fourteen, then twelve, and when he becomes an adult his sleep will be reduced to the smallest amount necessary, which varies, however, according to individuals.

Between the time when sleep was, in a sort of fashion, the natural state of the child, and the time when in adult life sleep is reduced to what is necessary, what has taken place? One of course thinks right away of the lessened organic expenditure of the adult. It is probably true that this phenomenon plays a rôle, and that to a certain degree sleep is proportionate to the organic expenditure. But for certain individuals, and particularly for adults of the same age, this expenditure may be considered as a constant factor; nevertheless, sleep varies according to the individual. Still further, with the same organic life, sleep may vary in a given individual from one day to another. It seems to us, therefore, that this element of organic expenditure must be eliminated. On the other hand, in those animals which from the day of their birth are capable of living by themselves, particularly birds, this difference between the sleep of the new-born and that of the adult is much less marked.

In reality, what seems to us the essential thing that leads to such a variation is the progressive development of mental life.

Sleep henceforth seems to us to be limited by three orders of facts, —namely, the demands of bodily life, peripheral stimuli, and what we might call mental stimuli.

These three factors have a different importance according to different individuals. With the farm laborer, accustomed to hard work, and with scarcely any tendency toward meditation, it would chiefly be the peripheral stimuli which would affect his sleep. He falls asleep at night and wakes with the returning day. With an intellectual man, sleep will be limited by psychological stimuli. The sleep of some individuals will be more particularly affected than others by the demands of their bodies, and they will find it very difficult to fall asleep if their stomachs are not satisfied, and will wake up because they are hungry. But with all, the laborer, the savant, and the epicure, sleep will remain a necessary function, an irresistible need of the body. Whence comes this need of sleep?

When the necessity for sleep appears, two different kinds of facts come into play. On the one hand, habit seems to step in, and arranges it so that at a certain hour, under the usual circumstances of life, after we have passed through the same daily succession of deeds and movements, the idea of sleep comes to us.

Often the need of sleep appears earlier than is habitual, when the day has been fatiguing, or when our daily duty has necessitated great mental tension. Inversely, all causes of mental excitation delay the appearance of the idea of sleep. Emotion, preoccupations, and the cerebral tension of the present moment, not of some past time, inhibit the need of sleep.

Up to what point may this need be inhibited? It is one of the characteristics of man to be able to act upon his functions by his will. This is the very basis of the psychic origin of so many objective disturbances. Man may control his own sleep, and in certain circumstances he may delay it indefinitely. Does not one see people going for weeks, even months, without sleeping while caring for some relative,—a sick father, a mother, or a husband? Their psychic tension and their devotion are sufficient to inhibit sometimes all desire, even all need of sleep.

It happens, however, that, in spite of the person's will, he may be taken with what one would call an imperative desire to sleep, which he is incapable of resisting.

What we conceive as happening to such a person as we have just described, who is nursing another, is that his will at a given moment becomes deficient, and that the instinctive need gets the upper hand. He does not resist it then, any more than the starving or thirsting man could resist the need of taking food or of drinking.

In other cases, after intense physical work, having gone far beyond what one habitually does or is capable of doing, one may be, as it were, overcome by sleep. The work, in order to be finished, has necessitated a considerable expenditure of energy, and the invincible need of sleep marks the limit of possible voluntary tension.

On the other hand, sleep may, to a very large degree, be a matter of education. Just as an individual who has restrained himself from eating may, even though he be the most normally constituted of beings, gradually lose his appetite, in the same way a subject who allows himself only a limited amount of sleep, or goes without sleeping at all, gets to the point where he is no longer able to sleep.

To sum up, the moment at which the need of sleep appears is determined by habit, whether settled or accidental. If the need of sleep appears to correspond to an organic demand, this demand may be retarded by the intervention of the will, by some mental stimulus, or more simply by distraction, which is here only a form of excitement. The need of sleep only becomes imperative when the "psychic tonus" is exhausted.

If we go back to the comparison already made between the succession of waking and sleeping and the succession of contractions and relaxations of a muscle while working, we see that all the terms which rule the one may be applied to the other. In a given subject a definite number of contractions creates the need of rest. The will may prolong the effort, but there comes a moment when it itself fails, and where it becomes a physical necessity to stop work.

With education and training, or on the contrary with a too prolonged muscular rest, the limit of possible work, which on the other hand has personal voluntary energy as well as a factor, will either increase or diminish.

If, now, we take a subject who has yielded to the normal non-imperative need of sleep, how does he pass from his waking state to the state of sleep? This passage is performed in an infinite variety of ways, according to the subject, and in the same individual according to the circumstances. There are some people who fall asleep the moment their heads touch the pillow. There are others, and a very great number, who do not fall asleep without having gone through a certain amount of *mechanical* intellectual work, during the course of which they feel themselves "gradually getting off to sleep." To this group belong the great number of people who cannot go to sleep without reading. A question of habit one will say, but this habit is often legitimate. If, on the one hand, reading induces sleep by letting down the psychic tension, its object on the other hand, is often to dull consciousness progressively in subjects who are habitually excited, and whose psychological automatism is continually introducing new combinations of ideas into the mind. Here we are also on the frontiers of pathology, and the very people who in the ordinary course of life feel the need of coaxing sleep, find it spontaneously when they are away on a vacation in the country, and at rest and free from all preoccupations and cares.

Normal sleep, therefore, is spontaneous sleep, constituting, as Claparède has said, a true reaction of disinterestedness. But it cannot occur without the loss of voluntary or involuntary psychologic consciousness.

Now that our subject has fallen asleep, his sleep will either be deep, slight or heavy, calm or restless. By what will these qualities of sleep be determined? It is evident, after what we have just said, that either painful or simply instinctive demands upon the body and slight or marked peripheral stimuli will have a very decided bearing upon the quality of sleep. But what will also affect it will be the demands made upon consciousness by the psychologic automatism, which preserves its independence in sleep. These demands are the dreams which one does not remember, as well as those which one does remember, and also nightmares. There are also dreams which come to order, which enable certain people to wake up at the time that they have fixed. But it is very certain that, in all this ascending gradation, sleep may be more or less affected by incursions of the psychological automatism into the domains of consciousness, which may be so slight that no traces of them remain in the memory, except the impression that the subject has on waking that his sleep was not as restful as it should have been. The rôle played by these "doings in dreamland" seems to us under certain circumstances to be fraught with great importance.

Now for awakening. This may be sudden or, on the contrary, gradual. It varies according to constitutional or acquired conditions. There are many people who are so made that from their earliest childhood they are never really wide awake and actively conscious until a certain time after waking. There are others in whom the same phenomenon is an acquired habit. These are those who are stimulated by life, and who as the day goes on gradually reach a state of complete physical and intellectual activity. It is cruelly hard for them to wake up, and they have to, as it were, lash themselves to go about, to work, to think, even to make themselves get up. It is really a question of an abnormal symptom. But it exists in a great many people whose lives taken as a whole are perfectly normal, and in this lies the interest of the fact, as we shall see further on.

Such being our conception, not of the intimate nature nor, of course (which goes without saying), of the physiology of sleep, but rather of some of the conditions which control it, we may pass on to the study of the disturbances of sleep which may be seen in the course of the psychoneuroses.

First of all, we must make one reservation. It is self-evident that the act of sleeping presupposes a certain number of organic conditions, and that organic afflictions of various kinds may disturb the sleep of the neurasthenic as it might any other individual who was attacked in the same manner.

A neurasthenic could quite evidently be a neurasthenic and something else besides. He could be arteriosclerotic, a victim of Bright's disease, a cardiac, an asthmatic, etc. He could even be merely strung up or intoxicated, and for that reason have his sleep affected. We would not dream of denying this. But we believe that it is the exception, and that, in the great majority of cases, sleep disturbances presented by this class of patients belong wholly and exclusively to the neuropathic affections from which they are suffering.

Insomnia is the most frequent symptom of which neurasthenics complain. It constitutes in itself an extremely variable phenomenon. Sometimes the insomnia is absolute. Whole nights will pass without a moment's loss of consciousness. Sometimes it is the need of sleep which is lacking. The patients feel themselves to be excited and nervous and cannot fall asleep. At other times the patient has a great desire to sleep. He goes to bed, but cannot really go sound asleep for several hours. One sees patients of this kind going to bed at ten or eleven o'clock at night and falling asleep toward four or five in the morning. Two phenomena may then occur. Sometimes the sleep will be simply out of place, and the patient once he has fallen asleep will rest for a reasonable length of time. Sometimes he will awaken at his regular time, and will thus have considerably reduced his daily allowance of sleep, when there was no necessity, so far as his day was concerned, for him to waken and get up, and when he would have liked to prolong his rest.

There are patients who fall asleep easily, but who awaken in a very short time. There are some who get into the habit of waking in half an hour, an hour, or two hours. Once awake they cannot go to sleep again.

Certain subjects complain of broken sleep. They get to sleep with more or less difficulty, only to waken shortly afterward, and to have trouble in falling asleep again, and waking again, and so on. Under other circumstances patients say that it is the quality of their sleep which is disturbed. This one complains of sleeping too lightly, that one of sleeping too heavily, while another is too restless in his sleep. There are some people who even find that they sleep too much and too soundly!

Perhaps the commonest of these daily observations consists in the statement made by patients that "their sleep is not restful." They wake up as tired as when they went to bed, if not more so.

Briefly put, these are the troubles of which patients complain. As to the pathogeny which they attribute to them and the morbid relations which they establish, they are numerous and most fantastic. Although it goes without saying that sleep may be better or worse, according to the surroundings, the air, the temperature, or according to what one has just been eating, or to the kind of bed, etc., yet one can not imagine how much may be made of these causes and associations by patients. Changing the position of the bed or couch by an angle of a few degrees, a slight modification of temperature, imperceptible barometric or hygrometric variations,—these would be enough to prevent them from sleeping or to make them sleep poorly. The slightest change in their diet or modification in their night clothes or in their bed covering is enough to establish insomnia. We might go on indefinitely with the list of "causes." This enumeration only proves one thing—namely, that insomnia has a moral as well as physical effect upon the patients who suffer from it. It haunts their imaginations, and they have no peace unless they can attribute it to some external cause, which consequently is, according to their idea, modifiable. It is true that the cause is susceptible of modification, but it is mental.

Different mechanisms may come into play. Insomnia may be the result of education. A woman has, we will say, been taking care of her parents or an invalid child for years. The beloved one finally dies, taking with him, as far as our patient is concerned, all interest in life. She feels herself alone in the world and is lost and discouraged. She eats very little, becomes depressed, and grows thin. She feels that in order to regain her strength she is in need of restful sleep, which would at the same time be a sleep of oblivion. But, in spite of all she can do, she keeps for a very long time, sometimes indefinitely, the habits of sleep that she formed during those years.

In the case of indefatigable workers and trained nurses who have ascetically deprived themselves of sleep, the same facts may be observed.

The interesting fact lies less in the acquisition, which is easy to conceive, of a bad habit formed through years, than in the acquisition of this habit, which is sometimes very rapid, under given conditions. We have seen patients of this kind in whom, the rhythm of sleep having been voluntarily modified for only a few weeks, seemed to be almost definitely changed. This was because a new mechanism intervened.

Here, for example, is a man of some forty years, who during six weeks nursed his wife, who died of a severe case of typhoid. During this period he took only two or three hours of rest each night, and always at the same time, between two baths given to the patient at ten at night and two o'clock in the morning. After the death of his wife, for several months he was not able to get to sleep except at the same hours and for the same length of time. It would really seem that the time which he had spent in sitting up at night had been too short to have permitted education or habit to be the cause. One could understand it if after his wife's death he was afflicted with absolute insomnia by the obsession of memory; but he did nothing of the kind, for, as a matter of fact, he would fall asleep at a comparatively early hour and without much difficulty. We think that here we have to do with facts in which the psychological automatism is the cause. Our patient was very much in love with his wife. He nursed her with absolute devotion. He was absorbed in every detail of the care which he gave to her. His mind was continually in a state of tension, so that he should forget none of the treatment which was to be given or of the observations to be made. It is very evident that there was established in his psychological automatism a whole series of strong associations, of which a certain number had to do with the appeal to his consciousness, which wakened him at the end of two or three hours. The thing that seems to us to act in cases of this kind is the recall of consciousness due to functioning of the psychologic automatism. It is a mechanism identical to that which makes a healthy man, in the immense majority of cases, no matter whether his sleep has been sufficient or insufficient, waken every day at the same hour. But, while in a healthy man this mechanism may easily be set aside to allow him a chance to take compensatory rest, it is firmly established in our patient, and this is because all the automatic ideas which had to do with his waking are bound up in the memory of his wife, and in ideas connected with her, and that he thinks continually all day long of the loss which has come to him.

Here it is a question merely of a habit which is in some respects organic, of the quantitative diminution of the need of sleep; it is, if one might so call it, a psychological habit which is at the bottom of it, and which the thoughts and memories of daily life only tend to reinforce.

Outside of cases where the patients sleep less because they have formed a habit of needing less sleep, it is the intervention of the psychological automatism which seems to us to play an important rôle in the early wakening, the broken sleep, or the restless sleep of which so many neurasthenics complain. These, for reasons that we shall have to analyze further on, while they may at the same time suffer from depression from the point of view of consciousness are nearly always excited from the point of view of the subconscious automatism. Ideas penetrate consciousness involuntarily with the greatest facility. It is the same mechanism of certain slight obsessions which one may discover in them, and what goes on during their waking hours continues to occur while they are sleeping; hence the broken sleep, the numerous dreams, and the restlessness.

In certain people, who have been accidentally awakened once by phenomena of the same kind, the fear of being awakened again which they have been nursing all day, is enough to furnish the cause and the explanation of the tendency to wake.

This is a fact which occurs very often among those who have sleep phobias. They do not sleep because they are afraid that they will not sleep. But what we find most often in these cases is the difficulty that the patients have in getting to sleep. And if they cannot get to sleep it is because in their case and from the fact that their thoughts are continually focussed on the idea of wanting to go to sleep, that the impossibility of succeeding in losing their voluntary consciousness which, as we have seen, constitutes an essential condition of sleep, occurs.

Here are two examples:

Mr. X., fifty-two years of age, a musician of parts, when we saw him for the first time had passed fifty-six nights without sleeping. All hypnotic medications—morphine, opium, chloral, bromides, etc.—had been given without producing anything more than a passing drowsiness. He had been looked upon as a toxic case or one of hypertension, and treatment and medicines had been ordered with this in view.

The starting-point of this prolonged insomnia went back to some disturbance of sleep caused by very strong emotions. But when we saw the patient these emotions were no longer a causative agent, and it was only the persistence of his insomnia that disturbed him. The day after our first interview with this patient, we received a card from him on which he had written, "A miracle, doctor: I have slept a little."

He was modest in his appreciation, for upon inquiry we learned that he had slept soundly and well for ten consecutive hours, without waking once.

Now, what had we done? We had ordered nothing, and we had been content to suppress four things,—namely, his medicines, his treatment, his electricity, and—his sister.

What happened in fact in his case was extremely simple. When he had had his accidental insomnia, our subject was in the act of "composing." It goes without saying that his sleep disturbances naturally affected his power of creation. He had been very much concerned by this and was extremely upset. His sister, who lived with him, had shared his uneasiness. Our patient, from that time on, always went to bed with the same idea, "Am I going to go to sleep?" He would go to bed, read a few minutes, put out his electric light, and wait. Naturally sleep could not come so quickly. At the end of a scant quarter of an hour, he would turn on the electricity, read again, and turn it out again, and would repeat this performance all through the night. Meanwhile his sister, who occupied the adjoining room, hearing him move, would come every once in a while to open his door, and ask, "Joseph, aren't you asleep?" and then would condole with him on receiving the inevitably negative reply. Once removed from his sister and deprived of all means of lighting his room, and also, let us add, reassured concerning the mechanism of his insomnia, this patient was able to get back the sleep which he believed lost to him, in the manner we have described.

Another patient whom we have seen complained of insomnia which was nevertheless very irregular. He had established a very curious series of systematizations. His sleep at night, he said, depended on impressions of the day. He could tell in the morning whether or not he would sleep the next night. In this way, when he went to bed he had a conviction of his inability to sleep, or the possibility of its coming, which determined his condition for the night. When he was sure that he would not sleep, he would walk up and down his room, read and think about things, and would thus get through the night without too much discomfort. When, on the contrary, he knew that he was going to sleep, he would tranquilly go to bed, and would fall asleep comfortably. Otherwise his health was excellent, and he was in perfectly good humor. He was a good liver and practised no privations, and, when the chance presented itself, he thought nothing of taking a good long sleep in the daytime to make up for his loss.

One thus sees that in cases of this kind conscious preoccupation may come in to disturb sleep. If in this instance the preoccupation was of the kind that concerned sleep itself, under other circumstances it would be all the emotions and obsessive thoughts which would arise, and which as soon as the patient was in a more or less voluntary state of consciousness would hinder sleep from coming. Here we have the chief reasons for insomnia in neurasthenics. Either the emotional cause itself which has engendered their neurasthenia persists, or else it is the idea of their condition which haunts them.

Thus, in patients suffering from insomnia the return of sleep is one of the chief signs of improvement, not so much because his recovered sleep permits the patient to improve, but because its return proves that the patient is less preoccupied and less uneasy about his health, or, in a word, that his moral state is better.

To sum up, outside of the phenomena of habit which are apt to be to some degree superadded, the neurasthenic does not sleep because he has lost the faculty of being able to either voluntarily or involuntarily stop thinking. He does not sleep because he thinks, and, if his thought is often involuntary on account of appeals made to his consciousness by a psychologic automatism which is no longer under restraint, his thought also is often voluntary because the pessimistic moral condition of these patients makes them abnormally interested in all their depressing preoccupations.

The act of waking in these neurasthenics may be the origin of all sorts of disturbances. The impression which they get at that time may fix their mentality all through the day, and thus play a rôle in the persistence of the appearance of many secondary troubles. We are not at all sure but that the fatiguability of certain patients may not be due in part to the impression of fatigue which they feel on waking.

This fatigue on waking may, in some cases, be legitimate. When, under the influences which we have tried to bring out, the patient's sleep has been poor, broken, or restless, it is not astonishing that our subject should feel when he wakes that he had not had sufficient rest. But there are neurasthenics who sleep well, and who nevertheless experience the classic feeling that they are more tired in the morning than at night, and who henceforth will pass their whole day under this impression, which is peculiarly inhibitive to every kind of effort. Now, generally, if one questions these patients about the periods of their life before they developed this neurasthenic condition, they will tell you that this sensation is one which they have felt always or at any rate for a very long time before they became avowed neurasthenics. We have already said that this was in fact nothing but an affectation, which was sometimes constitutional and often acquired, by people who had fallen into the habit of doing so little that their chief interest in life resolved itself into thinking of themselves. It is very certain that the conditions which bring about this state of being—preoccupation, care, emotions, obsessions of overwork which force patients to take up their life, get hold of themselves, and to be in a state of continual excitement in order to preserve their existence along its normal lines—are the very conditions which frequently bring on the neurasthenic state. There is nothing astonishing, therefore, in the fact that such a phenomenon—either for constitutional reasons, or for accidental reasons, or depending on the manner of living—should be found almost constantly in neurasthenics. But, outside of legitimate fatigue, in connection with insufficient sleep, the thing that becomes abnormal in these patients is the conservation of the impression. Formerly they did not even take it into consideration, they would go on just the same, and they could do their daily work just as well or better than others. Now, however, their minds have become fixed on this impression of fatigue, they are obsessed concerning it, and can make it a factor of every succeeding stage of the day.

It is in this way that the neurasthenic's fatigue on awaking resolves itself into two kinds,—namely, true fatigue caused by disturbed sleep for psychological reasons, on the one hand, and, on the other hand, the fixation of the patient's ideas on impressions which have existed for a long time.

Disturbances of sleep as hysterical manifestations are no less numerous. Insomnia may exist among hysterics as among all neurasthenics, but its mechanism is generally quite different. Without his being able to bring into play the rôle of education or of habit, the hysteric loses his idea of sleep for a time, which, however, is generally quite brief. He does not feel the need of it, he does not pursue the sleep which evades him. He simply does not try to sleep. He is in a condition of continued wakefulness. Sometimes his insomnia, we must not fail to add, is purely subjective, and he pretends not to sleep, and, when we inquire a little more particularly, we find that in reality he is not sleepless. Is this a question of simulation? It does not seem so to us. It is simply an erroneous conviction.

On the other hand, when it comes to not sleeping in the cases of neurasthenics or hysterics, or even accidental insomnias in healthy people, the hours when they do not sleep, when every one else is sleeping around them, always seem peculiarly long. The human mind is only conscious of time through association of ideas. In the domain of pure subjectivity the idea of time is quite uncertain, and is only measured by the number of impressions experienced or the successive states of consciousness which are registered. Therefore, during hours of sleeplessness, in the absence of all external interests and the absence of all voluntary choice of ideas, the domain of consciousness is confused with that of the psychologic automatism which is on much greater tension than usual. Thus, without order and without cohesion, following the type of automatic psychological associations, ideas come rushing in and out of the mind during the hours of insomnia. It seems as if one had lived through whole days when only a few minutes have gone by.

The physician will therefore always do well to be on his guard, for the patient who pretends that he "has not closed his eyes" has often slept soundly all night. This is true for a normal man; it is also true for the neurasthenic, and even more apt to be the case with the hysteric, by reason of his great involuntary tendency to exaggerate everything.

The hysteric may manifest other disturbances in connection with sleep than those which bear upon insomnia. Narcolepsy consists of sleep attacks which come on suddenly and wholly out of season, and only last for a short time, perhaps from ten minutes to half an hour. The frequency with which they occur may vary from several times a day to once a month. The waking from these is apt to be slow and more or less difficult. Nothing differentiates the narcoleptic condition from the condition of sleep. Its pathogeny is very difficult to understand. The most characteristic thing in this state is the sudden loss of consciousness,—its paralysis, as it were. The function of consciousness is suddenly arrested, just as the motor function is abruptly inhibited in the production of an hysterical paralysis. Without insisting too strongly upon this, we think it very possible that the phenomena may result from identically the same mechanism, and that inhibition of consciousness in the hysteric may be brought about in the same way as motor inhibition.

Lethargy is another hysterical manifestation affecting the function of sleep. Sometimes suddenly, and sometimes after a premonitory aura, a person is abruptly overcome by sleep. Once fallen asleep the patient's face may be pale or retain its color, the muscles, particularly the masseters, are contracted, the eyes are fixed, and disclosed by the eyelids which flutter rapidly. Respiration is calm, superficial, sometimes slower, sometimes more rapid, and sometimes panting, or, as in a case of Achard's, of the Cheyne-Stokes type. The pulse is regular. The temperature remains about normal. There may be present generalized psychosensory anæsthesia; nevertheless, and this is the important thing, there is no loss of perception. There are subjects who in a lethargic state are conscious of everything that goes on around them.

Certain of these sleeping attacks are sudden and short, pseudo-syncopal. Others are prolonged for weeks and months. There are cases where lethargic sleep has lasted for years. Generally they are brought to an end by a convulsive attack or by passing over into some other hysterical symptom.

These conditions—which, moreover, are very closely allied to hysterical crises—are of very great theoretical importance, for, as a matter of fact, the majority of instances which have been found of people who were buried alive must be attributed to lethargy. Now, the most ardent partisans of the purely suggestive nature of hysteria would undoubtedly find that it is going a little too far to admit that a subject would push suggestion so far as consciously to allow himself to be buried. One might offer as an explanation the possibility of errors in retrospective diagnosis. One will say that the real hysterics have always managed to arrange it so as to wake up in time. Nevertheless, there are some who have pushed the joke pretty far, even up to the point of interment. Among those who have wakened in time, there are some who were in their coffins and already under the earth.

However this may be, the psychopathology of these conditions is variable. Sometimes it is no more than a prolonged narcolepsy, with absolute loss of voluntary or involuntary consciousness. Sometimes it is voluntary consciousness only that is inhibited. The psychological automatism remains intact and introduces passively in the field of consciousness a great number of images, of which the subject is aware as in a dream. Voluntary reaction alone then is absolutely wanting.

If such facts are interesting because they permit us in a certain degree to make landmarks of successive psychological functions, they are still more important from the same point of view not as disturbances, but as the peculiar conditions which hysterics may present in the course of sleep. Hypnotic sleep and somnambulism, which is quite closely allied to it, are not, properly speaking, pathological phenomena; they are peculiar psychological conditions.

B. Headache.—Headache is a symptom so often observed in the course of the psychoneuroses that it deserves to be studied alone.

It is met with so frequently in neurasthenic states that, according to Charcot, it formed one of the primary symptoms. Nevertheless, the very peculiar headache which Charcot described under the name of "helmet headache," consisting of a feeling of pressure localized principally at the back of the head and the nape of the neck, does not by any means seem to us to be the only form under which the symptom is manifested.

Patients who are "well read" are very apt to use the term "helmet" to describe their pain. Others, and even a great number of those who are well informed concerning their malady, use particular epithets to describe their headache and its very variable localizations. A band around the forehead, sensations of emptiness, throbbings of pain which every movement exaggerates, feelings of heaviness, an undefined torture which they cannot exactly localize, are the symptoms of which our subjects have most often complained.

They say to us, "It seems to me as if I had a weight of several hundred pounds upon my head," "I feel as though my head were held in a vice," "My brains actually beat in my head," etc. Other patients complain of sudden sensations of heat; they feel as though their "head were on fire." Others complain of sharp or shooting pains.

But what we have met most frequently is perhaps less a real pain than a distressing sensation of discomfort, or emptiness, or sometimes, on the other hand, a tension or the feeling that one's mind would not work, sometimes accompanied and sometimes not by feelings of dizziness. Many patients compare these sensations to those which they have had normally after having pushed some intellectual work, and very naturally they attribute what they feel to symptoms of exhaustion.

What interpretation could one give to these various forms of headache? It seems to us that this manifestation has extremely diverse origins. First of all, there appears to be no doubt that in a large number of cases the headache may be a purely subjective symptom. It is a form of localized pain. Patients who are struck by their lack of brain activity or the difficulty they have in working are apt to refer the impressions they feel to the periphery. Their headache is only a subjective excuse for the deficiencies of which they complain.

Under other circumstances, the headache is subjectively encouraged, and continued, so to speak. It has really existed, but in a transitory fashion. Afterward it persists as a state of memory which is more or less continually evoked. The patient's pain is really only a reminiscence.

Sometimes the headache is explained by the extreme malnutrition of the patient; it then belongs to the same mechanisms as those by which we explained the headaches of anæmics and certain convalescents.

Finally, and this probably rather frequently occurs, the headache may be the expression of a real cerebral exhaustion. As a matter of fact, although the intellectual work of the neurasthenic may have no objective realization, the pain may be none the less real for that, and the constant absorption with preoccupation, obsessions, and emotional conditions and being always exploring one's mental recesses is at least as fatiguing as the most abstruse geometrical problems or the most subtle metaphysical meditations. It is from this mechanism in particular that there seems to us to proceed those diffused feelings of headache with vague feelings in the head from which so many people suffer. One does not have to push the analysis very far to find out that these are people who are preoccupied and obsessed, and whose preoccupations and obsessions allow them very little rest.

Insomnia may also play its part, and help to determine what is described to us as that sort of continual feeling of soreness of the head or scalp which is the despair of so many patients.

A transference to the periphery of a sense of intellectual weakness, a reminiscence which is obsessive or caused by real fatigue—these are in fact the various mechanisms which seem to us able to interpret all kinds of headaches in neurasthenics.

In hysterics one may meet with nearly all the symptoms which we have just described. But in these last patients the rôle of auto-suggestion or of hetero-suggestion is predominant, above all when their troubles are associated with phenomena of contracture or paralysis.

These are often patients in whom one has tried to discover a possible organic origin of their symptoms, and who have become gradually convinced of the existence of the headache which has been previously sought for. The hysterical *nail*, which consists of an extremely sharp pain in a very limited area on top of the head, has often no other origin.

In fact, in these patients painful subjective disturbances are frequently accompanied by localized or diffuse hyperæsthesia of the scalp.

C. Disturbances of the Reflexes.—These troubles, which are of very slight importance from the clinical point of view, involve, on the other hand, from the theoretical point of view, a whole series of important questions. We are far from solving the problems which are offered by the modifications of the reflexes, and we by no means pretend that we can offer here any definite interpretation of the facts which clinical observation has enabled us to establish.

We shall take up successively the tendon and skin reflexes in the course of neurasthenic and hysteric conditions.

The tendon reflexes in neurasthenic conditions are very frequently modified. The knee-jerk may be found perhaps somewhat exaggerated or somewhat diminished in such patients. But exaggeration is a phenomenon much more frequently observed.

We feel it necessary to point out a certain number of distinctions. It may happen that one has to do with patients who are extremely run down and emaciated, in whom the reflexes act as they do in all conditions of grave denutrition. One knows that in these conditions there is sometimes exaggeration and sometimes diminution of the reflexes, and that this is the first mechanism of change in the reflexes during the course of neurasthenia.

On the other hand, we know that the reflexes vary according to individuals. Cases have been shown where there is congenital absence or at least diminution of the knee-jerk. We even know subjects who in their normal state have very strong reflexes. In the absence of any idea concerning the previous condition of the reflexes, it becomes very difficult to say whether the exaggeration or diminution which one has discovered has or has not anything to do with the actual symptomatic expression.

Under other circumstances we may find ourselves in the presence of morbid associations. A subject may be tuberculous, or diabetic, and also neurasthenic, and under these conditions the disturbances of the reflexes may be attributed to the associated disease rather than to the psychoneurosis itself.

Finally, there does not seem to us to be any question that the exaggeration of reflexes in particular may be in a great many cases considered as a symptom peculiar to the neurasthenic condition. But how shall we interpret this phenomenon?

First of all, clinical observation has shown us that these exaggerations of the reflexes are found particularly marked in all the cases in which the patients are in an extremely emotional state. By repeated examinations we have even assured ourselves that this exaggeration would to some degree vary with the emotional condition itself, more particularly when our subjects would say of themselves that they felt "more nervous," and less markedly so when, on the contrary, from the mental or moral point of view, they felt themselves calm and tranquil. So much so that from the start one can be sure that these changes in the reflexes have no relation to any organic disturbance or any modification of nutrition.

The interpretation which it seems to us should be adopted is as follows: The various functions which devolve upon the cerebro-spinal axis cannot be isolated from the anatomical point of view any more than from the physiological. There is reciprocal action of the phenomena of the automatic life on those of the conscious life, and *vice versa*. In the same way that a given idea is able to provoke vasomotor and secretory actions, etc., so a given mental condition is capable of modifying a whole set of reflex phenomena. Concentration of consciousness (obsessions) or diffusion of consciousness (emotions) may in this way act upon and disturb the inhibition or the tonus which the different stages of nervous functions receive one from the other. Such is the hypothetical explanation which an examination of the facts suggests.

Among hysterics, excluding accidents, one may see various conditions of the reflexes. But the interesting problem is raised by modifications which the reflexes may undergo in the course of hysterical symptoms, and particularly in the case of paralyses. One may note in hysterical paralyses a more or less considerable exaggeration of the tendon reflexes. May this exaggeration of reflectivity go so far as to produce, as in organic paralyses, ankle-clonus? As a matter of fact, one of us has been able to observe, without any organic association and without the slightest possibility of any simulation, actual cases where this phenomenon was produced in hysterics; but it is something which happens very rarely. Hysteria, either directly or indirectly, would thus be capable of setting the medullary automatism at liberty.

Cutaneous reflexes may also be modified in the course of a psychoneurosis.

Ordinarily, in neurasthenia the modifications that these reflexes undergo are very slight, and depend upon the condition of general reflectivity. When the tendon reflexes are strong, it is rare that the cutaneous reflexes are not also accentuated, and, inversely, any diminution is apt to be found in the tendon reflexes as well as in the skin or mucous-membrane reflexes.

Nevertheless, there is no absolute law, and it has seemed to us that in the zone of localization of their functional manifestations neurasthenics may present remarkable exaggerations of the cutaneous reflexes. Peculiar irritability of the abdominal wall in gastro-intestinal fixations, exaggeration of the pharyngeal reflex, fixations in the regions of the upper digestive tracts—such facts we have been able to demonstrate on several trials.

In hysteria, in the course of paralyses or hemianæsthesiæ we have been able to establish unquestionably disappearance of the cremasteric reflex in a certain number of cases. As for the plantar cutaneous reflex, we have never found dorsal extension of the great toe (Babinski's sign). On the contrary, we believe that the cutaneous plantar reflex, as well as the tension of the fascia lata, may perhaps be absent in these patients on the hemianæsthetic side. One of us has observed three examples in his service during the last year. In these three patients, afflicted with absolute hemianæsthesia, two women and a man, the sole of the foot did not respond to any stimulus whatever, and the reflex of the fascia lata was likewise lacking. On the well side the reaction of the toes and the fascia lata was normal. Two of these patients were cured of their hemianæsthesia, and then recovered their plantar and fascia-lata reflexes.

We shall not dwell any longer upon this question of reflexes. The only theoretical point which really matters to us is to know that purely psychic influences are capable, to a considerable extent, of bringing about modifications in phenomena which are habitually regarded as purely automatic.

This, however, is not at all astonishing, if one considers the evident existence, as functional manifestations of psychoneuroses, of disturbances which, like spasms and contractures, are really only reflexes which have become permanent, persistent, or stereotyped in some way.

D. Disturbances of Speech.—One may sometimes find in the hysteric a symptomatic *ensemble* which more or less approaches motor aphasia. But writing is, as a rule, wholly unaffected. When it is a question of agraphia, which rarely occurs, it is total, and exists for all kinds of writing.

On the other hand, a very few cases of sensory aphasia and of pure verbal deafness have been noted in hysterics.

A thing which is much more frequent in the hysteric is mutism. Mutism strikes hysterics at every age; nevertheless, it is rare after forty. It may come on after an emotional attack, and take place suddenly, or, on the other hand, progressively, preceded by stuttering, then by the impossibility of speaking aloud (whispering), before it becomes confirmed. Once established, it makes the patient absolutely dumb, incapable, in spite of the integrity of his phonetic muscle, to utter the slightest sound or even a cry. It is really a purely motor disturbance related to all the psychological functions. In some cases mutism is not absolute: the patient may make a few sounds but cannot utter them in a loud voice.

When once established, hysterical mutism lasts sometimes for hours and sometimes for years.

It is very evident that of all hysterical manifestations mutism is perhaps the one which most easily permits simulation. It is none the less true, however, that we know a certain number of cases where the possibility of this could not for a moment be considered. One of us has seen a case like this, a teacher who was extremely devoted to her pupils and in love with her profession, who was suddenly struck mute as the result of a violent emotion. This patient was a woman of upright character, and, in spite of her very strong desire, had been mute for four years when she came into our wards. She was only cured after several months, and then by exciting a very strong emotion in her.

It does not seem to us that such cases should be any more difficult to grasp than many other functional manifestations. Does not everybody know that emotion will "make the voice break" and render one incapable of uttering a sound? The hysteric, as we have already seen, fixes himself in his emotional symptoms. These become crystallized in him, as it were. When in phenomena of this kind suggestion comes in as a secondary element, the thing is very possible. Persuaded of his inability, the patient may continue his auto-suggestions, and the symptom will last as long as the suggestive action persists, and will only give way to some new emotional influence or an opposite suggestion. But the emotion will, nevertheless, be always the main agent. When it comes to a question of a disturbance of speech, the patients who have lost their voice by reason of an emotional crisis very probably do not know how to recover it, because their hopelessness hinders them from making any effort in this direction.

This was particularly so in the case of the teacher of whom we have just spoken, who, every time that one tried to persuade her that she could speak, would reply in writing that she was convinced that she would never be able to speak again.

Among neurasthenics one sees other disturbances of speech, which the patients express by saying, "I can no longer find the words I want to use," "I can hardly understand what people say to me." "I do not understand what I read." In reality these disturbances correspond to two kinds of phenomena. There is, on the one hand, a purely ideational disturbance, which we shall take up again when we study the affections of psychological functions; and there are, on the other hand, phobic manifestations, which we shall consider with all the disturbances of this kind which affect the nervous system.

E. Acquired Disturbances of Psychological Functions.—The disturbances of psychological functions which one may come across in the course of the psychoneuroses are extremely varied.

We may, from the start, divide them into antecedent disturbances and consecutive disturbances. We place under the term antecedent disturbances those which, whether constitutional or acquired, were present before the development of the psychoneurosis with its symptoms. We shall take up their study in the second part of this work. The consecutive disturbances, which are the only kind we shall consider here, are developed secondarily, and give rise to a whole series of manifestations which did not form an integral part of the previous mentality of these patients.

Such a distinction may appear subtle. It is, however, a very important one. Neurasthenics may in fact accidentally present a whole series of psychic troubles which one would find constitutionally established in certain subjects belonging to a family whose mentality was different. We are alluding to the psychasthenics of Janet in particular.

Can one say that acquired psychological troubles exist in the hysteric? If in their case some psychic medium may have been accidentally inhibited,—such, for example, as the various forms of language, as is the case, as we shall see further on,—then the mental disturbances in these patients are essentially constitutional. Therefore, they would not be described here.

The same thing is not at all true of the neurasthenic. In his case, in proportion as his affection develops there appears a whole series of secondary disturbances, holding a capital place in the subjective and objective symptomatology of these patients.

The immense majority of neurasthenics complain of not being able to fix their attention on any intellectual work whatsoever, no matter how hard they try. All work, they say, at the end of a certain time, which varies according to the individual nature and on different days, fatigues them. As a rule, it will be their necessary occupations which will fatigue them the most and the quickest. More or less rapidly, they will find themselves obliged to give up either the daily routine by which they live or the intellectual work which interests them.

Is it a question here of what might be called an organic intellectual deficiency, tending to some particular form of fatigue, or an exhaustion which takes place more rapidly than what might be called the psychic contraction? Not at all, and more often it is the patient himself who furnishes you the proof of this. If certain subjects are sufficiently logical to attribute their rapid fatiguability to all kinds of attention, there are certain others who forget themselves. One sees patients who declare themselves to be exhausted at the end of a few minutes' attentive work, and who devote hours to the solution of problems in chess or geometry. But, above all, the time when logic is wholly lost from sight is when the patient finds himself with his physician. With him, the very individual who has just said that he was incapable of any intellectual effort will be able to bear up through discussions which last for hours, exhausting the doctor, but from which the patient sallies forth fresh and cheerful, provided he has found some consolation.

This intellectual incapacity may be interpreted objectively and subjectively. Sometimes the patient is able to fix his attention only for a short time, a time during which intellectual activity is normal. It is not then a question of rapid fatigue. Under other circumstances it seems that the elementary psychological functions may be the ones which are troubled. The patient is quite capable of fixing his attention for a time, often fairly long, but the work that he would have accomplished formerly in a few minutes will take him hours. Simple operations, mental calculations, will seem very difficult to him. Nearly always, however, not to say always, the work or the calculation will be right. That is to say, in other words, the elementary psychological phenomena remain qualitatively unharmed, and what is affected is the faculty of association.

Other patients complain of distractions, involuntary flights of mind. "They are not there," they say, but when they are "there," the work is accomplished in a normal manner both as to quality and quantity. Others again say that their memory is affected, particularly for what concerns recent events. "I am obliged to make a note of everything," they say, "because if I did not I never would remember anything."

Certain others do not complain of their memory, properly speaking. They can remember things, but their power of recall is slower than usual; whence arises a series of secondary disturbances in the imagination and in ideation.

There are subjects who, on the other hand, suffer from recall, from memories too numerous and diffuse which present themselves to consciousness. Ideation is affected because in the multitude of phenomena of consciousness the patient can no longer choose; he therefore becomes a sort of psychological automaton; he sees, he says, "as if he were in a dream," and he feels incapable in various degrees of any cerebral control, or of forming any judgment. All the phenomena of life appear to him as on the same plane. He is like a person in the theatre who cannot distinguish between the actors and the "supers." He has in some way lost his sense of proportion. He will magnify some trifling detail to such a degree that the important facts lose their relief. Thus, one will often see a patient whom an insignificant thing will preoccupy just as much as an important thing. It would not be exact to say that he wholly neglects the latter. It often only appears to be so on account of the relation between the mentality of the observer and the real mentality of the patient. The physician, conscious of his own mentality, sees this lack of proportion, and is inclined to accuse the patient of taking no interest in the most important things of his life. This is not exactly true. He does not lack interest, but, rather, he is interested in too many things, a number of which are futile.

These reactions of failing interest may occur at any time, but it is when any new psychological phenomenon has appeared that it is necessary to know whether any systematization has taken possession of the patient.

These systematizations are phobias and obsessions. It would be a mistake to believe that manifestations of this kind do not belong to neurasthenia, and, on this account, to classify such patients in another pathological group, as psychasthenics. We should be tempted, on the other hand, to say that it is a characteristic of the neurasthenic to have obsessions and to be liable to them. This is easy to conceive; for is an obsession anything else than an involuntary and irresistible apparition in the field of consciousness, phenomena of psychological automatism? Any individual who is not "master of himself" is practically phobic or obsessed. The neurasthenic, having no longer his cerebral control,—that is, his judgment,—has accidentally lost the mastery over himself, which the psychasthenic has never had except in the most relative degree.

Still further, while the psychasthenic recognizes his obsessions, and while he is vainly trying to drive them away, the neurasthenic is complacent about them. Here we enter into phenomena of another kind. It is here that along with obsessions are found what are called preoccupations, having a very different psychological mechanism. These are, if you will, voluntary obsessions, depending directly on the moral condition of the patients. In neurasthenics pessimism is evidently at the bottom of this condition. They also entertain voluntarily all the depressing ideas, all the hypochondriac preoccupations that the psychological automatism may have introduced into the field of their consciousness either as an incident or as an obsession. Here we must take into consideration the fact that the passing moral condition either inhibits or excites—it comes to the same thing—psychological automatism. If we are gay or sad, our automatism will not introduce into our field of consciousness—or our field of consciousness will not permit the entrance of—any ideas but those which are gay or sad. More or less influenced by his condition and more or less weak, the neurasthenic will, therefore, have hardly any but pessimistic ideas, which will crystallize in some way into a state of preoccupation or obsession.

An example will help to make our thought clear: We see a firearm, a revolver or a rifle, or perhaps a sword or a knife. Among the many ideas which might be associated with these things there are some which are pessimistic, like those of suicide or the possibility of a criminal action. A healthy person will pay no attention to these ideas. A neurasthenic, on the other hand, by reason of his moral condition, will lay hold of the idea and cling to it. He will think that he might be "tempted" to commit suicide, that he might "conceive the idea" of injuring some one. This idea disturbs him, and remains persistently in his mind. He will think of it for a long time. He is henceforth caught in a vicious circle. In fact, the more he thinks about it the more there will be registered in his psychological automatism many vivid impressions, which, as a result, will have all the greater opportunity of running through his field of consciousness again and again, and all the more so because at the same time, by the simple fact of circumstances, associations of ideas, which are capable of recalling them are multiplying qualitatively, so to speak. Thus, step by step, the neurasthenic, who has at first been merely preoccupied, becomes finally, by the very reason of this common intellectual mechanism, the subject of obsessions. A voluntary obsession, if one might so call it, directly creates an involuntary obsession, or a true obsession. But the latter, and this is the important point of diagnosis, is secondary.

We shall not dwell upon this just now, but we have already seen that this is the key-stone to the whole construction of visceral symptoms in neurasthenics.

However it may be, when the neurasthenic has gotten an obsession it goes without saying that his mental incapacities are multiplied and aggravated, because by one road or another he can always return to his obsession. Obsessions may take a variety of forms, but it is especially hypochondriacal obsessions which are met in these patients. The phobia of suicide, the phobia of harming some one else, and other such scrupulous obsessions are also found, but much less frequently.

As to the mechanism which produces the mental disturbances on which these accidents are grafted, it depends altogether upon the emotional state in which the neurasthenic is indulging, or in which he finds himself. We shall take up this question further along. But it is evident that the succession of emotions, intellectual disturbances, preoccupations, and obsessions which we have established do not appear in regular succession, so that one would be able to say that there were three corresponding neurasthenic periods developing as time goes on.

In reality, and almost from the start, the phenomena are complex. On examining patients, one finds that obsessions or preoccupations and intellectual disturbances are, as a matter of fact, reciprocally conditioned one by the other. At this period, if one did not take into consideration the way in which the symptoms started, it would seem as if all intellectual disturbances were directly caused by preoccupations or obsessions.

In fact, if in those patients who complain of intellectual disturbances of every kind one pushes the analysis a little further, one will readily perceive that all these disturbances, or at least the majority of them, are due to diffusion of the attention toward the obsessions or preoccupations.

Of a patient who complains of tiring rapidly during any intellectual work, of being distracted, or of finding it impossible to fix his attention, ask, "What do you think about when you are working?" He will invariably reply, "I think of my illness, or of such and such a vicissitude that it has brought about," and, if your patient reads without understanding what he reads, if he lingers a long time over some work which does not advance, if he experiences difficulties in formulating his ideas, it is not because he is incapable of working or of thinking, but it is because he is thinking of something else, something which is particularly dear to him, that is his ill health.

There are some patients who manage to get hold of themselves, but, in order to become absorbed in their occupation, they are obliged to do double work,—the labor of fixing their attention upon the undertaking in hand, and the labor of struggling against distraction caused by the obsession or the preoccupation which is always flooding their conscious mentality. They thus plunge into heroic struggles which cannot help but produce fatigue which this time is real. Here again is one of these troubles belonging to the mechanism of disharmony, like so many others which we have already met.

Under other circumstances, and among those whom we have already described as "neurasthenics who have arrived," the intellectual fatigue is real, and in direct proportion to the emaciation and weakness of the subject, who may at the same time be physically as well as morally depressed. In these patients a very curious phenomenon sometimes occurs which resembles a periodic psychosis. It is not at all rare, among such subjects, to find that for short periods of time intellectual work becomes almost too easy for them. This is because a new element has come into play,—namely, the psychic excitement which may be met with in all conditions of psychic depression. This is a phenomenon of organic nature, but secondary. It is of great practical interest to recognize it, because, if the patient makes use of his excitement and profits by it to do any rather arduous work, he becomes rapidly exhausted for often a considerable time.

All these psychological troubles are apt to be followed by rather peculiar sensations, due to the fact that, under the influence of the very considerable—though wholly abnormal—development of their inner life, these patients lose, so to speak, contact with the outer world, and, their consciousness being incumbered by former incidents and every kind of preoccupation, they get to the point where sensory stimuli produce nothing but diffused or remote images: they listen without hearing; they look without seeing. In a word, they are "somewhere else." When by chance, or because it is keener than usual, a sensory stimulus mounts into conscious perception, it surprises the patient. It wakes him up, so to speak, but before he completely resumes his relations with the external world more or less time has been lost. With the patient who is absorbed in his reflections all communications with the outer world have been, as it were, cut off. The stimulus which he has perceived has reëstablished one of them, but it takes a moment's time before he can make connection with all the others, and these are the subjective impressions felt during this period of getting hold of one's self which patients express by saying that they have what they describe as "empty brains," or again when they complain of sensations of dizziness.

In a normal condition all our functions of relation and balance in our environment are assured by sensory stimuli which are more or less consciously perceived, so that the outer world is continually projected upon our minds. The neurasthenic finds himself in exactly the situation of a healthy individual who is suddenly wakened from a sound sleep. The latter, before coming to himself and being aware of exactly what has happened to him, and of his surroundings, will, in the same way, lose a moment's time, in the course of which he will force himself to connect his actual impressions with the previous sensations whose continuity sleep has interrupted. He will feel exactly as the neurasthenic does, that his "brain is empty." He will be under the impression that he cannot walk straight. As a matter of fact, he may even start off in the wrong direction, stumble over obstacles, etc.

Such, then, is the origin of these sensations of emptiness in the brain, and impressions of dizziness, which make such an unfortunate impression upon patients, who may manufacture from them a whole series of secondary phenomena, such as we shall see in a moment. In reality the sensations of cerebral emptiness, expressing in the psychic domain the same facts as vertigoes in the physical domain, may be included in one and the same definition: they are phenomena of awakening and of regaining consciousness of the external world.

The disturbances of will and character which we meet in neurasthenics seem to us to be directly dependent upon their mental state.

According to writers on the subject, it would seem as though abulia constituted a most important psychological symptom of neurasthenia. This is a great error, coupled with profound injustice. When they bring such a judgment to bear upon the patients, they confuse two essentially different things. The will does not act in a void or in space; and there are, as a matter of fact, two kinds of will,—the will of itself, a psychological faculty which supposes in the patient the disposition of a quantity of given energy, and the practical will which consists in making this energy move along certain definite paths. The neurasthenic very often possesses a storehouse of energy which he, moreover, expends, but expends unwisely and unprofitably, without any practical result. He makes a brave struggle, but for nothing. His will is there, but it has nothing to rest on; what it accomplishes is of no value.

In other words, he always is in possession of this instrument, but he does not know how to use it, because, in the very nature of things, on account of the intellectual and moral difficulties in which he finds himself, his activity—the practical expression of use of the will—becomes unequal to his demands. We say of a healthy man that he has a "strong will" when we see him using any considerable amount of energy in attaining some determined end, and when he concentrates all his activity along the line which he has laid out for himself. There can be no will where there is no rational systematization. It is this rational systematization of which the neurasthenic is incapable because he has lost the sense of proportion.

Then other elements come in, which, however, are secondary and acquired. The neurasthenic may preserve what is virtually a will, which he no longer uses, because previous experiences or his weak moral condition have impressed him with his sense of helplessness. He has reached the point where he does not make any effort, because he is certain beforehand that no result can be obtained. Now, as far as the practical will is concerned in its application to external things, one can very well see that preoccupations and obsessions which lead to a life of self-absorption may peculiarly inhibit it. One really cannot be too self-absorbed and at the same time pay proper attention to external things. The neurasthenic lives wholly in himself, and hardly permits any interests concerning outside activities to cross the threshold of his consciousness.

All these elements may be added together and combined. They explain the appearance of being abulic which our patients acquire. They explain why their wills are never the same; why they are variable, irregular, and essentially wavering. They make us see how the neurasthenic susceptible of phobic manifestations or obsessions may be incapable of impulses.

Just here we ought to give our attention for a moment to a certain small secondary point which, nevertheless, is important. Hardly a day passes but what in the literature of current events one reads that Mr. or Mrs. X. has committed suicide during an attack of neurasthenia, or has perpetrated some criminal act. We have seen that the reading of such facts provides a starting-point for preoccupations and phobias. Now, a neurasthenic never commits suicide and never hurts anybody. He is wholly incapable of it. In his case it is purely a question of stopping and drawing back, and if the conscious progression in any determined path is extremely difficult for him, all the more so is any impulsive decision contrary to the very nature of his condition. Such a thing would be absolutely contradictory to all laws.

All the disturbances of the will in the neurasthenic come back to this fact, that he reasons badly. It is not that he is lacking in reason, but that he reasons too much, all the time and on every subject, and yet is incapable of following out a single idea if he is not helped toward it.

But let some outside element come in, in particular let something really important that would seriously move him call him back to his normal life, or let a psychotherapeutic influence make a definite path for his efforts, and immediately this man, whose will was thought to be so inefficient, will find himself capable of an energy which certainly no one ever suspected in him. To appreciate this fact, one has only to see what one can get out of the will of such patients the moment one has gained their confidence. There is no one who will show more tenacity or a firmer will, or more vigorous discipline. The neurasthenic is no more abulic than he is asthenic or exhausted. If he appears to be all this objectively and subjectively, it is because everything is retained in his psychological and physical mechanism, and that he is essentially lacking in coördination, because under the influence of his moral condition the end and aim of life escapes him. It would seem that each of his psychological functions was evolving on its own account—only on the ground of pessimism and discouragement, because here everything falls into line—the instruments agree and harmony is established.

As to the modifications of character which one finds in neurasthenics, they are extremely numerous according to what people around them say. They are egoistic, self-centred, touchy, peevish, complaining, very irritable, and extremely sensitive, weeping at the slightest thing, and overwhelming the family with their complaints. Such is the none too flattering picture which is given of them, in order to make one understand how disagreeable their presence is; and, as a matter of fact, to superficial observers these changes in character seem to be real. But often this is only the case with their intimate friends, with those in whose presence "they do not care how they behave," and not with others. Does this mean that the personality of the patient has been affected, and that his qualities and failings considered intrinsically have been wholly changed? We do not think so. Our good qualities and our failings only appear objectively as so many reactions of our personality to outside influences. These reactions, for a given individual, under definite circumstances, may be considered as constant. Nevertheless, in the most sound-minded individual these reactions differ according to the day and to the time. Are there not days when one feels nervous, irritable, easily upset, and disagreeable? This is why the same excitation does not always produce the same impression, and why the reaction varies with the impression itself.

This depends, first of all, upon a mental, intellectual factor. In the impression there is an element of judgment, and by this very fact the impression is falsified in the case of a neurasthenic. As we have seen, he has lost to a more or less marked degree the sense of proportion, so that the same thing may make either too great or too little an impression upon him. Our patient may appear to be moved out of all proportion by some trifling thing, and react emotionally in a susceptible or irritable way, while, on the other hand, one thinks he is lacking in feeling, because he has not responded sufficiently to some exciting event which would normally have disturbed him. In reality, it is not that he has become more peevish or more selfish. He has reacted to the impressions which he has received in a manner which is wholly in keeping with his previous character; it is the impression which has been modified by the mental condition of our subject. Still other phenomena come in. It would be a psychological error to imagine that, in the mentality and moral condition of an individual, an impression and its consecutive reaction may be separated one from another. In consciousness, or in the moral condition of the moment, if one so prefers it, the impression finds an element of reinforcement or of inhibition. If you are very preoccupied and very much obsessed, an impression which would otherwise have made you quiver in response will leave you perfectly indifferent. If you are sad and discouraged, you will reinforce by this fact all sorrowful impressions. Exactly the same thing is true of the neurasthenic, whose moral condition, being peculiarly pessimistic, helps to magnify and exaggerate all disagreeable impressions and their consequent reactions, just as the preoccupations which are obsessing him may be of such a nature as to inhibit and mask the altruistic tendencies which a certain given stimulus would have called forth.

Another thing which strikes us is the opposition which exists between the integrity of the psychological organ and the disturbance of function. The whole problem, of the distinction between neurasthenic conditions and other conditions which border upon them in certain of their symptoms which are but partly of an organic nature, finds its solution here.

F. Phobic Manifestations.—If one sketches rapidly a picture of the functional manifestations,—headache, vertigo, disturbances of psychic functions, disturbances of sleep, disturbances of equilibrium, pain in the kidneys, etc.,—one can easily see what a large number of patients may be persuaded that they have some organic affliction of their nervous system.

The fear of madness—and in the neurasthenic this is not the beginning of wisdom—is perhaps one of the most frequent forms under which these phobic localizations are expressed. This is because the patients have no difficulty in perceiving that they are not quite as well under self-control as they were. The modifications of their emotional condition as well as their intellectual state do not escape them. "I have a dread of becoming mad," they will tell you, repeating it until you are weary of it.

Certain phobias, such as the fear of committing suicide or some particular criminal deed, encourage them in this conviction. They have then all the greater fear of losing their self-control because they are in dread that their theoretic unconsciousness will lead them to perform some dangerous act, either to themselves or to others.

But under the influence of these preoccupations a whole series of secondary phenomena appear.

On the one hand, it is the moral condition which is still depressed. On the other, as a direct result of autoöbservation aroused by autosuggestion, it is a peculiar aggravation of all psychic manifestations. Being anxious to know that his intelligence is normal, his comprehension intact, his manner of speaking natural, and his explanations sufficiently clear, the patient will by this very inquiry inhibit the majority of his faculties. One can easily see that this is not the method one would choose in order to sharpen one's comprehension or make one's conversation brilliant, to be continually asking oneself if one is able to understand, and if every word which one uses corresponds exactly with the thought which one wishes to express. Patients in this way get into a vicious circle. Their uneasiness as it grows at the same time increases the various objective and subjective manifestations which formed its starting-point. Things may go on in this way until matters have been pushed pretty far. By his preoccupations the patient withdraws himself from his daily environment—from his business, from his circle of friends. The most sinister resolutions may run through his mind.

We must hasten to add, however, that he never carries them out. However, he is none the less profoundly miserable and worthy of pity.

Sometimes the only thing that has been necessary to bring about the lamentable result is a medical examination which has been a little too pointed in its special direction, and which has served to centre the patient's mind upon the conditions of his faculties for much too long a time.

Nevertheless, things do not usually go quite so far. It generally happens that patients, instead of becoming uneasy about their mental condition taken as a whole, become interested only in one or another of their faculties. There are some who in this way, and by the very mechanism of inhibition under the influence of preoccupation, will get to such a point where they will more or less practically cease to use this or that cerebral function of reception, elaboration, or transmission.

Attention deafness and attention blindness may thus be created by a process inverse to that of distraction, which we have already pointed out. A certain patient, convinced that he does not understand very well what is said to him, will really have some trouble in following an explanation or a lecture, because he will pay too close attention to it. He will no longer perceive words, but rather sounds, like an individual whose ears are strained to catch the slightest noise who will not grasp words which may be addressed to him quite near by. In the same way he may be able to see signs whose signification he does not understand for the same reasons.

Other patients declare that they are incapable of connecting their ideas. Some pretend that this or that creative faculty is peculiarly restricted. This one says that it is impossible for him to make any calculations; another avers that he cannot write a business letter; another claims to have lost his memory; a fourth will state that he can no longer express himself clearly and that he stutters and stumbles when he speaks. One may see every variety. There are no cerebral functions which may not become effective either alone or with the most varied associations. "Not here," because under the influence of preoccupations of another kind the patient's attention is wandering, and he is put "somewhere else," as we said before. The phenomenon in this case is quite the opposite. It is one of concentration on the function itself, from which results a peculiar disturbance in the exercise and in the objective and subjective practice of this function.

Less frequently, but still very often, one meets with patients whose attention has become side-tracked concerning the existence of some organic affection of the brain. General paralysis, congestion, hæmorrhage, softening of the brain, and cerebral arteriosclerosis are among the affections with which certain patients actually believe themselves to be afflicted or are on the verge of contracting.

And although there are a certain number of pseudo-neurasthenics who are merely weak by reason of vascular insufficiency, there is a much greater number of patients who, either spontaneously or from hetero-suggestive influences, take care of themselves in order to ward off or to cure purely imaginary maladies.

The psychic orientation of the patient responds to various mechanisms. Medical intervention plays a by no means negligible rôle. We have seen a great number of subjects who, being simple neurasthenics, have had their psychological troubles cast up to the account of precocious arteriosclerosis. The clinical diagnosis is confirmed by the therapeutic measures to which they have been submitted,—lacto-vegetarian régime, treatment by iodides, arsonvalization, etc.,—so much so that at every hour of the day the patient was obliged to recall that he was arteriosclerotic, which was hardly the best thing to improve his moral tone and to distract him from his condition.

Sometimes medical practitioners have aggravated matters, for they have not refrained from speaking to the patient of congestion, and hæmorrhage, and paralysis which is lying in wait for him if he does not take care of himself regularly. Is anything more needed to fix a neurasthenic's mind and give him obsessions?

In other cases, it is the symptomatology itself which becomes the starting-point for preoccupations of our subject. Vertigoes have always seemed to us to play a preponderant rôle along this line. Sometimes it is a slight congestion which follows a meal, sometimes insomnia, sometimes the disturbances of psychological functions themselves which play the rôle of *primum mobile* for this fixation. Elsewhere it is the memory of an unfavorable heredity of some more or less remote ancestor which haunts the patient. Sometimes it is syphilis, either established or merely possible, which, in an individual who knows the cerebral consequences which may follow this affection, attributes the symptomatic neurasthenic sensations experienced by the patient to a slowly developing general paresis. Such a mechanism is also frequent among physicians themselves, and we have seen very well-educated colleagues of excellent intelligence spend whole hours in examining their pupils, testing their knee-jerks, or listening to themselves speak, to see if they were not dysarthric. Old syphilitics who are accidentally over-fatigued are seized by the idea of a possible general paresis, and it is in this way that they gradually get into a neurasthenic condition which in such cases is secondary.

It is hardly necessary to say that, once the patient's mind has become fixed in this way, the symptoms of localization will grow and multiply. The attacks of dizziness will become more frequent and occur at any hour of the day; patients will begin to complain of disturbances which they attribute sometimes to anæmia and sometimes to congestion. All the little congestive pressures which are so common even in healthy people will receive the most careful consideration.

Briefly speaking, the patient will be in a fair way toward establishing a complete systematization. He will live for his malady, and his very existence will centre upon it. He will think that he is going to die soon, and dwell upon the possibility of sudden death, in view of which he will put his affairs in order. He will behave really like a hypochondriac. But once again we must insist that none of these manifestations, any more than all the others which we have studied, are signs of hypochondria, properly speaking, for the patient's mind is always fixed on positive phenomena which really exist, but which are interpreted in a fictitious way.

All these patients are false cerebrals. They are also false medullaries. We do not allude here to the hysterical paræsthesiæ which are mistaken in diagnosis for medullary affections. We only wish to consider the phobic manifestations which a neurasthenic shows under various influences.

An old syphilitic will be in dread of the development of tabes. A genital neurasthenic will think that his spinal cord is in some way affected. Any sharp pains in the kidney or rapid fatigue on walking will be enough to turn the patient's mind toward the idea of the possible existence of some affection of the spinal cord.

Asthenia alone might be interpreted as a myelopathic phenomenon. The feeling that one cannot stand alone, as seen in the phenomenon of stasobasophobia, may sometimes be the cause as well as the effect of such a fixation.

When the patient's mind once becomes settled on such an idea, he sees visions of himself ending his days in a wheeled chair. The more his attention is drawn to his limbs, his fatiguability, and his genital functions, the more he brings on himself distinct disturbances of equilibrium, he grows tired more rapidly, and his sexual impotence really appears.

Other phobic manifestations, which are really much more frequent among people who are slightly disturbed mentally than even among pronounced neurasthenics, seem, however, to be easily produced in this latter class of patients, but in an episodic fashion. We refer here to agoraphobia, and the various phobias connected with open spaces, crossing streets, and danger of carriages. They may have a common origin in the fear of accident. The patient who thinks that he has some congestions and who is afraid of suddenly losing consciousness, or who knows himself to be liable to attacks of giddiness or sudden exhaustion, grows more and more unwilling to run any risk by going out of doors. First of all, he will assure himself of the possibility of help in case of accident. He will take every precaution that his identity could easily be established if such an accident should occur. Under these conditions he will dare to go for a certain distance. But he will not be able to accomplish this without very great uneasiness, which will quickly exhaust his strength and make him still more fearful about his next walk. Little by little he will get to the point where he will no longer go out of his house, or at least will not dare to walk anywhere except upon grounds which are surrounded by walls. Thus limited in all his activities and more or less continually in a state of anxiety, it will not be long before he is profoundly depressed.

We do not wish to close this chapter without remarking that it is almost impossible to make any artificial distinction which would separate these nervous or psychic symptoms from one another. Clinically they react upon one another and are reciprocally created and strengthened. Finally, they may get to the point where they form a very full and complex symptomatology, and it is extremely difficult to establish the exact course which the successive manifestations take. And it seems to us that it is often because of this difficulty of the psychological analysis of things that so many neurasthenic troubles are attributed to phenomena of an organic nature. If they were better followed out, their psychic origin would be very clearly apparent. The neurasthenic who, looked at synthetically, may appear to be an organic will always on analysis reveal himself as a psychic. The whole thing is to push the analysis sufficiently far so as to be able to get at the true nature of things.

CHAPTER XI.

FUNCTIONAL MANIFESTATIONS AND ORGANIC STATES.

THE relations between functional manifestations and organic states are relatively very complex. Many questions arise in fact. In what measure are functional manifestations liable to create organic conditions either directly or indirectly?

First of all, there is emotional shock which may act in two different ways, either by creating of itself the succeeding organic condition or by acting only as an occasional cause in such subjects as are predisposed to the appearance of this or that symptom.

It is thus that, among those who are predisposed, emotion may be the occasion of the first attack of angina pectoris, or a first attack of hepatic or renal colic, or of a cerebral hæmorrhage, in subjects whose heart, liver, kidneys, or brain are far from being immune. By reason of the vasomotor phenomena and the spasmodic contractions that a strong emotion brings in its train, certain symptoms may be started up which had hitherto existed potentially in the individuals thus afflicted.

Exophthalmic goitre and jaundice, under certain circumstances, appear to be direct and immediate results of strong emotion. Emotional jaundice has been known for a long time. Rapidly developing blindness has likewise been established as following emotional shock.

Although the pathogeny of these latter cases is still very obscure, it is no less certain that the emotion and the organic upsetting which it causes may really be expressed by conditions which last for a long time, and which take organic expression. This is because there are in emotion certain organic factors, certain somatic modifications, which are really functional, but which are susceptible of having many objective consequences. Emotion, in other words, is capable of acting on the organism like an infection or an intoxication. The rôle of emotional shock in the determination of a rather large number of organic symptoms is admitted by nearly everybody, although they are scarcely aware of the fact.

What action prolonged emotional conditions may exercise on the organism is more open to discussion. The immediate expression of these conditions appears, as a rule, in functional manifestations of every kind. We have already studied the majority of these. It now remains for us to know whether functional manifestations may more or less slowly arrive at the point of becoming organic conditions.

It is certain that, if we refer to statistics, emotions which have been nursed along seem to come in as an etiological factor in a considerable number of affections. It is not merely a figure of rhetoric when it is said, as it often is, that there are people who "die of grief." The popular expression corresponds to an objective reality. One must needs be a very poor observer or to have never known life if one has not seen people who seem to have been unable to "pull themselves together" after experiencing some great grief. But it seems to us that in such cases the emotion does not act directly; more often it is by the intermediary steps of more or less marked malnutrition that such people, having become less resistant, easily fall a prey to disease. As for those conditions of malnutrition themselves, there is no doubt that they are directly due to emotional conditions. We have already said that nothing is so easily influenced by emotion as the appetite. It is also true that people who are preyed upon by grief, emotions, and cares no longer take enough food, and this is the mechanism of malnutrition which affects them, and the diseases which follow.

We would like to go still a little further along this line. It seems to us that, under psycho-secretory influences and because there is a feeling of disgust for food while one is eating, there may be in certain people a condition of insufficient assimilation. Such individuals may eat in vain, and, as one commonly says, "their food does them no good." They continue to grow thinner as long as they are preoccupied and obsessed, and this is a second mechanism by which, in a mediatory way it is true, but none the less effective, continued emotional states may be the accompanying condition of a great many affections. Might we go still a little further, and imagine that the emotional condition in itself renders the individual less resistant to acute diseases, that, in other words, the combination of organic reactions which struggle against the disease are found to be too weak to conquer in the presence of an emotional condition? If we are to believe popular tradition and read certain stories of epidemics, we would be tempted to reply positively. But it is more than probable that it is by the intermediary steps of mental disturbances—that is to say, the condition of moral depression—which bring with them emotion or preoccupation, that such phenomena will be sustained. When one is worried or preoccupied, one is in no mood to fortify oneself against disease, and against all the external and modifiable causes upon which it may depend. The history of armies conquered and decimated by disease is another instance that shows us the importance which the moral tone plays as a factor of physical resistance.

On the other hand, in such a domain it is not to be hoped that we can ever find cases so distinct that they would bring conviction. For our own part, we think that it is essentially by the intermediary steps of malnutrition which continued emotions (or preoccupations, if one so prefers to call them) bring about that they are able to exert such an influence on the eventual development of serious organic affections.

On the other hand, there seems to us no doubt that a whole series of bad habits, vicious attitudes, and disharmonies of all kinds, which the various functional manifestations are able to create and develop, may in a large measure come in to help the development of organic affections. It is very evident, for example, that a person who is under the influence of some continued oppression of emotional origin breathes badly, and by this fact alone will more easily become the prey of tuberculosis, against which he would otherwise have been better protected. In all the domains of functional manifestations which we have successively examined, we may find analogous examples.

We do not insist upon this, and we must content ourselves by saying that from the organic point of view a continued emotional condition or a preoccupation is by no means a trifling thing, and that in all cases it is a factor which must not be systematically neglected.

The most interesting of these, it seems to us,—because it is much the most positive,—is the grafting of neurasthenic conditions, or hysterical manifestations, on to antecedent organic states.

We do not attach much weight to hystero-organic associations. We know what they consist of. An individual is attacked by an organic hemiplegia. A homonymous hysterical hemianæsthesia is superposed on a paralysis; there may be besides a contracture or hysterical paralysis complicating a neuralgia, etc. The association is only of interest from a diagnostic point of view. As far as the psychogenesis of the symptoms is concerned, all the elements which we have already studied, reinforced by the existence of some real thorn in the flesh, will find themselves there in full force. In these associations we must say the part played by simulation or suggestion is much greater than in the hysterical symptoms due to an emotional traumatism.

On the contrary, the organic neurasthenic association seems to us very important. It is one of the most frequent, and, moreover, is of considerable theoretical interest.

It is a very curious psychological study to understand the minds of a great many physicians who are wholly engrossed with organic disease. The very men who are treating pure neurasthenics by the most complex medical therapeutics and without paying any attention to their mental condition, if they have a patient who is tuberculous or a cardiac, will impress upon him the necessity of rest, moral calm, and a life free from care and emotions and preoccupations. They freely admit that all these factors are able to modify and aggravate an organic condition. Why do they not perceive that it is the same thing as admitting that these cares, emotions, and preoccupations are likely to create outside of all organic associations a symptomatology of their own? As a matter of fact, when does a physician ever say to his patient who is a cardiac or tuberculous, etc., "Now, see here, you are not going to become neurasthenic over this?" Is it when he has detected some disturbance of internal secretory glands, or a dilated stomach, or intestinal fermentation? Is it even when he has noticed an unreasonable amount of fatigue, or too rapid exhaustion in his patient? Not at all. It is always—whatever may be his particular idea of isolated neurasthenic conditions—when he sees that the moral condition of his patient is growing weak and his emotionalism is increasing. The same physician who feels that the bodily mentality may be explained by the associated lesion will make an appeal to the patient's energy, to his will, to his reason, to his self-confidence. He will strengthen it and reinforce it; but, if he is in the presence of a pure neurasthenic in whom he finds no organic lesion, he will give him arsenic, phosphates, lecithin, and will exhaust the whole medical arsenal without paying the slightest attention to the patient's state of mind. So much for the logic of things.

But let us return to the objective study. First of all, by what mechanism does a person's body gradually become neurasthenic? There is only one constant and necessary intermediary. This is preoccupation. It may be connected with the patient's state of health and be centred around his fears for his life or for his future. It may be fixed on any symptom whatever of the affection in process of evolution.

Any painful symptom is particularly apt in this way to become the starting-point of obsessions. Then the consequences of the disease may become factors of the preoccupation. One feels that one is a care to one's family, one's business has come to a stand-still or is in jeopardy, or one is fearful of infecting the people around him. Sentiments of a less praiseworthy nature, such as conjugal jealousy, may come in to play their rôle.

From thenceforth, under the influence of neurasthenic association, the organic affection which is developing may be singularly modified.

Let us take, in order to press these ideas home, a tuberculous patient—and upon this subject Renon has written very wisely—who has become neurasthenic. His appetite, which has already often been affected, will become still poorer. He will no longer eat as he should, and will add disturbances of true mental anorexia to the disturbances of appetite caused by the disease itself. We can readily see that under these conditions he will fail much more rapidly and that the prognosis will be distinctly less helpful. If he has a fever or an obstinate cough, or intercostal neuralgia, he may become obsessed upon one or the other of these symptoms. He will cough much more often than is necessary, because he will be listening to see how bad it is. His neuralgia, which until that time had been intermittent and not very troublesome, will become intolerable and continuous, because he will think of it all the time, and he will suffer from it in memory as he would suffer from the actual pain.

Let us take a convalescent recovering from some acute disease. Instead of his being able to regain his health completely in a few days or weeks perhaps, it will take him several months. The asthenia of the neurasthenic is superimposed on the asthenia of convalescence. His first steps will be much more hesitating and wearisome if he is afraid than if he starts forth deliberately. Whatever habits he has contracted during the course of his disease will be hard to get rid of. Long after he has been cured of his organic trouble he will still remain a functional.

Here is a cardiac who knows that he has heart disease and who lives in terror of the idea of sudden death. It is very evident that the emotional tachycardia which he will show on the occasion of the slightest palpitation will not improve his cardiac contraction and that his moral condition will not be any the better for his feeling his pulse all day long.

A urinary, who thinks of his prostate or of the contraction of his urethra, will graft on to his organic condition superadded functional manifestations. In this way he may add a great many complications to his organic symptomatology. As retention of the urine is often the result of unconscious contractions, it may also be the result of contractions due to a phobia, because the patient does not dare to urinate or because, being convinced of his lack of power, he inhibits the need he may feel.

It is a mere commonplace to say that in all organic affections of gait a functional element is always superimposed upon the troubles which are there "by right." It is on this principle that elsewhere all the so-called re-educational methods have been based. There are innumerable subjects attacked by spasmodic paraplegia, for example, who, though able to walk very well in their apartment, feel their limbs give way from under them, or, so to speak, find them, on the contrary, rooted to the earth, as soon as they have to walk in the street without being supported by some one. One often sees patients of this kind in whom at least the half of their motor helplessness is purely phobic in its origin. The same thing is true in many ataxics. In all these cases motor re-education combined with psychotherapy gives very good results.

There are no organic conditions which may not be multiplied or diffused in some way by the addition of functional manifestations, as there are no functional manifestations which one may not find superposed upon an organic defect.

A very interesting point to study is the future of these morbid associations. Organic affection may by the very force of things become cured, and the neurasthenic condition persist in its functional manifestations. Numerous topalgias and pains *sine materia* seem to us to be of such origin. There are individuals who for months, even years, continue to suffer in some organ or some region or point which is no longer the seat of any real morbid disturbance. These are subjects who have grafted an obsession on some passing disturbance, and who, so to speak, continue to suffer in memory. Among the very theoretic "painful adhesions" a great number seem to us to spring purely and simply from this mechanism.

Other persons who have long since been cured continue indefinitely to nurse themselves. It is not that they are still suffering from any pain or persistent morbid disturbance: it is a habit which they have formed and from which they cannot free themselves.

Finally, there are people who after a disease, and because they have established a neurasthenic association, preserve the mentality of illness. They have left their energy, and their will, their physical, intellectual, and moral aptitudes, behind in their illness, because they have formed the habit of auto-observation, of lack of confidence in their strength, and the conviction that all their efforts are useless, and they do not know how to get rid of these impressions.

It is by phenomena of this kind that we ought to interpret all the neurasthenias which follow illness. In these cases the condition that follows some organic disease, such as typhoid fever, or anything like that, is not due to any material disturbance of functions; it is a modification of the moral and physical condition.

Setting aside all reserves on the possible existence of lesional troubles of an emotional origin, the thing that constitutes the great interest in the study of these organic and functional associations is that it is very clear that neurasthenic symptoms are only superposed upon the organic symptomatology when there are changes in the moral and psychic state of the individual.

CHAPTER XII.

GENERAL DIAGNOSIS OF FUNCTIONAL MANIFESTATIONS.

It is evident that functional manifestations do not exist independently. They are closely bound up with the neurasthenic or hysteric condition which has engendered them. There is, therefore, no doubt that in many circumstances it is a neurasthenic condition or the hysterical mentality of the subjects having such symptoms which is the chief sign that points to the diagnosis. But this is not the point which we wish to consider now: we shall return a little later to take up this broad question of the diagnosis of hysteria or neurasthenia.

For the time being we shall consider functional manifestations in themselves. We shall seek for their principal characteristics of diagnostic value, and we shall study how with the help of these characteristics we can differentiate a fixation of psychic origin from a morbid organic disturbance which may be found associated with a neuropathic condition.

The first diagnostic sign is of a negative nature. If it very frequently happens that nervous people are taken for those who are organically afflicted, the opposite error is also possible. Sometimes the whole symptomatology may spring from an organic affection in process of development. Sometimes there exists some organic difficulty, on which functional manifestations have been subsequently engrafted. The real trouble is often insignificant, and of such slight importance as hardly to amount to anything. Nevertheless, it is very important to discover it, as any misconception concerning it may bring about disaster, for the patient, convinced that in spite of his best efforts he has not been able to get rid of some definite symptom, would rapidly lose confidence and be completely demoralized.

This is why, before even pronouncing the word neurasthenia, or referring to any neuropathic symptom in words which to our ideas carry in themselves the requirements for an exclusively psychic therapy, one should examine his patient from head to foot, and find out whether or not a rheumatic pain, a painful hæmorrhoidal growth, a varicocele, enlarged veins, or even a corn on the foot may not be the starting-point of an almost purely psychic asthenia. Though the organic part may be almost infinitesimal, nevertheless it must be taken into account.

A small patch of eczema, a slightly painful cheloid, a neuralgia, or a slight synovitis may sometimes serve as a starting-point for very serious and complex functional manifestations. And, if one does not take into consideration the organic element, it goes without saying that therapeutically speaking one can have absolutely no success.

We are now speaking of persistent organic manifestations, which not only might be the starting-point of other symptoms, but which also, by continually recalling the idea and by attracting the patient's attention, may set up and develop a functional fixation.

Under other circumstances, it would be necessary to make a retrospective organic diagnosis, and to remember that the patient originally had real organic difficulties, and that the functional manifestation is a memory, reinforced and diffused, it is true, but, in spite of all, a memory of a real thing.

As to differential diagnosis with an organic affection playing the capital rôle in the production of the symptomatic *ensemble*, it is clear that it is a simple question of objective examination. But sometimes this examination will leave one in doubt, and then in order to make an accurate diagnosis it would be necessary to refer to the positive characteristics of functional manifestations. These latter are, moreover, sufficiently distinct for one to be able in the greater number of cases to make a diagnosis by questioning the patient.

A very curious phenomenon of medical mentality is the fact that physicians hardly ever find out under what circumstances a certain symptom appeared. It would seem as though they regarded the moral and emotional life on one hand as separated by an absolute barrier from the physical life on the other hand. In the presence of any symptom, such as fatigue, gastro- or enteropathic pain, cardiac or urinary disturbances, the physician will ask his patient when this symptom appeared for the first time. He will try to locate the exact place in which it was felt, he will study its characteristics carefully, he will make all sorts of inquiries about the physical conditions under which it appeared and its relations to all the organic functions; but, when it comes to looking for any coördination whatever between the symptom and the moral condition of the patient, that is quite another matter. One of us has seen thousands of patients, of which the majority had consulted usually several physicians. We have known individuals who had been to as many as twenty or thirty doctors. One of our patients, of whom we have already spoken, was able to give us a list of fifty-five physicians whom she had successively visited to consult about her ills. But when we try to find out whether any of these patients had had any questions asked them concerning their moral condition as related to their physical condition, not merely do the majority but every single one of them give us a negative reply.

This was the response which was called forth; it was always the same: "Doctor, you are the first one who ever spoke to me of my feelings and mental state, or asked me about the griefs or misfortunes which have come to me in my life." Some patients would add, "They often told me that it was merely that I was nervous, that my nerves were out of order, but that was all."

There was never any moral inquiry made, even by those who most carefully and conscientiously made a thorough physical examination. Now, the moment that one has the slightest suspicion that one has a neuropath to deal with, the first question to put is one which will try to find out whether there is any possible relation between the symptom or symptoms of which the patient complains and any upsetting event in his moral or emotional life.

Any symptom which appears along with an emotion or grief or a strong material preoccupation is very apt to become a neuropathic symptom.

As we shall see a little further on, the great majority of functional manifestations are produced on bad moral soil. Question a false gastropath, or a false enteropath, and go to the bottom of things with him, and you will always find as the starting-point of his symptoms either the loss of money or of a situation, or some grief. "I have had trouble with my stomach ever since my wife's death," this one will tell you; "I have suffered in this way," another one will say, "ever since I lost my position." Among women who are peculiarly sentimental and scrupulous, it will sometimes take a long time to ascertain the moral cause. Feelings of jealousy, or scruples concerning incomplete coitus, infidelity, whether real or simply in thought, is often enough to start the neuropathic condition going with all its secondary functional manifestations.

Here, for example, are a series of false gastropaths treated by one of us during a short time, with the moral cause of the difficulty appended in each case.

A young man, twenty years of age, a law student; genital preoccupations.

An officer, thirty-six years of age; preoccupations concerning his career.

A woman, fifty-six years of age; preoccupied with the future of her son.

A woman, fifty years of age; false gastropath since the death of her husband.

A woman, thirty-two years of age; false gastro-enteropath; conjugal cares.

A woman, twenty-one years of age; false gastro-enteropath; preoccupations concerning her mother's health, domestic troubles arising from misunderstandings between the husband and mother-in-law.

A man, fifty-five years of age, a political writer; false gastropath by reason of genital preoccupations.

A woman, thirty-six years of age; false gastro-enteropath by reason of conjugal worry.

A man, fifty-four years of age, a manufacturer; a false gastropath with acute depression, both as the result of his financial losses.

A woman, thirty years of age; a false gastropath as a result of conjugal unhappiness.

A woman, thirty-seven years of age; false gastro-enteropath as a result of deep grief.

A man, forty years of age; false gastropath following the loss of his mother.—Etc., etc.

We might continue this series indefinitely. The moral cause is always to be found. Sometimes the patient, being too reserved or lacking in confidence, will not reveal it at once, and especially when, with women in particular, it is a question concerning preoccupations connected with the genital sphere. But it is not necessary to have had a great deal of experience with such patients to enable you to feel that they are holding something back when you question them. But when you really get hold of your patient, he will acknowledge the cause which ofttimes he will have hidden.

The first step in a diagnosis, therefore, consists in finding out the moral cause. This of course is the main element in the diagnosis, but the study of the functional manifestation which has been established furnishes us with many others. One of the most important seems to us to be the variability of the symptoms, but it is a very peculiar variability, being so closely connected with the moral condition of the moment.

One of the chief psychotherapeutic procedures, as we shall see further on, consists in turning the patient's attention away and distracting it from his functional fixation. Often this may be accomplished for a time by regulating one's manner of life, but without therapeutic intervention this does not last long. There cannot help but be considerable variation in the intensity of the neuropathic manifestations, and once these are brought out they are often useful in the diagnosis.

Here, for example, is the case of a false cardiac who complains of palpitation, throbbing of the heart, and slight pains. During a certain month, he will tell you, things went better with him, and then he was taken worse again. Do not follow this up immediately, but a little later bring your conversation round to the subject of how he spends his days, try to find out the schedule of his life during the weeks and months that have preceded. You will almost always find that the period of improvement coincided with some greater activity, or some joy which came to him. How often it happens in the same way with false gastropaths, and false pathies of every kind, that a happy marriage, an improvement in business affairs, or some success has caused these symptoms to disappear for a time, varying with the degree of fixation on the one hand and the duration of the "distraction" on the other hand.

Inversely, let a new emotion, an added grief, a moral preoccupation become established, and the symptomatology will be intensely increased. "My husband fell ill six years ago," one of our patients told us. "I lived continually between hope and despair all through his illness. During all that time I suffered more or less with my stomach, but since his death it has become intolerable."

A magistrate, who was a false enteropath, had suffered for twelve years with indigestion. Five or six years before we saw him, he had had a period during which he was greatly relieved; but for the last two years the symptoms had become much sharper. As a matter of fact, at the time of his improvement he had been very satisfactorily advanced, while for two years he had been seeking in vain for a more suitable post.

We could go on enumerating these examples, but these that we have given are enough to illustrate our idea, and to show that the functional manifestation varies with the moral condition. This is the second point in diagnosis. But there are still others.

The illogical combination of the sensations described plays a rôle which from this point of view is by no means small. However well instructed a patient may be in medical or surgical pathology, it is very seldom that he gets to such a point that he may not deceive himself. Study an algia in a neurasthenic. Everything makes it worse,—cold, heat, movements, and rest. To bring this about the patient needs nothing more than to be constantly noting all the modifications which his pains may undergo, and thus fix his attention on them. To pay attention to them is inevitably to aggravate them. A false gastropath will suffer from a test breakfast, and will tolerate a hearty dinner providing he has been amused while eating it. A false urinary will be able to urinate easily at home, but only with difficulty away from home, and more easily in the morning than during the day. A false cardiac will feel his heart beating rapidly when he is sitting by his fireside and examining it. If he is prevailed upon to go out and get a little exercise and tire himself, his heart will be forgotten and will be quiet. All functional manifestations offer us a study of similar phenomena. The lack of logic is, moreover, always apparent. It is this lack of logic relating to what one knows of those organic manifestations, by which one is aided in making a diagnosis. But when one knows that in a functional localization everything that fixes the patient's attention leads up to or reinforces the symptoms, one understands that this lack of logic is so necessary and inevitable that the patient who is the most organically suggestible will be taken in by it. It furnishes at the same time an excellent aid to diagnosis to the physician who is examining him.

Too many symptoms is another thing which one finds almost constantly in the picture of functional manifestations. Patients who have read and who have picked up a considerable number of ideas concerning medical pathology in doctors' offices progressively practise auto- and hetero-suggestion. There is no symptom which a doctor has tried to find in them but that they finally experience, and, although this symptomatology is more often apt to be quite illogical, combining characteristics of different affections which could not belong to one another, it also happens that it may be too logical and too classic when, for instance, a physician has been called in and has given a precise diagnosis. The case then rapidly becomes too perfect and typical to be true. When you find yourself in the presence of a patient who recites his symptomatology as glibly as a medical student would rattle off symptoms in a quiz, if no objective symptoms are experienced, in the majority of instances it is apt to be a case of functional disturbance.

A false gastropath, or a false enteropath, who has been treated by a specialist will present quite too precise a symptomatology, but if he has been under the care of a physician who was less informed he will offer a more diffuse and rather cumbersome symptomatology.

Functional associations constitute still another element of diagnosis. It is rare in fact that these patients are monosymptomatic. The digestive symptoms perhaps are the only ones that often occur independently. Nearly all the other functional manifestations are grouped together and increase and multiply.

Digestive disturbances are apt to become coupled with genital fixations, and the latter may become complicated by urinary symptoms. Cardiac disturbances and respiratory troubles lead to general asthenia, etc. Every simple and complex association that exists may be found in these cases.

We shall have finished with this chapter on diagnosis when we add that we have omitted the most important factor,—namely, the moral and mental condition of the subject in whom the neuropathic symptoms are manifested. But we shall take up these conditions at much greater length further on, as well as the peculiar habits or mannerisms that they give to patients, and which often give us the cue at the start, so that during the first examination of the subject we are often convinced that we have a neuropath to deal with.

There remains one last point for us to study. It concerns the differentiation to be made between hysterical symptoms and simulation. Some authors avail themselves of a very simple solution, for, as all hysteria, according to them, is due to a more or less conscious simulation, it follows that it is impossible to make any diagnosis between an hysterical symptom and simulation. The whole difference would lie in this fact, that simulation is voluntary, conscious, and reasoning, while an hysterical symptom is but half voluntary, semi-conscious, and semi-reasonable. This distinction is evidently subtle and would hardly serve as a basis for a differential diagnosis. According to our way of thinking, although we are convinced that suggestion plays a large rôle in the production and persistence of certain symptoms, yet we are, nevertheless, persuaded that there are hysterical symptoms which cannot be simulated. If mutism, deafness, and paralysis may be conceived as being of a purely suggestive nature, which is, however, far from being always true, it seems to us that it would be very difficult to attribute such symptoms as contracture and anæsthesia to the same cause. The strongest and most vigorous man would be able to maintain only for a very short time a contracture such as one sees persisting in hysterics for weeks, months, and even years. The most stoical individual would be able perhaps to bear pain sufficiently well to utter no cry, but he would never be able to prevent his face from showing some sign of suffering and to preserve an appearance of complete indifference.

It is our opinion that all the phenomena which emotion and shock are able to create may be recreated and maintained by hysteria.

That is to say, it is very possible that the phenomena which are simulated are those which emotion of itself is not able to produce. The majority of the trophic symptoms of hysteria which we have elsewhere entered tentatively among the functional manifestations are symptoms open to simulation.

For the other symptoms, such as contractures, anæsthesias, etc., is it possible to trace the simulation which may evidently exist? A most profound inquiry on the mode of producing functional fixations, a study at first hand of the symptoms themselves, would seem to us to permit the solution of the problem in the great majority of cases.

First of all, the hysterical symptoms which are produced at the same time as the emotional shock without any period of development, and a large number of examples have been quoted, hardly admit a pathogeny of simulation. But these symptoms are, as a matter of fact, rare.

As a rule, the symptom, in order to express itself in all its fulness, needs some time to develop completely. But this period of development, from the symptomatic point of view, has to be absolutely blank in the cases where emotion comes into play; but the symptom is already outlined through the course of this period. Before he becomes paraplegic, for example, the patient will not feel quite sure of his limbs. If the trouble becomes progressively worse, he will at the start have no more than a virtual hint of its existence. The patient who describes to you such a progressive coming on of the symptoms is no simulator.

In the presence of a symptom once established, the great point in diagnosis seems to us to rest in the persistence of instinctive acts in the injured region in the hysteric, and in the absence of these acts in the simulator who is on his guard. The instinctive movements of defence will persist in the hysteric, while they will disappear in the simulator. In other words, in created functional troubles the true hysterical symptom is always less logical than is the simulated symptom.

But the most important element undoubtedly lies in the mental state with which the patient regards his symptom. The true hysterical symptom does not worry the patient. He manages to accommodate himself to it in some fashion. With the simulator there is nothing of the sort. He always appears to be extremely concerned about his functional fixations, and this is one of the commonest facts in those whose symptoms "interfere with their work." Certain reserves, however, must be made. It is true that there exist certain morbid associations called hysteroneurasthenic which belong chiefly to traumatic hysteria, and in which the patient takes considerable interest in his condition. But if one examines these patients rather carefully when they are not simulating, one will find that they are disturbed about everything except their symptom, considered in itself. They proclaim themselves exhausted and unable to work. They see themselves reduced to misery. But they will never say that they are afraid that they will always be paralyzed, or have this contracture, or that they will have more serious symptoms. They are obsessed on the results of the symptom, but not on the symptom itself. The simulator behaves quite differently, for in his case the functional fixation occupies the most prominent place in his mentality.

Under some circumstances, however, the question of diagnosis becomes more delicate. It is, as a matter of fact, by reason of their very mentality that certain hysterics are simulators. But in these cases they are hysterical in character; they are not cases where the mental condition has been unhinged by an emotional shock, but where it has always existed. This is no longer, properly speaking, hysteria; it is mythomania, and there is no doubt that a certain number of patients—though certainly not all, nor even the majority—ought to be struck out from the nosological picture of hysteria and put into that of mythomania.

However it may be, with the sudden onset or distinctly progressive symptoms, with the persistence of instinctive actions and with psychic indifference in the presence of the symptom, it seems to us that we have enough cardinal characteristics to permit us to differentiate a true hysterical symptom from a phenomenon of simulation.

As for the diagnosis between an hysterical symptom and an organic symptom, that is nearly always very easy. It may be necessary, under some circumstances, to employ laboratory methods (lumbar puncture), principally when there is difficulty in walking; but in the great majority of cases the clinical characteristics alone are sufficient to establish the differential diagnosis, all the more so that for a certain number of years the semiology has been enriched by so many positive signs of organic affections that it is hardly possible now to make an error. In the hystero-organic associations alone it may sometimes be a rather delicate matter to distinguish between functional troubles and troubles with an organic cause.

There is, however, one last test for neurasthenic functional fixations as well as for hysterical symptoms. This is the treatment. All functional symptoms may be cured by psychotherapy, which naturally is powerless in the presence of the results of an organic lesion. This is a diagnostic procedure which one should not call in except as a last resort, after a thorough examination, in which one has examined every possible organic source for the symptoms presented.

For ourselves, who have a rather broad conception of neuropathic pathology, we consider it a very bad mental attitude, and one even more dangerous than that of viewing everything as organic, when the physician acts in the opposite way and inconsiderately says to his patient, whom he is examining for the first time and who complains of his various troubles, "This is a case of nerves." It is the right and duty of such a man to tell the patients this while developing the therapeutic consequences of their illness, but only when he is sure that there is no organic trouble.

SECOND PART

Synthetic Study of the Psychoneuroses and Their Functional Manifestations

The first part of this work has been devoted to the analytical study of the phenomena of which patients complain when they are afflicted with functional nervous troubles. For every one of the objective or subjective symptoms with which they may be attacked, we have offered an interpretation. We have thus been led to perceive how great a rôle emotion, attention, and suggestion have played in the production of the symptoms and as incidents in the evolution of the psychoneuroses. The object of the second part of this work will be to bring together these individual analyses, into a conception of the whole, to show what we think the psychoneuroses are, the manner in which they are caused, and the general mechanism which gives rise to particular symptoms.

We wish, above all, to attempt to give a distinct and precise conception of neurasthenia, to isolate neurasthenia, with its general characteristics, from the whole series of physical and psychic conditions which are too apt to be mistaken for it. It seems to us that neurasthenia is really, in spite of all that has been said, an independent psychoneurosis, connected perhaps by an intermediary series with other psychological conditions, but having nevertheless characteristics which are so sharp that it may be considered as a true morbid entity.

We shall pass a little more rapidly over hysteria. Almost everybody agrees, concerning it, at least practically though not theoretically. The comparisons between hysterical and neurasthenic manifestations cannot help but be extremely instructive, and it is for this reason more than any other that we shall devote a few pages to a conception of the general picture of hysteria and of its symptoms.

CHAPTER XIII.

NEURASTHENIA AND ORGANIC CONCEPTIONS CONCERNING IT.

EVERYBODY agrees that neurasthenia is a neurosis,—that is to say, a nervous disease without any known lesions. It is very natural that there should be engrafted upon this general idea a great many peculiar conceptions in the endeavor to interpret the pathogenic mechanisms of a neurasthenic condition. By the very nature of things, neurasthenia ought to pass through the same phases which have progressively diverted from the list of the neuroses a certain number of affections whose true organic nature has been brought to light by the progress of science.

It is quite to be expected that in a period where all medical progress sprang from pathological anatomy and from the laboratory, where one was able to see a certain number of diseases which had hitherto not been classified become anatomically and pathologically defined, that the medical mind should rebel against the idea of any disease without lesions, without at least the slightest of all lesions, such as represented by some humoral change, a disturbance in secretions, or some reciprocal effect of the blood-vessels upon the functions.

If, as all that has gone before has very clearly shown, it is our conception that one must take out of the class of neuroses, those diseases with indetermined lesions but which are not indeterminable, the psychoneuroses whose chief characteristic is that the trouble is purely psychological, we do not feel that we should be astonished at the opposition which our point of view must receive from many excellent thinkers. As a matter of fact, among all the authors who have attempted to interpret neurasthenia, by far the greater majority of them attribute this affection to some organic trouble. This, however, is only a question of the mental attitude, of the times and of methods, and one can easily see how neurasthenia or ''psychoneurosis'' runs counter to the most legitimate and well-established medical conceptions which have been built up in the course of centuries.

One cannot help but be struck, at the very start, by the multitude of organic interpretations which have pretended to furnish a sufficient explanation of the facts observed. Neurasthenia might be essentially polymorphic and multisymptomatic; it is none the less curious to see the essentially different positions taken by the various authors in their pathogenic conceptions. Never perhaps has any disease lent itself to so many discordant interpretations.

We hold neither to the genital theory nor to the vasomotor theory. The latter could by no means possess more than the merit of interpreting certain phenomena presented by neurasthenics. It retreats from the problem without furnishing any solution of it. We shall simply mention the theories of acid dyscrasia, of demineralization, and various chemical disturbances of nutrition; we shall cite the theory of neurasthenia of hepatic or polemic origin, of neurasthenia by visceral ptosis, and neurasthenia of cerebellar origin. The simple mention of the thyroid theories and the theories attributing neurasthenia to a complex disturbance in the functioning of the blood-vessels we feel is enough.

As a matter of fact, two broad doctrines sum up almost completely all the modern organic interpretations of neurasthenia,—namely, the theory of intoxication and the theory of exhaustion. These two theories, moreover, are not incompatible, and, according to certain authors, neurasthenics may be either suffering from exhaustion or from intoxication, or from both at the same time.

The partisans of neurasthenic disease by intoxication do not exploit it any more often than intoxication of endogenous origin,—namely, auto-intoxication. The facts upon which this doctrine seeks to found itself are of various kinds. First of all, there is the frequent existence of digestive troubles in neurasthenics. At the period when the doctrine of dilatation of the stomach was dominant, it was to the latter, by the intermediary of gastric fermentation and secondary toxic reabsorption, that was attributed the capital rôle in the production of neurasthenic conditions. It goes without saying that the absence of neurasthenic conditions in major organic dilatation of the stomach, as well as the frequent absence of any digestive disturbance in neurasthenics, does not permit us to attach any serious importance to such a conception. Similar theories based upon the insufficient elaboration of albuminoid material by vitiated digestive functions are open to the same objections.

The modifications of the urine found in neurasthenics have served as a basis for a whole series of diathetic theories. The unfortunate thing is that the variations observed are extremely inconstant and different between one subject and another. The urines of this neurasthenic are hyperacid, of another hypoacid. The urine is sometimes scanty and sometimes increased, as is also the uric acid. The urinary relations undergo every possible variety. The accidental and rare presence, however, of pathological products in the urine, such as sugar, urobilin, indican, and the various albumins, is nothing but an epiphenomenon, without any pathological relations to the neurasthenic condition which is in progress. Briefly, there is no urology of neurasthenia.

Arterial tension has also been invoked. But this again is so variable that the very authors who have attached a certain importance to it have been obliged to divide neurasthenics into two classes,—those with hypertension who would be suffering from intoxication, and those with hypotension who would be suffering from exhaustion. They fail to mention the existence of an intermediary class which is by far the most numerous, that of neurasthenics whose tension is normal.

Does there exist any positive sign whatsoever of an auto-intoxication to which neurasthenic conditions might be attributed? To tell the truth, there does not seem to be any single one which will apply to a sufficient number of patients for any theory whatsoever of neurasthenia by auto-intoxication to be founded upon. And it is really too simple a supposition to suppose or admit, as some have done, a multiple pathogeny in the absence of any definite pathogeny. Neurasthenia, certain authors practically say, is a syndrome having its source in the most diverse auto-intoxications and manifesting itself inherently by a great variety of phenomena.

Would it not be much better to acknowledge frankly that any theory of auto-intoxication in neurasthenia cannot at the present time be maintained with any show of truth? One might just as well try to uphold the toxic origin of hysteria. Some authors, it is true, have thought of this, but very few have lingered long in the way. And, as far as neurasthenia is concerned, they have very poorly grasped the reasons why physicians have set themselves against establishing a pathogenic path which does not seem to lead anywhere.

The theory of exhaustion becomes confused in a certain degree with the theory of auto-intoxication. But here it is a question of a very special auto-intoxication, of an auto-intoxication caused directly by overwork and by the waste products of this assimilation which have been produced in excess.

By the partisans of this theory, neurasthenia is an exhaustion of the nervous system, just as the individual who has made any very considerable physical effort has exhausted his muscular system, and is in need of rest before he is able to take up his work again.

But the great difference between the neurasthenic and the person who is fatigued or exhausted is that the latter will spontaneously recover his energy after he has had a chance to rest, while the neurasthenic will not recover it. At least it will take considerably more time for the latter patient. The nervous system being exhausted, there will be a very low state of functional activity of all the organs, which will be expressed in a feeling which will penetrate the consciousness and even affect the mind of the patient. In this way the mental condition of the neurasthenic is created.

This theory, which does not explain much, and which is nevertheless much more etiological than pathogenic, has at least the merit of being based on a certain number of clinical facts.

First of all, in the etiology of neurasthenia, it is the rôle of physical, intellectual, or moral overwork which has probably been the important starting-point of this conception. Now, this rôle seems to us doubtful, at least. Overwork in itself has never created neurasthenic conditions, and we shall learn further on to distinguish between the conditions of fatigue which overwork really brings on and neurasthenic conditions which follow only under very special circumstances.

This is because when one is overworked there is generally some special reason for it. Those people who are always rushing themselves to death for no reason and without any aim or object are already virtual neurasthenics, having an antecedent psychological trouble which existed before their overwork, properly so called. Those, on the other hand, to whom such overwork is a means to neurasthenia, and it is the general rule, constantly add to their intellectual and physical work all kinds of preoccupations. As one of us had already written in 1886, "It is brain work doubled by worry and anxiety which creates neurasthenia." In one case it may be the future which comes into play. There it is one's *amour propre.* In another case it is the family fortunes, the bread for one's children, that one is striving for. There is always added to overwork such psychological elements of preoccupation.

We shall see a little further on that it is some such element, and not the overwork in itself, which creates neurasthenia. As a matter of fact, to speak only of physical overwork, one has but to question army physicians to be convinced of the reality of what we are setting forth. During manœuvres or wars, whatever may be the fatigue imposed, not only upon young soldiers, but also on the reserves and the volunteers, one never sees any neurasthenia,—that is, according to the idea of fatigue conditions which cannot easily be repaired, or states of true exhaustion. On the other hand, one frequently sees men who are completely used up, who require a rest of several hours, or perhaps of several days, to put them on their feet again.

We do not believe, moreover, that we could cite one case—not a single case, we repeat—of a neurasthenic condition coming on as the result of tranquil intellectual work wholly free from anxiety. The overworked accountant only becomes neurasthenic through fear of losing his place. In the whole list of men who accomplish great intellectual work, neurasthenia is extremely rare if only it is unaccompanied by any of those various elements which start up psychological disturbances of any kind.

The fact—forming another element of the theory, and which cannot be contested,—namely, that there are neurasthenics who are really exhausted,—cannot be denied. In other terms, there are people suffering from fatigue in whom no amount of rest in proper proportion to the fatigue is enough to put them on their way; this cannot be denied. There are a great number of such patients. But we must make this clear. In such cases we do not have neurasthenics simply to deal with; we find ourselves in the presence of patients in whom the exhaustion is a secondary phenomenon connected with the first stages of mental anorexia to which so many of these patients are susceptible.

It is very true that a rest of a week, a fortnight, a month, would not be enough to give back strength to a patient who for weeks, months, or years had not taken sufficient nourishment, and who had practised, from a moral and intellectual as well as a physical point of view, the most deplorable hygiene. These are the patients whom we have already described as neurasthenics who have "arrived." Their history is of no value in building up a pathogenic theory of neurasthenia, because the structure here is too complex. In order to understand neurasthenia one must apply one's self to the beginning of the neuropathic condition, when the patient was still free from any superadded trouble.

Again we must not let ourselves be deceived, for in the very exhaustion of these "arrived" neurasthenics the psychic factors perhaps play a much larger rôle than has been thought, and one much more important at all events than the upholders of the organic theory have proposed. We will not dwell upon this, but merely refer the reader to what we have written concerning the asthenia of neuropaths.

To sum up, the theory of exhaustion, with or without secondary intoxication, does not correspond to the reality of clinical facts any more than the theory of the primary disturbance by intoxication.

We hold that neurasthenia is due wholly to psychological factors, and that these psychological factors are essentially, if not exclusively, determined by emotion. It is to this thesis that we will devote the following chapter.

CHAPTER XIV.

THE RÔLE OF EMOTION AND EMOTIONALISM IN THE GENESIS OF THE PSYCHONEUROSES.

In the first part of this work we have frequently brought out the important rôle which is played by the emotions in the production of the functional symptoms of neuropaths. We have seen that a great many of them might be considered as the crystallizations of emotional phenomena. We would like now to push our study a little further, and to draw from the facts that we have already set forth the conclusions to be derived from them, and to show also in what degree emotion may be responsible for the establishment not only of the symptoms of the psychoneuroses but for the very genesis of the mental condition on which these symptoms are engrafted.

But first of all we must get a little more precise conception of emotion. Just how far does it extend? What are the phenomena which enter into its make-up? To what mental and physical reactions does it lead? What is emotionalism, under what influences is it developed, and to what does it respond? You see how many problems there are, and how singularly complex, which we must attempt, not to solve, but at least to explain.

First of all, so far as the production of emotional stimuli is concerned, it seems to us that a very important division ought to be made. Emotion may, in fact, be of external or of internal origin.

Emotional Stimuli of External Origin. Emotional Shock.—A person may be caught in a railway accident, or be abruptly told of the death of a relative, or find himself suddenly ruined; these are examples, taken at random, of a whole series of external emotional stimuli, creating what we have called emotional shock,—that is to say, a sudden intense emotion, coming on without any preparation to a subject who is perfectly tranquil in mind. But an emotional shock does not belong only to the negative events of life. A great joy, the unexpected success of some plan which is dear to one, a fortune which one had not dreamed of falling into one's hands, may in the same way constitute an emotional shock. The common factor in these phenomena is, therefore, making the subject pass by a shock or surprise from one moral, material, or affective situation into another wholly different one, for which he is insufficiently prepared and to which his present mentality is by no means adapted.

One must not imagine, however, that external emotional actions are limited to the great shocks of life. Between a great emotional shock and a slight emotional stimulus there is every shade of intermediary gradation. If one takes this fact into consideration that there is no necessary relationship between the intrinsic gravity of the emotional stimulus and the reaction which constitutes the emotion, one can immediately see how much interest there may be in recognizing in a patient the existence of emotional stimuli which although sometimes very slight in themselves yet may cause considerable reaction.

Will he be indifferent to this disagreeable surprise, or that little unexpected event? Some slight wound to his feelings or to his self-conceit, the bringing into play of certain sides of his personality which sometimes are considerably exaggerated and wholly out of proportion,—all these are so many trifling causes which may call forth slight or even great emotions. On the other hand, emotional reaction, but of a peculiar order, may be brought about by certain stimuli, such as a keen artistic impression, the discovery of a wonderful view, something moving that one has read, or some slight triumph obtained either by one's self or one of the family.

Speaking generally, there are two kinds of phenomena in life. On the one hand there are those which are regulated, foreseen, and expected, to which one is adequate and for which one's life is adapted; on the other hand there are those which one does not expect, which surprise, astonish, and jar one. The former never produce emotional reactions, while the latter are always likely to provoke them. It is no longer a question of stimulus; it is the circumstances under which the emotional action is exercised which comes into play, with all variations. As we shall see further on, in order to create the same reaction, the intrinsic value of the emotional action, on the one hand, and the emotionalism of the subject, on the other, are two factors which vary in an inverse relation one to the other.

Emotional Stimuli of Internal Origin.—Emotion has not necessarily any external cause. We would readily say that, as far as numbers are concerned, if not intensity, emotional stimuli of internal origin play a preponderate rôle. Sometimes it will be the recollection or the memory of a previous emotional shock, which will be the starting-point of the emotional reaction. Is it not a common thing to hear a person say that he cannot recall a certain thing without being affected by it? But it is not even necessary that one should have previously experienced an emotional shock. One can become emotional over a simple idea which knocks at the threshold of consciousness. Think of the death of some one who is very dear to you, or that ruin is lying in wait for you, or of some possible dishonor, or of a threatening illness, and without these thoughts having any objective foundation whatsoever they will be enough to create emotional reactions.

As a matter of fact, it is very difficult to separate exactly what belongs to interior emotion from what is likely to be created there. What difference is there between a sentimental state and an emotional state? The emotion is certainly not very sharp. The religious emotion of the person who prays, the esthetic emotion of the artist who creates, the intellectual emotion, if we might so call it, of the thinker who evolves something, are all emotional phenomena, but which are singularly remote from internal emotional shock. Even a dream might in some cases, if it introduced sufficiently vivid pictures into consciousness, be regarded as an emotional stimulus.

We would readily go still further, for we hold that all manifestations of individual psychological activity which do not belong to the domain of pure consciousness may, after all, appear as touching the domain of emotional stimuli. The idea itself only draws its creative value, its force of action, from the emotional reinforcement which it may undergo, and from the fact that it may be attached in some way to some intimate, profound, unconscious or unreasoning phase of our personality.

In a very general way, emotion is a reaction of the personality. It is called sthenic when the emotional excitation acts in the sense of development of the personality. It is called depressing when, on the other hand, this stimulus arrests or reduces the action of the personality.

What are now the psychological modifications produced by emotional stimuli? These modifications are evidently variable according to the nature and intensity of the stimulus. They vary still further according as to whether they are regarded as immediate or as later results of it.

Immediate Psychological Modifications Produced by Emotional Stimuli.—Emotion may completely overthrow the equilibrium of the subject who experiences it. Under the influence of an emotion he will become incapable of any conscious action or judgment. He will act like a crazy man. This is the peculiar quality of intense emotional shock, which can suddenly completely overwhelm, as it were, individual consciousness. Deprived of his most elementary perceptions, feeling nothing, seeing nothing and hearing nothing, the subject is transformed into a simple automaton, and is plunged, as it were, into a state of psychologic syncope.

Although this modification may in a few rare instances be lasting, and the psychic disorientation which follows the emotion may become fixed in the form of some characteristic mental affection, more often this does not occur, and the syncope is followed by a gradual coming back to one's self. But the regaining of conscious judgment is far from being regular. It is attained only after successive relapses. The subject at first manages to get hold of himself for a few moments, then his emotion sweeps over him again. He thus passes through successive waves of emotion. Although the moments of conscious self-control will in the majority of cases lengthen, and finally the time will come when the individual has regained complete mastery over himself, yet this does not always come to pass, and it may happen that for weeks, months, and even years, the same succession of moments of self-control and periods of emotion will continue to be produced. This is when the emotion is continually being renewed by the mechanism of memory. But independent even of memory, this series of oscillations, which tend toward equilibrium, may be prolonged for a very long time.

It would not be exact to say that emotional excitement always produces this immediate and sudden upsetting of conscious control. It sometimes happens that even the most profound emotion requires a certain amount of time to produce this result. It would seem as though to gain its full effect the emotional stimulus needs to be reinforced by the addition of internal emotion, and that the external stimulus grows, as it were, like a rolling snowball, to greater proportions by contact with internal emotions.

The action of slight emotional shocks—that is to say, of emotional excitations of comparatively slight importance, coming from outside—varies from one subject to another. There are some people who behave in the same way over emotions which are trifling in themselves as they would behave under one of the most serious shocks of their existence. The quality of the emotion comes in here, in a peculiar way, and each individual has his realm of special susceptibility. Here, again, the emotional shock does not assume its full importance until, after being reinforced by interior emotion, it has sounded, under the emotional influence, the more or less profound depths of personal individuality. The latter will react sharply to an emotional shock which even lightly touches the affective domain, and will not react at all, or very slightly, if attacked from the point of view of material things or ambitions. The importance of the personal coefficient increases in direct proportion as the intrinsic importance of the emotional shock decreases.

External emotions, even the most trifling, may produce considerable effect, perhaps less upon the intellectual function properly so called than on the morale. It constantly happens that under emotional action a person's mentality will completely veer about. All of us in differing degrees are more or less susceptible to alternate moods, passing rapidly from more or less pronounced states of depression to more or less marked excitement. Without any transition, these emotional excitations may make us pass from one condition to another, and this is just as true for slight emotional surprises that are positive as for those of a negative nature. It is quite frequent to find that some unexpected pleasure will make us sad and pessimistic. This fact, moreover, has much more therapeutic than pathogenic value in the history of the psychoneuroses.

In a general way, all the little depressing emotions are translated into that peculiar moral condition in which we are aware of various sensations of insecurity or more or less marked anxiety,—the so-called feelings of incompleteness, to use Janet's expression. It would seem that when one has experienced one emotional shock, one is always expecting another. As we shall see further on, emotion begets emotionalism.

As for the immediate psychological effect produced by those emotions which we have described as internal, it does not differ from that which is produced by the emotions of external origin. The essential thing which distinguishes an external emotion from an internal emotion, though the latter may sometimes be a residue of the former, is chiefly the lesser continuity of action. As a matter of fact, the internal emotion being closely allied with the mentality of the subject and secondary to it, it naturally has every chance to be reproduced, and reinforced by itself, with great frequency. The internal emotion created in fact by unintermitting emotional conditions, whose action becoming dissolved in the mentality, instead of being abrupt as in an emotional shock, cannot help, in the long run after being subjected to a whole series of added phenomena, but become finally established.

After having seen what are the immediate psychological actions, we would like to continue this discussion by inquiring into the later psychological actions exercised by the emotions.

Later Psychological Actions Exercised by the Emotions. Preoccupations.—In the domain of pure consciousness, the acquisitions of the mind pass through a certain number of stages. There is the stage of reception, the stage of judgment, or, if one so prefers it, the adaptation of our mind to the new idea introduced, or that phase of acquisition, properly so called, where the idea becomes an integral part of our psychic personality. It is a peculiar characteristic of emotional actions that they cannot be judged. This is because, as a matter of fact, they differ essentially from phenomena of pure consciousness. They run counter not only to our intellectuality, but to our intimate personality and our deepest feelings. They act upon domains which include such profound ideas as the vital instinct and our affective tendencies, for example. It is impossible to introduce emotional phenomena into consciousness. One cannot—or it is with great difficulty that one can—bring one's self to embrace the idea of illness or of one's near death, of the idea of danger or of ruin, or of the death of some one we love. Let us put it in other words—which have already become classic—one does not adapt one's self to emotional ideas, because they strike at the very foundation of things, at the entity of our being. The intelligence does not adapt itself any better to ideas which hurl themselves against the make-up of one's consciousness. An emotion which is judged and which has become an integral part of acquired consciousness is by this very fact no longer an emotion.

If the emotional upsetting of our intimate personality may be expressed by violent reactions, such as anger or sudden impulse, will it not at least show itself by the persistence of the emotional idea in consciousness? However much we may mentally revolt against an emotional idea, it will nevertheless remain to form a mental state which we then call a preoccupation. Here we enter into the very mechanism of the genesis of psychoneuroses, and can conceive how important a rôle is played by the emotional factor of preoccupation.

But emotion acts in still a different way, and precisely because it makes those subjects who are its plaything lose their faculties of judgment and intellectual control. The moment that a conflict is set up in us between our intimate feelings and actions of an exterior or interior origin, our intelligence loses the upper hand. Every individual in an emotional condition becomes by this very fact auto- and hetero-suggestible, because suggestibility consists in the possibility of the admission into consciousness, of ideas and notions which are not under the control of one's reason. It is by this mechanism that emotion again plays the most important rôle in the history of the psychoneuroses.

What has gone before enables us to understand the exciting and stimulating action of certain emotional excitations. These are those which adapt themselves easily to our inner feelings, strengthen them, and which instead of diminishing our personality rather increase it. We shall take up these emotions again a little further on, and shall place a great deal of importance upon them when we come to discuss the treatment of the psychoneuroses. For the present moment we only ask you to bear them in mind.

Let us remember as the most important thing this fact, that, outside of emotional shocks, which throw one off one's balance for the moment, one might say that the field of emotion occupies nearly the whole realm of human life. Let us remember also that among the emotions there are some which adapt themselves to our inner feelings, and that there are others more or less violently opposed to them. It is these latter which as factors of preoccupation and suggestibility dominate the pathogeny of the psychoneuroses.

Physical Phenomena Produced by Emotion. Anguish and Hysterical Attacks.—We have now come to the physical phenomena produced by emotional excitations. These phenomena are innumerable, and produce as passing phases nearly all the manifestations which when prolonged and established constitute the majority of the functional troubles which we have studied in the first part of this book. However, we shall not dwell here either upon digestive, cardiac, or respiratory troubles, nor upon motor or sensory inhibitions, nor on the vasomotor actions or secretions which, either directly and immediately or after being worked up for a more or less prolonged period, may be created by the emotions.

But there are still two other troubles which are very important in relation to their cause and effect upon emotional stimuli which we have not yet taken up. There are, on the one hand, the symptoms of anguish, and, on the other, the phenomena of hysterical attacks.

Anguish is a physical feeling which corresponds to the psychic feeling of anxiety. It sometimes consists of bodily sensations of thoracic constriction, with the sensation of smothering, sometimes by feelings of dull, deep-seated, boring or stabbing pain, which is very frequently localized at the pit of the stomach, and which may become crystallized in the form of nervous pain.

Anguish is much less frequently created by emotional shock than by progressive internal emotional stimuli. It is a physical diffusion of the psychic emotion, which is gradually amplified in consciousness, and which psychically creates the anxiety with which anguish is often bound up.

Let us take, for example, an idea of ruin, or death, or dishonor, which might involuntarily pass through our minds. This idea may merely flit through one's brain, producing a simple disagreeable impression. But in certain subjects, if we may use the expression, the idea is going to hang on to them, and remain in a condition of progressive preoccupation, which soon becomes anxiety. When consciousness has been completely invaded by this idea, and when the individual has lost, as it were, all cerebral control, he finds himself in the grip of the idea, as he will find himself seized by its realization, and this is where physical anguish is born. Under such circumstances it is nothing more than a physical expression of psychic anxiety. An emotion which one is dreading, and for which one feels one's self more and more unprepared, creates anguish by an analogous mechanism. As for emotional shock, it hardly ever creates the feeling of anguish until much later, when the subject recalls the emotional phases through which he has passed, and when he lives over again the distressing moments which he has formerly experienced.

On the other hand, feelings of anguish may become fixed in the form of a more or less continual memory, or memories which are more or less frequently recalled. The memory of anguish recreates anguish, because the agonizing impressions are so painful that merely to recall them brings back the anxious emotion, and because also, under certain circumstances and with certain individuals, the remembrance, from the point of view of subjective impression, is equivalent to the thing itself. These are the phenomena which we have already seen when we studied nervous pains. Phenomena of anguish, in whatever way they may be interpreted, may become the starting-point of a whole series of secondary functional manifestations, gastric, respiratory, intestinal, etc.

We cannot expatiate at any length upon hysterical attacks. Attacks with regular phases, such as they used to have at the Salpêtrière in the great days of educated hysteria, are no longer to be seen in our time. But what always exist are nervous attacks with emotional discharge, of every degree and aspect. They are made up of elements of various orders which may or may not be associated with it, elements of anguish, elements of motor agitation with tonic or clonic convulsions, spasmodic attacks of laughing or weeping, dyspnœa, and syncopal elements with more or less complete loss of consciousness. In the majority of cases the attack starts off with feelings of anguish, followed by symptoms of syncope, and ends up with various forms of motor agitation.

When relieved of all the elements which are superadded and due to cultivation, such as passional attitudes, etc., an hysterical attack is by no means a phenomenon of suggestion or simulation. It is directly bound up with emotion, and often comes to subjects who have never known what it was to have a nervous attack, who have never seen one, and who once the emotional shock has passed will never have another in the course of their entire life.

An hysterical attack more usually occurs after an emotional shock, but not always as an absolutely immediate result. It sometimes takes time for the emotion to develop to a sufficient intensity, or, as we have already said, it requires a greater or less length of time to come to a head, and the attack could not occur until the emotion which was in progress had reached its highest point of intensity. It is a gross psychological error to think that there is always a direct relationship between the emotional cause and the individual emotional reaction. A fact, as a cause of emotion, may first of all be accepted perhaps by the subject as a simple matter of knowledge only to become later a causal fact of emotion. There is a primitive adaptation to the fact in itself, but as its recognition grows deeper and it affects one's inner feelings it becomes a factor of emotion. We could cite numerous cases of this kind. We have seen individuals, who were overcome by domestic troubles, caught in an accident and not reacting at all to the emotional shock until a very long time afterward. If you want an example here is one, of a man sixty-five years of age, an old soldier who had been in many campaigns, decorated on the battlefield in 1870, and who had many times been in great danger without having felt the slightest emotional phenomenon. On his return to civil life his occupation took him upon a dredger. He was accidentally caught by the machinery of the dredge, which was stopped just in time to save him from being crushed. As a matter of fact, he escaped from his accident without being hurt at all, and was only slightly upset by it. But, little by little, the memory of his danger gradually worked upon his emotion. He became anorexic and lost considerable flesh. As a matter of fact, he experienced very belated emotional phenomena which made him profoundly neurasthenic.

All those authors who, in order to establish a theory of suggestion or simulation for hysterical symptoms, have wanted to bring up as an argument the time that often passes between the emotional shock and the appearance of the symptoms, seem to us to be wholly in the wrong in not taking into account the internal emotion which, in the genesis of neuropathic symptoms, plays quite as great a rôle as that of external emotion, if not a greater. We thus place in emotional pathogeny a whole series of facts which it seems to us wrong to try to separate from it.

Is there any relation between the modality of physical disturbances brought about by the emotion and the nature of the emotion itself? As we shall see further on, we feel that this is chiefly a question of individual reaction, varying more with the individuals than with the emotional causes themselves. It always seems to us, but without being able to lay down this proposition as a general thesis, that internal emotion gives rise chiefly to phenomena which are dependent in various degrees upon the feeling of anguish. The psychic manifestations of being wholly upset and of intense excitement and inhibition arise chiefly from emotional shock, and more often follow it immediately; but let us repeat that we do not lay this down as a rule. As for vasomotor disturbances, digestive, cardiac, or respiratory troubles, they seem to us to belong indifferently to one emotional form or the other. We might say as much of genito-urinary disturbances, and perhaps only the phenomenon of fainting and phobias of walking belong almost exclusively to emotional shock.

Relations between the Psychical and the Physical Disturbances.—Is there any relation between the psychological and the physical disturbances of emotion or any superposition whatever?

It would seem to us that the reply ought to be in the affirmative, for we feel that there is a very close parallelism between these two kinds of phenomena. There are no acute physical disturbances without simultaneous psychic disturbances. A reciprocal statement would not always be true, for in certain subjects emotion may produce only purely psychical reactions, without having any physical disturbances immediately associated with it. A psychical disturbance, however, is constantly antecedent to physical troubles. Even in the most upsetting emotions loss of psychological consciousness comes before the loss of physical consciousness. The fact that psychological consciousness is the first to be attacked is demonstrated objectively. We see people who are about to faint making vague movements which are gestures of defence and which show their vain efforts to get hold of themselves or defend themselves. We would readily say that psychical disturbance is the very condition of physical disturbance. Although emotion, particularly in its vasomotor reactions, may appear as a bulbar disturbance, it is, however, only a secondary phenomenon. Will not a mental representation be sufficient to produce vasomotor disturbances, such as blushing or paling? One may, to use a popular expression, "turn scarlet" merely on thinking of something. This brings us to conceive—a purely hypothetical idea, but more reasonable than probable and extremely important from the point of view of the pathogeny of functional manifestations—that the fields of intellectual consciousness lie very close to the fields of organic consciousness, and this explains why and how an emotional preoccupation concerning a given organ affects the function of that organ. This is also the explanation of the fact that phenomena of excitation or diffuse psychic depression are able to influence the general progress of organic function, and this naturally in a more marked manner in those functions which are more particularly subject to nerve reactions.

Emotions Varying According to Individuals.—There is no doubting the fact that we all react in different ways to various emotional stimuli. Each one of us, according to his individual mental make-up, responds or fails to respond to emotional reactions, with more or less ease. These emotional reactions themselves, both of a psychological as well as of a physical order, vary in nature and intensity according to the subjects. The degree of individual emotionalism measures the intensity of the reactions for given emotional stimuli. How and according to what laws quantitatively and qualitatively does individual emotionalism vary?

First of all, there is one fact that is very evident,—viz., there is no emotional stimulus which has an absolute intrinsic value, and which is able to arouse the same reaction in all individuals. All emotional reaction is the function of the particular personality. This may resolve itself into tendencies of different kinds. Some are instinctive, congenital, hereditary, common to the great majority of people springing from the same stock. Others are acquired and special, resulting from eccentric developments of the personality, and are individual. Here, for example, are such instincts as the instinct of self-preservation, the maternal instinct, even the sexual instinct, which enter as an integral part into the great majority of the mental constitutions which we have been accustomed to consider. It is a fact that anything that attacks these instincts creates in a general way, although with quantitative and qualitative variations, the same emotional reactions.

Here, on the other hand, are a miser, a man who is jealous, and one eaten with ambitions. It is certain that each will react in a very special way to the emotional actions which may affect that particular domain in which his personality is hypertrophied. Harpagon is in despair over the loss of his strong box, but is quite indifferent to his matrimonial disillusions. One man will take the loss of his money with perfect *sang froid*, but will be wholly upset at anything that touches his affections. The other will be unmoved when death has separated him from some member of his family, but will be beside himself at the loss of some position which he had coveted.

That is to say, in other words, the emotional reaction varies according to the personality of the subject and with the domain in which the emotional excitation occurs. But this means also that all development of the personality in a certain sense inhibits in some way emotionalism in other domains, on the condition always that in the zone thus hypertrophied the personality be entirely respected by the emotional stimulus which was the cause.

Therefore, given two opposite poles of mental constitution, there are those individuals whose personality is more diffuse, and less specialized, and those again whose monoideistic personality is more marked, but who will react less frequently to common everyday emotions. It goes without saying that these latter will on the contrary react with extreme intensity if they are touched in the sphere of their particular development; thus it is that the soldier who believes that he is marching to victory laughs at danger and death, but in defeat loses his head, and is overcome with extreme fear.

But there are some monoideisms which life hardly touches.

Such are the religious, and moral or philosophic monoideisms, which are so absorbing that individuals whose lives are filled with some such ideas, or who, in other words, have an ideal, are able to fortify themselves both against emotions, and against the psychoneuroses which proceed from them. The life and death of martyrs of a faith, and of idealistic philosophers, furnish many striking examples of this. They possessed a serenity of soul which as applied to the psychoneuroses is one of the best prophylactics.

There are, on the other hand, people whose mental make-up is such that they are able to defend themselves against the invasions of emotional stimuli, even when they conflict with their intimate work. We are thinking of those individuals who are quite able to feel emotional shocks, but who do not prolong them by the mechanism of internal emotion. They know how to externalize them, and render them objective, and how to transform them rapidly into conscious ideas. With them emotion resolves itself into an intellectual problem to be solved. Such people are rare it is true, and instead of giving them credit for the solid basis of their mental constitution, we are apt to reproach them, however vigorous their active or passive intelligence may be, for not being able to feel things, because they do not seem to know how to suffer, as though their personality were colorless and something below normal. It is none the less true that this mechanism, if it be not exalted into a system of life, opens a path which should not be neglected in the treatment and prophylaxis of exaggerated emotionalism.

As a matter of fact the clinical study of psychoneuroses brings us face to face with patients whose emotionalism is peculiarly exaggerated and progressively diffused in all domains. We shall now take up the various factors which create this exaggeration and this diffusion of the emotionalism.

Emotionalism and its Factors.—In a great many cases emotionalism is constitutionally exaggerated. Even among very young children one will find differences already established in that there are some that become excited over nothing, who blush or pale, or are disturbed or upset over the slightest trifles, and others who, being more resistant, seem to know, at the very start of life, how to live sanely. We shall see further on the part that must be attributed to physical conditions under these circumstances, but there is no doubt that heredity comes in, and that there are constitutions which are naturally emotional, or at least constitutions which show by physical phenomena of all kinds their emotional reactions. But it is extremely rare that this excessive emotionalism does not bear a direct relation to some peculiar and often very marked trend of the personality.

These are the children of whom we say that they have "a sympathetic nature," and who even though very young seem already to "take things to heart."

This inner stratum in the child is very susceptible to modification by moral and physical education; unfortunately modern education is too apt to encourage it when it does not develop and amplify it.

From the physical point of view we accustom children to be watched and observed. We want to protect them of course. They are taught to be afraid of things, and to feel a certain sense of physical insecurity; in a word, we are too apt to bring them up "wrapped in cotton." This is particularly dangerous. It has often seemed to us that it is in just such practices that we could trace the origin of emotional uneasiness concerning the health which later becomes a hypochondriacal preoccupation, and the source of neurasthenic conditions which are often very serious.

From the moral point of view the same thing is true, and if one urges children to be excessively sentimental, and to pay great attention to moral scruples and questions, one runs a great risk of preparing them to be restless and overscrupulous, and subject to excessive emotionalism. The adaptation to normal life, to its shocks, to the deceptions which it brings, and the limitations and obstacles that go with it can only be achieved later, provided the child has learned early enough to be conscious of his personality and to be sustained either by some moral direction, external to himself, or by sufficient confidence in himself. It is only too true that modern education fails to satisfy either one or other of these desiderata.

Sometimes education leads to a very different result, and it is because the child has heard personality excessively discussed, and because he has too much confidence in himself that at the first disillusion the whole structure will be pulled down. Thus, by different ways, one may arrive at the same result.

But education is really prolonged through one's whole life, and the individual, at a given stage of his existence, is no more than the result of the relationship between his previous personality and the successive events which have modified it. But even the individual who feels most sure of himself will not be able to resist indefinitely the shocks of life if they multiply and hurl themselves upon him, with too much force, for on the day when he loses his feeling of self security he will become truly emotional. That is to say that he may have emotional states, leading even to a psychoneurosis, which, outside of any previous mental make up, may be laid wholly to the storm and stress of life.

But outside of these cases, unfortunately too numerous, there are others where, either on account of their surroundings, or by the moral trend of their thought, or often also—we might almost say generally—through unfortunate medical advice, which has brought about a sense of secondarily acquired physical or moral insecurity, a preoccupation or scruple will be born, and the emotional state will follow.

All these later developments may be summed up, by saying that emotional reactions are directly proportioned to the way in which the personality is affected and inversely proportioned to the degree in which the subject can keep his physical control. It goes without saying that the loss of self confidence and the feeling of physical insecurity and moral uncertainty which lessens for the individual the value of his intellectual control bear in themselves a direct relation to all the emotions which have previously been felt.

Already we can see the vicious circle into which our patients may be swept, who being less intellectually strong because too emotional become more emotional in proportion to their lack of intellectual strength. It is the very same mechanism which presides over the evolution of the psychoneuroses in their neurasthenic forms which is almost sure to become progressive unless some saving element intervenes.

Physical Conditions which Exaggerate Emotionalism.—The functions of physical life and the functions of psychic life are not in human nature separated by air-tight compartments, and, although we consider, contrary to what is usually admitted, that a great many troubles in physical life are brought about by antecedent disturbances of psychic life, we also are not blind to the fact that there are a great many circumstances where modifications of organic functions are likely to bring about psychological disturbances. Although we refuse absolutely to admit that fatigue, overwork, exhaustion, and organic disease are the immediate pathogenic factors of the psychoneuroses, yet it seems to us very evident that these elements may play an important etiological rôle in the development of these affections. But it is always through the intermediary of psychological disturbances that these take effect, and on ground that is predisposed, and in the presence of superadded emotional causes. We do not know any cases of individuals who without some emotional cause have been made neurasthenic by that kind of overwork which might be termed passive. We have never met, outside of more or less justified hypochondriacal preoccupations or of superadded emotional causes, with subjects who became neurasthenic while convalescing from serious fevers. These are ideas which we have already developed. But it is none the less true that the various causes above mentioned, in the presence of an emotional cause, are capable of increasing and reinforcing a neurasthenia.

In order to understand this, it is only necessary to notice what happens in one's own case. What person who is tired and over-strained will not be more irritable and have less self-control and be likely to become obsessed on some subject? Especially one sees how cerebral fatigue, which by the very nature of things diminishes the value and duration of intellectual control, may be capable of playing an effective etiological rôle in the genesis of the psychoneuroses.

But here again an emotional cause must come in somewhere, to have given the person some reason for being preoccupied and obsessed. As we shall see further on, simple fatigue or over-tire, or so-called states of exhaustion, can never in any degree be confused with neurasthenic conditions, any more than they can engender them. They may, in the way which we have just indicated, contribute to the genesis of these conditions, which can acknowledge no single true pathogenic factor except emotion. Overwork and fatigue are no more a cause of neurasthenia than they are of tuberculosis. They create a condition which predisposes to tuberculosis, and which favors the sowing and the proliferation of the tubercle bacillus which remains the only true pathogenic cause. In the same way, by the lowered psychic and physical tone to which they subject the patient they may become factors of a greater emotionalism on the one hand, as they also constitute by themselves true causes of emotion on the other hand. But without emotion there are no psychoneuroses.

We would like again to draw attention in passing, but without dwelling further upon it, to the frequent relations which exist between the increase of individual emotionalism and disturbances of the genital life. If these latter act generally through the intervention of disturbances of a psychological nature, it has seemed to us that in certain cases there may be a direct connection, in some way physical, between genital disturbance and emotionalism of the subject. In particular, and often without there being any question of scruples, regret, or remorse, we have been convinced that the practice of incomplete coitus, as also certain abnormal sexual practices, may produce a direct effect upon the emotionalism of individuals.

Individual Physical Reactions of Emotional Origin.—The physical modes of emotional reactions vary according to individuals. This is a very important fact, because it is the key of the mechanism by the aid of which the various functional manifestations are produced. Each person reacts to an emotion in a way which is peculiarly his own. Some have vasomotor disturbances, they grow pale, or become flushed, another will break into perspiration or have a copious secretion of saliva, a third will vomit, while his neighbor will feel constriction of the throat and dryness in his mouth. One subject will find his appetite grow less and his digestive functions upset, and another under some emotional influence will have an attack of diarrhœa. Another will have a sensation of perineal tension with a desire to urinate frequently, either with or without excess of urine. This individual will be taken with palpitations, and this other will have a tendency to faint. There are some in whom the emotion is physically expressed by motor agitation, or, on the other hand, by a sensation as if the limbs were giving way, or paralyses of the limbs or arms.

Every kind may be seen and observed. But the most curious and important thing connected with such phenomena lies in this law, which seems to us to be very general,—namely, the persistence of the orientation of the emotional reaction.

We mean by that that in the given subject, whatever may be the nature of his emotion, every time that this emotion is reproduced it will bring on physical reactions which are always qualitatively, if not quantitatively, the same.

A subject in whom an emotion has once been manifested by some gastric, respiratory, or cardiac disturbance, etc., if he experience some new emotion, or if he is simply internally upset and encourages the memory of the emotion which he had, will experience again or will continue to experience the same phenomena which he felt the first time. We have seen a great many examples of this. We have heard subjects who were affected by hysterical paraplegia tell us that, regularly and constantly when any emotion comes over them, they "feel it in their legs." A great number of our false gastropaths have told us that in their cases indigestion was the only way, and the same old way, in which they felt any emotional reaction.

Are these phenomena of auto-suggestion? We certainly do not believe so, at least not the first time that these manifestations occur. Should we refer them to individual predispositions? The thing is possible; but what we want to bring out is that these physical reactions to emotion are wholly subconscious when they occur for the first time. It is very important that this fact should be recognized, for it throws peculiar light on the why and the wherefore as well as on the manner of the localization of functional disturbances.

THE EMOTIONS. HYSTERIA AND NEURASTHENIA.—Although in the genesis of hysteria and its accidents, great emotion or emotional shock seems to us to play a preponderant rôle, this is very rarely true so far as the development of neurasthenic conditions is concerned. Here it is almost the rule that emotional shock, as far as its immediate action is concerned, has but slight effect; even when in the preceding history of a patient one finds some considerable emotional traumatism, it is not always and necessarily to this traumatism in itself that the development of the attack of neurasthenia must be attributed. The individual who in perfect health is surprised by some emotional shock very rarely falls immediately into a neurasthenic condition. This happens only after a long time, and because he has not been able to free himself from the memory of the emotion which he experienced. The sudden mental disintegration which the emotional shock creates may lead to an hysterical symptom, but, as far as neurasthenic conditions are concerned, the mental and moral dislocation of a subject only takes place progressively, as a rule. This is because the hysteric has a very peculiar mentality, and his moral condition is relatively little modified. The neurasthenic, on the other hand, whose mentality it is true is affected, is, nevertheless, chiefly affected in his moral condition. Now, if the error in mental representation, or the emotional discharges of any kind which properly speaking constitute the symptoms of hysteria, may be established, as may easily be conceived, at the very start, the modifications of the moral state, on the other hand, necessarily come very gradually. A great shock does not at once produce that general pessimism which forms the basis of the neurasthenic's moral condition. To create this condition it is necessary for the emotional phenomena to be long drawn out, to be continually coming back again and adding to and multiplying their action. As a fact, when, roughly speaking, the hysteric presents the picture of one whose actions are inhibited, the neurasthenic always appears as one in preoccupation,—we might almost say, as one having an obsession, if this word did not have its own peculiar signification in mental pathology.

An example will make our idea clearer. Here, for instance, is a young woman who has suddenly heard of the death of her mother. On receiving the news, she might have an emotional discharge in the form of an hysterical attack. She might, either with or without progressive emotion, show the reaction either immediately or more slowly in some hysterical symptom, such as a paralysis or contracture for example, which, being fixed in her mind by an error of a mental representation, will, by reason of her intense emotional condition, be kept up for a greater or less time. Under the emotional action she has become a passive being, which registers and admits without discussion the various physical phenomena which resulted from the emotional shock. We have seen several cases like this.

But, on the other hand, let this same young woman be with her mother, who is seriously ill, and who is fading away day by day, let her feel every moment that the end is approaching, and very different phenomena would be produced—if at least her constitution was either congenitally or in an acquired sense sufficiently emotional. She would at first be uneasy and preoccupied, and, for no other reason than this, her intellectual control, her moral condition, and her energy would gradually become diminished or weakened. Then, the emotional excitation which caused the continuous preoccupation still pursuing her, she will have need of getting hold of herself and pulling herself up if she is to go on living in a way that is at all normal. Later, when the power to act is dissolved by the persistent emotion, she would no longer be able to get hold of herself, she would no longer have the power to pull herself together. The emotion of preoccupation would have entered as a constant inevitable factor into all her thoughts and into all her acts. Disoriented from a mental as well as from a moral point of view, she will have become a neurasthenic, having lost her intellectual control, and capable of presenting any functional manifestation. We must add, once again, this very important idea, that it is the emotion itself which is physically and morally so fatiguing, and that consequently the effective phenomena of intellectual and physical depression are going to complicate the situation.

This is a fact which, it seems to us, has not been generally sufficiently considered; and yet just here perhaps is the only real organic thing at the basis of neurasthenic conditions. Everybody knows that any emotion, if somewhat deep, and chiefly if at all prolonged, even when it is borne passively, will physically and intellectually wear out the individual who is suffering from it. Emotion is quite as fatiguing, and in fact much more so than the most violent exercise, or the most intense intellectual work. But the effect which emotional preoccupation brings about is still more marked. Intellectual work which, in order to be accomplished supposes a constant struggle against the obsessive preoccupation, becomes peculiarly painful and fatiguing. No action or decision, not even the simplest affairs of life, may be decided upon without the subject being able for the time to disengage himself from the emotional cause which unceasingly invades his mind. Anyone who, in any degree whatsoever, has passed through a condition like this cannot fail to appreciate the tremendous wealth of energy which certain people must spend when they are experiencing this weakness which constitutes the neurasthenic condition.

There is no clearer pathogeny of the neurasthenic condition than that given spontaneously by certain subjects who, being a prey to obsessive preoccupations, "feel at certain moments that they are on the brink of neurasthenia." This is because they realize that the power of their energy is gone, not, as a rule, because it was originally insufficient, —though that is a very effective factor in many cases,—but because it has been put to too great a strain. From the moment when the will, by which we mean the physical and moral potentiality of an individual, undermined by the effect of successive emotions and dislodged and disintegrated by the repeated efforts made to get hold of it,—from this moment his will becomes utterly powerless, the subject is ruled by his preoccupation, and can no longer control it; in other words, from the moment in which his reason is carried away by his emotion he is a neurasthenic, and contains within himself virtually all the symptoms of this affection.

To give a definition in a few words, neurasthenia is constituted by a general ensemble of phenomena, which result in the non-adaptation of an individual to any continued emotional cause, and the struggle of this individual to bring about such an adaptation. One can see how far removed such a conception is from the organistic interpretation of neurasthenia; but it would nevertheless be wrong not to take into consideration those very real elements of fatigue which are directly produced by emotional excitation.

What are the emotional causes which are found at the base of a neurasthenic condition? How are they prolonged, and why? What are the factors which reinforce the emotional action? These are the questions which we must now put to ourselves.

THE NATURE OF EMOTIONAL CAUSES WHICH ENGENDER THE PSYCHONEUROSES.—We lay it down as a general rule, which, according to our ideas, permits of no exception, that there is always an emotional cause in the genesis of neuropathic states. If you cannot find such a cause, it is because either your diagnosis is at fault, and that your patient is neither an hysteric nor a neurasthenic, or else your patient is deceiving you. Let us add that, unfortunately, too often—and this explains the lack of unity in the medical comprehension of the psychoneuroses—this cause is not even sought for by the physician, who is quite too ready to apply himself to the subjective or objective symptoms presented by his patients, and wholly to neglect the moral and emotional origin of things. Then it must be added, that—as the symptoms of the psychoneurosis continue (as we shall see further on) to go on evolving on their own account, even when the emotional cause has disappeared from the patient's field of consciousness—it will happen that even the patient, to whom its action appears to be ineffective, will neglect it, as not worth relating. Finally, although a great many patients are perfectly willing to unfold their whole past life to the eyes of their physician, and although they will relate without any discomfort the various unpleasant things that they have had to undergo, there are others who are naturally very modest, and who, though they might be willing to narrate all the details of their physical life, yet refuse to disclose the miseries of their moral life. This is often also because these things, necessitating the mentioning of a great many people, are of such an intimate nature that the patient quite naturally hesitates to confide them to a physician, whose province he does not think it to know all the affairs of his moral life. It is, therefore, quite an art for a physician to know how to draw out from his patients who are somewhat reserved, and sometimes even peculiarly stubborn, the real origin of their symptoms.

It is only by an extremely careful questioning, when feeling that the subject hesitates to reply to him, that he will get an idea of the particular ground from which he must keep back his questions until the patient has decided to confess what always must exist,—namely, the moral cause of his condition.

The emotional causes which it is hardest to confess are always those which have to do with some hidden sense of guilt or with the sexual life. We have seen people become neurasthenic because they were continually dwelling in emotional preoccupation concerning something which they had done at a former time in their life. These actions often dated back for years, sometimes to childhood or to youth, and yet had nevertheless pursued them during all that time, finally upsetting the patient's morale. A certain man had deceived his wife some ten years before, and had preserved in a peculiarly obsessive way feelings of remorse for what he had done. Another had masturbated when he was about fifteen or sixteen years old, and had retained the depressing ideas that he was in some way morally and physically deficient on that account. This patient became neurasthenic because, having some years before in perfect good faith drawn several of his friends into a disastrous business enterprise, he had preserved the stinging memory of the prejudice that they felt against him. That patient in marrying had neglected to confess to her husband some hereditary stigma existing in her family, and had reproached herself violently for having done so. This other had married her husband without having confessed to him that one of her brothers had been condemned to penal servitude. We might go on multiplying such examples, and one can readily understand how making such a confession might be peculiarly painful. How many others have been seen who preserved in some way, either as memories or as remorse, some failure of their former life. Nothing more is needed for a person finally to become wholly unstrung morally, physically, and intellectually, and fall into neurasthenia.

Often the emotional cause must be sought in the sexual sphere. It is an attack upon one's modesty, an attempted violation, a defloration which was never known, sometimes unsatisfied desires which the woman experiences perhaps as often as the man, the insufficiency or the excesses of sexual life, which come in, by reason of the moral importance which certain people may attach to them, as pathogenic factors in the very grave neurasthenic conditions which follow. We have seen women who, being anxious to have children, became neurasthenic because the husband insisted on coitus interruptus. We have seen—the fact is common among sexual neurasthenics—men whom some accidental impotence had completely depressed. In this domain also it is sometimes very difficult to find the cause.

Often it is in the realm of the affections that the emotional cause will be found. A disappointment in love, a home which is broken up, a child who is sick or one who turns out badly, a family lacking in affection,—any one of these may bring about neurasthenic conditions which will become all the more serious as the emotional cause persists.

Less serious perhaps, but no less efficient, are the memories to which one cannot grow accustomed. The loss of a child, or a mother, or a husband in the realm of affections, the loss of a situation or a fortune in the realm of material things, is enough for the individual who is haunted by the memory of something that is no more and can never be again, to become depressed and enfeebled.

Sometimes it is the future which comes into play, either one's own or that of some one who is very dear,—these are the situations in which one cannot see any outlook ahead, lives whose safety is threatened by material or moral cares.

Then again there are always the real or supposed conditions of poor health, which come in as factors of emotionalism and emotion. We have seen people very weary after some excessive work or prolonged strain become neurasthenic, not by reason of the overstrain itself, but by their uneasiness and restlessness at finding their existence so reduced and limited.

We might go on indefinitely with this nomenclature of emotional causes. There are all the accidents, even for people who are not inured to them, all the incidents of life which must be reviewed. We think that we have said enough to show how the apparent lack of constancy of emotional causes makes them difficult to determine. But we cannot repeat too often that an emotional cause, whether visible or hidden, always exists, and that the most important thing is to know how to find it.

Is it possible to establish any order of comparative frequency in these emotional causes? This appears to us a difficult thing, and the pathogenic importance of these causes varies essentially according to surroundings. Preoccupations of a social and material order are met evidently much more frequently in the poorer classes of society. Emotional causes due to obscure and subtle scruples belong much more naturally to the educated world. One can, therefore, see how statistics based upon these causes would vary according to the social status considered, according to race, according to countries, and the peculiar trend of the mentalities. Nevertheless, we have endeavored to establish some such statistics, and we give them for what they are worth. Not counting the great emotional traumatisms, our statistics give us the following table in the series of emotional causes:

Psychoneuroses where the emotional cause is due to—

1. Preoccupations of a physical nature	27 per cent.
2. Affective preoccupations	24 per cent.
3. Sexual preoccupations	22 per cent.
4. Scruples of all kinds	14 per cent.
5. Material preoccupations	13 per cent.

The only really interesting fact which seems to us to be contained in this list is the importance of the sexual factor in the genesis of the psychoneuroses. It is, on the other hand, quite as unexpected to see scruples of all kinds taking the precedence as emotional causes over preoccupations concerning material things. If we can believe our personal experience, a man thinks a great deal about his health, and a great deal about his affections, and a good deal about his sexual life. The material questions of life occupy him less. From the way we generally look upon life this idea is rather unexpected, and one which tends to raise the neurasthenic in our esteem, because it is a part of his personality to put his affections before his interests.

THE FACTORS OF THE PERSISTENCE OF THE EMOTIONAL IDEA IN CONSCIOUSNESS.—The expressions "Forget it," "Leave it alone," "Give it up," "Renounce it," "Make up one's mind to resign one's self," etc., express the manner in which normal subjects behave in the presence of the different things that happen to them in life.

In normal individuals, even the action of persistent preoccupation does not necessarily inhibit their activity. A subject whose mentality is well balanced tries and succeeds in distracting himself, we have already seen, according to the very quality of the emotion, and according to the personality of the individual having it, that it was more or less easy to prevent the total invasion of the emotions. But, whatever might be the particular direction taken by the mentality, and whatever may be the nature of the emotional causes which come into play, the neurasthenic presents, as we have already pointed out, a mental constitution which makes him particularly susceptible to emotional actions, in the presence of which he sometimes finds himself completely helpless. To a large extent constitutionally, and partly by reason of education, by the moral hygiene of life, and by the various experiences which may be scattered through it, the mentality of a subject which is capable of becoming neurasthenic may be summed up in two words, emotional and obsessionable. To what degree may these two words be considered as one? At first sight it seems as though they applied to very different phenomena. The hysteric who is very emotional is not, as a rule, obsessionable.

Nevertheless, one may easily see that the tendency to obsessions would be naturally inversed in a subject with a faculty of adaptation. It is true that ideas which do not become a part of the personality have a chance to persist in the field of consciousness. If, to return to the ideas of Janet, one looks upon emotion as a reaction of inadaptation, then the power to be obsessed in some way resolves itself into emotionalism. It is only one of the reactions—psychic this time—of emotion. And we would freely say that the characteristic of a candidate for neurasthenia is to respond to emotional actions under the particular form of obsessions.

Without dwelling on this rather delicate psychological problem, we would like to show what are the extrinsic circumstances of the emotional idea which favor its persistence in the field of individual consciousness. In other words, apart from the mental constitution itself of the neurasthenic which more readily than another makes it fasten upon a preoccupation and exaggerate it, apart from the psychological deficiency which emotional states cause in the long run, apart from the value—either intrinsic or relative in the personality of the subject attacked—of the emotion in question, what are the common mechanisms which in all individuals, neurasthenic or not, encourage an idea and maintain a preoccupation?

First of all, the question of time comes in. It is very evident that the longer an idea has occupied the field of consciousness the more difficult it will be to uproot it, and the harder it will be to forget it. This is because the preoccupation, being associated with all the mental acquisitions of daily life, will have all the more chance of being called up as these associations become more multiplied. It is thus that the surroundings, the list of details in which the preoccupation will have become developed, will constantly recall it, because all the pictures which its environment or this list may furnish have already been previously associated with the idea which has become obsessive. Now, this power of calling up people and things is by no means negligible, because a whole series of therapeutic regulations depend upon it, as we shall see later.

But as far as certain preoccupations are concerned, such as hypochondriacal preoccupations, it happens that among certain subjects the calling forth of these is in some way voluntary, and in direct relation to a badly organized moral hygiene. All individuals who, either by habit or education, are accustomed to observe and scrutinize themselves, both physically and morally, will encourage by those very means every preoccupation of a physical nature and every moral scruple which otherwise would have been nothing but a mere passing incident in their lives.

It happens again that such evocation may be provoked exteriorly to the subject himself. Here is an individual, a false gastropath or a false enteropath, whose physician has advised him to analyze his sensations and to examine carefully his excrement. With such proceedings how can it be otherwise than for the hypochondriac to become daily more fixed in his way of thinking? Here, on the other hand, is a man suffering from scruples, who is encouraged, by inadequate or badly understood moral advice, repeatedly to examine his conscience. His uneasiness concerning these scruples will of necessity increase. Furthermore, we will frankly say that, in certain subjects with rather weak mentality, such medical or moral treatments are capable of creating by themselves an emotional preoccupation which is a factor of secondary neurasthenic conditions. All these ideas, over which we are now passing rapidly, we shall take up later when we describe the prophylactic treatment of the psychoneuroses. They are of considerable importance for the physician as well as for the spiritual adviser, who would do well to take for their guidance the adage *Primum non nocere.*

CHAPTER XV.

WHAT DOES NOT BELONG TO NEURASTHENIA. WHAT DOES NOT BELONG TO HYSTERIA.

WE SHALL study, a little further on, the essential mechanism of various hysterical symptoms and various neurasthenic manifestations. But, before beginning this study, it seems to us that it would be wise to define exactly the breadth and comprehension that we give to the two terms hysteria and neurasthenia. It seems to us that a certain number of morbid conditions, whose relations to neurasthenia and hysteria are more apparent than real, have been wrongly and too often included with the psychoneuroses. In the description of these affections it has been perhaps too frequently forgotten that only those pathological phenomena should be classed as one which have a common pathogenic causation.

Now, there is no doubt that in the popular conception of hysteria, as in that of neurasthenia, one groups together all kinds of troubles with widely different origins, and which have no relation whatever to the psychoneuroses except through more or less occasional bonds of association.

First of all, so far as neurasthenia is concerned, there are all those phenomena of simple fatigue which we consider to have no pathogenic affinity to the neurasthenic condition. The individual who, physically or intellectually, overstrains himself in his work, especially if his feeling of overstrain is sudden and if he is not sufficiently in good training to stand it, will get to the point after a greater or less length of time where he is really exhausted, or "knocked out." Physical effort will become absolutely impossible or painful to him; intellectual effort will be distressing and often not adequate to the amount of work put forth. Between these extreme conditions, and the simple sensation of the subject who sees his vacation approaching with pleasure because he finds himself a little tired, there is every shade of gradation. But, just as we would never dream of calling a man a neurasthenic because he had worked hard and feels the need of rest, so it seems to us illegitimate to describe as neurasthenic a man who having worked *too* hard shows for the moment all the signs of intense physical and cerebral fatigue which have obliged him to stop work. Every transition may be found between slight fatigue and exhaustion. There is no reason why, basing it on a simple question of degree, one should put the patient in one nosological class or another.

The soldier who after prolonged marches or the sportsman who after repeated climbs had fallen exhausted are no more neurasthenics than the person who has read too much by artificial light or has used his voice to excess and who is obliged to rest his eyes or his vocal cords.

It may happen that, having abruptly passed the capacity for which he was trained, the subject may suddenly find himself incapable of continuing his efforts, because there have come in all those phenomena of intoxication due to excessive fatigue. It may happen that then he will be obliged to rest for a much longer time than he supposed would be necessitated by the work which he had accomplished. But, nevertheless, he is not a neurasthenic for that reason. He may become one if in addition to his feelings of fatigue there should be added any continued emotional state on which might be grafted obsessive preoccupations. That fatigue may play its part, in a certain measure, by reinforcing emotionalism, is understood, but, although it may in this way constitute an etiological factor of neurasthenia as of many other affections, it is not a direct pathogenic factor of it, it does not of itself constitute a neurasthenic phenomenon.

Does this mean to say that the phenomena which one observes either objectively or subjectively among those who are exhausted differ essentially from the so-called symptoms of exhaustion which may be found physically or psychically among neurasthenics? By no means. But the organism only responds to these different causes by a certain number of simple reactions. Whether the impression of fatigue comes from real and true overwork, whether it is in relation to some continued emotional cause, or whether it constitutes merely a purely subjective phenomenon, patients all express their impressions about it in the same words. In the same way, to make a comparison, a feeling of heat, whether it be due to outside temperature or to a fever, or is in relation to a simple autosuggestion, will be expressed in the same manner by the same or by different subjects.

We have already insisted several times on this fact, that overwork, whether followed or not by fatigue or exhaustion, does not enter as a pathogenic factor of neurasthenia. But we have also said that in a great number of cases the overwork is accompanied, as a matter of fact, by associated emotional conditions. This we think accounts for the explanation of the too great importance which one has attached to fatigue and to exhaustion in the genesis of neurasthenia. It is the associated emotional condition and not the overstrain in itself which is the cause, and the importance of the emotional cause is all the greater when, either intrinsically or on account of fatigue, the subject's emotionalism is more affected.

Fatigue, exhaustion, neurasthenia are therefore words which may be found associated in the patient's history. But, as there are a great many neurasthenics who originally did not suffer at all from fatigue, and as there is an equally great number of overworked people who will never become neurasthenics, it seems to us perfectly legitimate as well as necessary to wipe the simple phenomena of fatigue and exhaustion out of the neurasthenic picture.

In the discussion on the rôle of emotion in the genesis of neurasthenia,[1] we note the following lines by Babinski: "The typical form of the disease [neurasthenia] is represented by what is called constitutional neurasthenia, which appears in youth in subjects who until that time were able to work intellectually and physically in a normal way. The least effort tires them; they are exhausted after reading a few pages or writing a letter. This form of affection may be developed without there having been any preliminary overwork, and in individuals who are not especially susceptible to emotion."

The type of patient to whom Babinski alludes is well known, but it includes a great many different cases of which only a few are included in the true neurasthenic picture. There are people who, being constitutionally very emotional, are excessively and emotionally preoccupied over an examination or competition which they are going to pass. Such people may become true neurasthenics. There are others who excuse an inferiority which they have really foreseen by a purely subjective helplessness which is sometimes frankly put on. This is a neurasthenia which is fostered by teachers and parents and it is not so infrequently seen.

But the interesting point in diagnosis has to do with certain subjects who really, without autosuggestion or without simulation, without any marked overwork or without emotion, fall into a state of fatigue or exhaustion which nothing seems able to explain.

It seems to us that it would be rather a hasty solution to say, as Babinski does, that these young people, who often later in life bear themselves in an extremely energetic manner, are attacked with nervous exhaustion, and that it is a question of so-called constitutional neurasthenia. It seems to us that here it is a question purely of organic deficiency. These troubles come on at the age when young girls become neurotic, and often occur in those who are suffering from amenorrhœa. This is the age also when tuberculosis so frequently becomes established, or when mitral stenosis may become a true disease of the heart. It is the age in fact when all kinds of troubles occur which have nothing to do with neurasthenia, and which are troubles connected with growth and evolution. On account of constitutional debility or by some anomaly of development, the subject may not be able to stand the strain of organic growth which has taken place at that time, and which is expressed in other parts of the body by disturbances connected with the blood-vessel glands which may be detected by close observation. If, as a matter of fact, one examines such patients very carefully, one will find anomalies in the development of the pilary system, as well as heart troubles,

[1] Revue Neurologique, December 30, 1909, p. 1633.

usually in the form of tachycardia, and also vasomotor phenomena such as congestions, blushing, hot flushes, etc.

These are what we might call rather indefinite organic conditions. It would be wrong to consider them as an integral part of neurasthenic conditions, just as it would also be incorrect to make use of their presence to establish a theory of the psychoneuroses, based on a blood-gland pathogeny.

We would say the same thing concerning what has been called neurasthenia of the menopause and neurasthenia of the critical age of men. There is no doubt that this period, which separates maturity from what might properly be called old age, is really a period of some organic danger. Statistics prove it in showing an increase of mortality toward the fiftieth year, after which period it seems as though human beings took a new lease of life. At this time in life the oscillations of the organism which is seeking its equilibrium may be translated into feelings of depression, exhaustion, and fatigue; of that there is no question. Just now we have been considering organic disturbances of evolution; here disturbances of involution are the cause. It is quite possible that pure neurasthenic conditions by means of hypochondriacal preoccupations may become established at this period of life by reason of an exaggerated state of emotionalism. But we do not believe that we should consider these conditions of fatigue which disappear spontaneously when organic equilibrium has been reëstablished as an integral element of neurasthenia. This would seem to us no more logical than to regard as a neurasthenic a man in the early stages of general paralysis or arteriosclerosis.

Nevertheless, in these patients one may see the same physical exhaustion and psychic debility. One does not consider them as neurasthenics because there are superimposed upon their subjective symptomatology such objective signs as pupillary or reflex reactions in some cases, and arterial, cardiac, and urinary in others. One speaks of the false neurasthenia of general paretic or arteriosclerotics. It seems to us quite as legitimate to consider as autonomous, and without any relation to true neurasthenia, the false neurasthenias of either the masculine or feminine menopause. Their organic substratum is poorly defined. The blood-glands may also be involved; in fact all the conditions very closely resemble the analogous symptoms which one may observe in Addison's disease or exophthalmic goitre.

However, the development of these pseudo-neurasthenias of evolution or involution plainly reveals their nature. Sometimes they yield spontaneously and disappear completely after a greater or less length of time. Sometimes they disappear, it is true, only to make way for a distinctly defined depressive psychosis or an organic disease. But in a general way, during the whole course of their evolution, they show a symptomatic constancy which is never found in true neurasthenia, the variability of whose symptoms is one of its chief characteristics.

Many other patients are also considered as neurasthenic under the idea that they are suffering from exhaustion, who are in reality suffering from some purely organic trouble, which too often does not appear until much later. We would be obliged, if we were logical and wished to confine ourselves to the classical conception of neurasthenic conditions, to describe biliary neurasthenias, renal, suprarenal, and thyroid neurasthenias, etc. Descriptions of this kind have, as a matter of fact, been made. The man who is intoxicated by opium, or chloral, or cocaine might in this way be considered a neurasthenic when he is deprived of his poison, and the man who is suffering from lead poisoning and who is threatened with encephalopathy ought also to be put in the same nosological class.

These developments enable us to see that a state of exhaustion leading, as a rule, to extremely different phenomena can give but a very inadequate definition of the neurasthenic condition. Can one find its specific qualities in the mental condition of the patient? Must one necessarily be a neurasthenic because he is depressed, or obsessed, or has phobias? By no means, and yet just here there are errors made in diagnosis every day, due to the stupid confusion shown by even the most intelligent physicians.

In the same way very often a mild depressed mania is confounded with neurasthenia. We do not refer now to the custom by which, for politeness' sake, characteristic psychoses are described either as a serious or an acute neurasthenia. In the diplomatic language of the press, for example, not a day goes by but that one may read that some one has committed suicide in an attack of acute neurasthenia. It is evident that families would much prefer to include a neurasthenic among their members rather than a man who had a psychosis. But such an abuse of the term is really dangerous. We have seen a great many neurasthenics who have been oppressed by these facts in a peculiarly unfavorable manner. They have been thrown into an intensely emotional condition, and the phobia of suicide has followed.

What we have in mind is a slightly depressed condition without any great feeling of anxiety, without absolute insomnia, and without very extremely marked psychic or moral depression. To tell the truth, the diagnosis is sometimes difficult, and can be made chiefly only through the development of the symptoms and by the history of the patient. The existence of former attacks under a manic or depressed form will often enable one to detect the true nature of the trouble; but the real element on which the diagnosis, whatever it may be, depends lies chiefly in the constancy and continuity of the psychic symptoms presented by these patients. In their cases psychotherapy is purely illusory, for they are convinced of the incurability of their condition. And when one finds one's self in the presence of a patient whom it is absolutely impossible to infuse with any hope, who presents a mental or moral systematization through which one cannot penetrate, it is more than probable that this patient is not a neurasthenic, but that he is involved in a manic-depressive psychosis.[1] Often also the suddenness of the onset is characteristic of a melancholic condition.

A cyclothymic constitution offers material for a great many errors in diagnosis. But here one finds one's self confronted by associated conditions. There are subjects who, on seeing their mentality and moral nature suddenly changed, and feeling themselves constantly hindered and stopped in an activity which is inclined to be brimming over with energy in the in-between periods, become disturbed, preoccupied, and depressed. Here it is a case of the superposition of a continuous emotional psychoneurosis such as neurasthenia upon an organic psychopathic condition. To distinguish what belongs to one and what to the other of the two elements of this pathological complex can be accomplished only by referring to the patient's previous history.

There is apt to be confusion also in two senses between neurasthenic states and hypochondriacal conditions, whether one calls a true hypochondriac a neurasthenic or whether, on the contrary, one considers as a neurasthenic a mentality which is hypochondriacal. Although one would not be apt to make a mistake in a certain number of cases when the hypochondriacal obsession is very characteristic and gets to the point of frenzied ideas, there are, on the other hand, very often patients whose hypochondria is more diffuse and more difficult to define. Not but what there are numerous elements by which a diagnosis may be established. If one questions a minor type of hypochondriac who complains about his head, and if you assure him that his nervous system is all right, he will begin by doubting your veracity, and will put a series of questions to you, of which the majority will begin with these words: "But how does it happen then?" Such a one has nothing characteristic and may be found among the neurasthenics. But what is quite specific is to see a patient, without having passed through any emotional phase, abruptly abandon his cerebral systematization and say, "If it is not my head, then it is my heart, my lungs, my stomach, or my intestines which are diseased." He will thus run through the whole field of pathological possibilities, and, if you have had the patience to pursue him from one position to another, you will abandon the siege when, having completed his cycle, he returns to the starting-point and begins to tell you all over again about his head.

With the neurasthenic there is nothing of this sort. He may have one or several preoccupations, not hypochondriacal but organic, but these preoccupations have a true reason for existing. The false gas-

[1] Cyclothymia is a frequently used word for this state. See Jelliffe, Am. J. Insanity, 1911.

tropath has painful digestion, the false cardiac has tachycardia, the false pulmonary has dyspnœa, the false urinary has abnormal urethral or vesical sensations. The troubles felt by these patients are functional in their nature,—that is understood. They are of emotional—that is, of a subjective and psychic—origin: so much so that their systematization is sure to be sufficiently distinct, so that a false gastropath when once cured does not become a false cerebral, a false urinary, etc.

However, the most important element of diagnosis does not, to our way of thinking, lie in this. That element lies chiefly in the origin of the symptoms. It is true that, under the influence of emotions and the various experiences of life, hypochondriacal conditions may be exaggerated, but they are exaggerated as a whole. As for the hypochondriac preoccupation itself, it constitutes originally a purely intellectual conception, apropos of which, but secondarily, the patient may really work up an emotion, but which is not of emotional origin. With the neurasthenic things take place in the opposite way. The localization is always due to an emotional cause, and, if intellectual interpretations follow, it is they and not the emotional phenomena which are secondary.

In the same way, when we are told that our patients who are attacked with false pathies are hypochondriacs and not neurasthenics, we cannot but think that the patients have not been thoroughly examined, and that such statements can only be attributed to a very inexact conception of things.

There now remains a last category of patients to be described, which are classified by Janet in the same nosological list, the psychasthenics. In what measure psychasthenia may be confused with manic-depressive psychosis and Magnan's syndromes of mental degeneracy is a problem which remains to be solved. But under whatsoever title these patients may be considered as resembling neurasthenics, it is something which we cannot admit as a fact. We feel that to regard psychasthenia "as a psychic form of neurasthenia" (Dupres) is to want to force into this psychoneurosis phenomena which, in whatever way they may be interpreted, have nothing to do with it.

It is perfectly evident to us that a perversion or an obsession may serve as a continued emotional cause, and preside in this way at the establishing of superadded neurasthenic states. Nor does it seem at all doubtful that there are psychasthenics whose life has been injured by the mental disturbances which they have undergone, and who therefore may associate their more or less constitutional mental condition with a neurasthenic condition, or, in other words, that there are patients who have a mixture; we have seen numerous examples of such.

It is no less certain to us that the emotions which are directly created by mental disturbance may accentuate and reinforce various psychasthenic manifestations. But what seems to us the most important element of distinction is that the obsessions, the phobias, and the doubts of the psychasthenic are not in themselves either of an emotional origin or nature.

We know that psychiatrists have had long discussions on the intellectual or the emotional origin of obsessions. It seems to us perfectly legitimate to distinguish between an obsession as an intellectual phenomenon, and a preoccupation which is a phenomenon of emotional origin. Now, if the neurasthenic has preoccupations he does not have obsessions. As a matter of fact, the neurasthenic never presents those common obsessions of the psychasthenic which result in the association of hasty ideas which contain no element of logic but which persist in the patient's consciousness. Here, for example, is a psychasthenic who associates psychically some idea pertaining to her food or her toilet with the idea of death for herself or one of her family. Here is a doubting man who has given himself up to speculations and vain questionings. In what way do the manifestations presented by these patients approach those that we have observed in the neurasthenic? The latter may be haunted by the fear of death or the fear of harming some one, or he may become fixed upon some scruple. But all these preoccupations are frankly emotional in their origin and carry in themselves intrinsically, and not only consecutively as in the psychasthenic, some emotional element.

The psychasthenic may really have an emotional constitution, which is only one of the elements of his general psychological inferiority. But he has above all an abnormal mental constitution, while the emotional constitution is practically in a general sense only an exaggeration of a normal condition. Psychasthenia has its definite place on the ladder of the psychoses. But it is not a psychoneurosis.

If, now, however, we glance at hysterical manifestations, it will seem as though we ought to establish a few more distinctions. To tell the truth, there is only one which seems to us really important, and we think that it is perhaps pushing matters too far to place in hysteria the ensemble of phenomena which result from conscious or unconscious simulation. Can one consider those patients as afflicted with psychoneuroses who carry their really crazy ideas so far as to allow themselves to be mutilated, or to practice self-mutilation? These patients are really mental cases; they are mythomaniacs. It is very evident that their various objective organic symptoms spring from mental representations, and thus offer a clinical picture which closely approaches that of hysterical manifestations, just as we have recently seen that our exhausted patients, whether they were or were not neurasthenics, express their fatigue by the same subjective impressions and the same real impossibilities. But here again there is an element of differentiation which must be sought for in the very origin of the symptoms. No symptom whose origin does not lie in some emotional traumatism, and which has no relation to the various modes of physical emotion, or which is not due to the emotional inhibition of a certain number of mental representations, is, to our way of thinking, an hysterical symptom. That there may be associations formed, and that the mental frailty of the mythomaniac predisposes him to hysterical symptoms, we do not deny; but we do not believe that mythomania and hysteria may clinically be confused. To make our position perfectly clear, we will state frankly that the opinions of Babinski on hysteria refer to mythomania and not to hysteria, and that in no possible way could we confuse it with this latter psychosis.

Having now accomplished our work of disintegration, we feel that we can pursue our study, and show that these two autonomous psychoneuroses, hysteria and neurasthenia, are really, in themselves and in their various manifestations, both indisputably morbid entities.

CHAPTER XVI.

HOW ONE BECOMES NEURASTHENIC.

THE FIRST factor of the neurasthenic state whose rôle it is extremely important to define is emphatically constitutional predisposition. First of all, are there individuals who, by reason of their constitution, may unquestionably be regarded as being liable to neurasthenic attacks? It seems to us that, although certain subjects appear to be better armed, there are none who under repeated blows might not succumb sooner or later. We have seen a great many examples of patients who have all their life shown extraordinary resistance, who, although having led the most excitable kind of life that one could imagine, yet had always maintained complete mastery over themselves. Yet these same subjects, when attacked frequently in a way which at first sight might appear insignificant in comparison with former shocks, nevertheless become depressed or very emotional, lose their intellectual control, and sink into intensely neurasthenic states. But here a different element comes in, and we think that, along with constitutional predisposition, other elements may accidentally intervene to create transiently in a subject an affective constitution in such a way that he may become neurasthenic. In other words, we think that no neurasthenic state is possible without a peculiar antecedent psychological constitution. On the other hand, we are quite ready to admit that this psychological make-up may be either constitutional or accidental.

What, however, are the elements of this peculiar constitutional state? We are accustomed to saying, and it is a very true expression, that neurasthenia springs from what is called an emotional make-up. Here we must stop to understand the value of this term and to distinguish its characteristics. That the neurasthenic may be emotional in the physical sense of this word is a thing which cannot be denied, and we have already indicated our way of looking at this with sufficient distinction. It is this physical emotional constitution which dominates the pathogeny of the symptoms of the psychoneuroses, and which plays its part in hysteria or neurasthenia. It is by the necessary existence of this antecedent constitution in the neurasthenic, as well as in the hysteric, that we are sure of the relationship between these two psychoneuroses, which are considered by others as autonomous, because with this common constitutional element are associated, either in the hysteric or the neurasthenic, additional constitutional elements, which latter are peculiarly different according as they are considered in one or the other of these diseases.

The thing that appears to us to characterize the peculiar psychological constitution of the neurasthenic is the total absence of the power to be indifferent. Question a patient on this point. He will tell you that he has always taken things to heart. Although in the domain of pure consciousness he may be capable of close and exact reasoning, yet, when it comes to the application of everything that relates properly speaking to life, he feels more strongly than he reasons. Everything is personal to him. He thrills to excess, he responds in all cases much too strongly to be able to reflect without first being obliged to make an effort to control himself. His life is a perpetual struggle between his power of direction—or his will, if you prefer it—and his feelings. Very generally, however, and this is in the common sense of the word, the candidate for neurasthenia is over-sentimental. He has too much of what we are accustomed to call "heart." His affections are too strong, and sometimes a little jealous, and in the whole domain of affectivity he will feel special susceptibility. It would be both an error and an injustice to tax such subjects with a lack of will and faint-heartedness. They often have as much and even more courage and will than many others, and, in reality, there are hardly any but those who have a neurasthenic constitution who really accomplish anything in life. But if he has this quality which consists in taking life very seriously, the very excess of this quality becomes a defect in him and a danger to be avoided. This means palpably that his will, however vigorous it may be considered intrinsically, is, none the less, often put to tests which are too great and too frequently repeated. In so far as he is sentimental, he has a manifest tendency to play a passive part in life, and all action presupposes a preliminary struggle in him in bringing his will into play. Action, as far as he is concerned, is not an instinctive and almost unreasoning reaction. It is the result of the tension of his whole being in which his reasoning will comes in conflict with his feelings.

Such a mental constitution is a long way removed from the constitution of a psychasthenic. The latter is a weakling and a degenerate in many ways. It is rare for him to sin by excess of sentimentality. It is enough, in order to understand this, to call to mind the impressions made upon persons who have come in contact with psychasthenic subjects or individuals who have become neurasthenic. The latter have always been considered by those who lived with them as brave people, perhaps too scrupulous and too loyal, but possessing the power to attract strong, firm friendships; the former have given the impression of being selfish and indifferent, and incapable of arousing any sympathy. The difference is recognized even by the physicians who care for these patients; they become fond of the neurasthenic, but, in spite of all efforts they may make, it is rare for them to become friendly with psychasthenics. Reciprocally, the neurasthenic is a grateful patient, but one cannot always say as much for the psychasthenic.

This leads us to bring out into relief the difference which distinguishes the constitution of the emotions and affections which belongs and has always belonged to the neurasthenic, from the constitution of the psychasthenic. The latter may be of an emotional nature; that is understood. As a matter of fact, he generally is. Inversely, the neurasthenic, like the psychasthenic, may come to have, but more or less slowly, phobias and obsessions. But, as we have already said, while the obsessions and phobias of the psychasthenic spring from some fault of the mechanism, a fault which emotion may exaggerate, but which it does not directly create, quite the reverse is true of the neurasthenic. The latter does not become obsessed in the true sense of the word, but, rather, preoccupied, and only in a secondary way. When his intellectual control or his will has become deficient, he is invaded by impressions and sensations which he cannot prevent from becoming diffused in his consciousness, because he is unable to get hold of himself. It would be altogether wrong to look upon the neurasthenic as having the mental constitution of a man with phobias and obsessions. And likewise, as we have already said, it does not seem to us that we could consider psychasthenia as a peculiar constitutional form of neurasthenia. The future neurasthenic certainly has a constitutional predisposition, but this predisposition differs essentially from that of the psychasthenic in that from the start the latter is already sick, while at the start the future neurasthenic has only one fault, that of having an emotional nature accentuated by large-heartedness.

It is beyond all doubt that a manifest exaggeration of emotionalism, allied to a marked development of affected sentimentality, though not of sentiment, may accidentally break out in certain individuals and in this way favor the development of secondary neurasthenic states. This is all the more apt to happen in subjects who are organically affected in the general ensemble of their psychic faculty. Although exaggerated emotional states and tearful sentimentality form factors of these conditions, there are very frequently associated with them a more or less marked diminution of intelligence and an almost constant lack of will power. Such processes may be observed either as episodes or in a definite way. Here, for example, is a man fifty years of age, who previously had not shown any of the constitutional elements which one meets in future neurasthenics, but who nevertheless presents symptoms which are distinctly superposable to those of neurasthenia. However strongly inclined one might be to attribute the capital rôle to the psychological elements in the genesis of the psychoneuroses, it would be wrong to consider such a patient otherwise than one presenting mixed symptoms, functional symptoms in relation to psychological troubles which in themselves are of organic origin. Arteriosclerosis or insufficient renal development, etc., may be the cause of it; and the further one advances in the study of neuropaths the more one will find that, if among the so-called organics there are a great many functionals, among the nervous or those who pretend to be such there are also many who are organically afflicted. But in so far as the psychic defects may be constitutional or secondary, the results may remain the same. It is none the less true, from the pathogenic point of view, as well as from the point of view of prognosis, that there is a great distinction to be made between true neurasthenics all of whose symptoms are functional in nature and those patients who add a functional symptomatology to an organic symptomatology which often has every chance of becoming aggravated in consequence.

That like conditions of diffuse psychologic debility may be produced as the result of serious diseases is theoretically possible. Practically it appears to us quite exceptional.

What is more curious and less rare is a diffuse psychological modification which the uprising of a sudden and intense emotion may cause in an individual. We have seen subjects who up to a certain time had been remarkably resistant, but who, when caught in an accident or hurt in some way in their deepest feelings, underwent a change no less abrupt and intense than that which a great emotion might have caused. Serious neurasthenic conditions may follow and be developed as a result of troubles thus created. Such subjects, who up to that time had been calm, reasonable, with plenty of *sang froid*, sometimes even rather indifferent, have under the influence of emotion become extremely sensitive and emotional.

But the peculiar thing about all these conditions is the simultaneous attack upon intellectual control and the will, whereas in ordinary neurasthenia we have to do with subjects who have always been emotional and sentimental, but who have only lost control over themselves after a considerable length of time and heroic struggles. The self-control in such cases of neurasthenia following sudden emotion has been lost, at the same time that the character of the subject has changed in the way that we have just indicated.

It seems to us, therefore, that there is something peculiar in this, and that such affections, if we wish to preserve neurasthenia as a pathological entity, ought not to be included within the limits of our study.

Let us now study our candidate for neurasthenia with his emotional, affective, and sentimental constitution, and his tendency to exaggerate and magnify things, and to take them, as we have just said, too much to heart, and watch him in his struggle with life. When and how will he become neurasthenic?

It is evident that the different elements which we have studied in the preceding pages are going to come into play, and that his chances of becoming neurasthenic will be in proportion to the number of emotional shocks which he will experience, and the number of attacks upon his domain of peculiar susceptibility, and to the duration of each of his emotional preoccupations. They will be, on the other hand, inversely proportional to the degree in which he can conserve his intellectual control and to the resistance of his will. Here there is evidently a whole series of individual variations, and in the mastery of self in the subject who is constitutionally predisposed to neurasthenia one may find every degree. But it is the nature of one who is predisposed to be possessed of a limited resistance. No one who is predisposed may ever dare say that he will never become a neurasthenic; every chance is in favor of his becoming one if he undergoes any emotional excitement which is sufficiently strong and which lasts long enough.

The latter seems to us to be the chief factor in a certain number of given circumstances. Here, for example, is a subject having very great preoccupations concerning himself, which have, however, never made him lose his mastery over himself. Let a new emotional excitement come into play, and something very analogous to what occurs for a stimulated contraction of the cardiac muscle will then happen to voluntary consciousness. One knows that the muscle during its whole period of contraction does not react to any excitation by a new contraction. This is what has been called the law of periodic non-excitability of the heart. The same thing is true for the will of our subject, which, tense at the time when some new emotional excitation occurs, is incapable of opposing this new excitation by a new contraction. One can see then that under the influence of successive and different emotional stimuli, of which one is continuous and the other episodal, the subject who has resisted the former will become incapable of reacting to the latter, even though it in itself may be of mediocre value. It thus happens sometimes that even a slight additional emotional strain is enough completely to upset a mentality which has hitherto been resistant. This helps us to conceive of the mechanism of the action of slight emotional stimuli in the production of neurasthenia in those individuals whose will had been on a great strain for other reasons. This fact has its clinical value, because one is often astonished to see intense neurasthenic conditions attributed by the patients to very slight emotional causes.

On the other hand, this mechanism is comparatively rare, and it generally happens that life is quite able to furnish the predisposed with continuous exciting and emotional causes which are abundantly sufficient in themselves to overthrow the subject who after having held out for a greater or less length of time ends by finding himself completely overcome and dominated by some emotional cause.

It is not often that neurasthenic states make regular progress from the very beginning. Very often, on the contrary, they are produced in successive attacks occasioned by some continuous emotion. The subject will steel himself not to feel the emotion which he is aware is gaining a greater and greater control over him. But the duration of his voluntary resistance is all the shorter in proportion as the strain has been harder to bear and required the output of a greater effort. Just in the proportion that the emotional stimuli are repeated, so does the difficulty of getting hold of himself increase. Finally, the individual becomes incapable of reaction. He is no longer master of himself. His intellectual control has weakened. He is henceforth potentially ready to show all the psychic or physical manifestations of neurasthenia. He is already a neurasthenic, because he has entered into that condition which corresponds to the definition which we have given of neurasthenia,—namely, the whole group of phenomena which result from the non-adaptation of an individual to some emotional cause, and the struggle of the individual toward this adaptation.

It goes without saying that the moment the emotion, if it be of external origin, has reached the point where it dominates the patient's will and reason, it will establish itself as the leader of internal emotion.

All these ideas have been pointed out in the preceding chapters. What we must do now, starting from the point of view which we seem to have acquired, is to show how the various classic as well as the rarer symptoms of neurasthenic states have become established.

It generally happens that a physician pays very little attention to the mechanism which is present at the genesis of various symptoms presented by neurasthenics. This is because he more usually finds himself in the presence of patients belonging to that very special class of those whom we have already called "neurasthenics who have arrived." These latter present such a crowded and complex symptomatology that a pathogeny as unequivocal as a psychic pathogeny seems very difficult to accept. This is because the physician very rarely sees the neurasthenic at the beginning of his affection. In fact, the subject who has some real cause for continuous preoccupation and allows his mind to become invaded by emotion is already virtually and even actually a neurasthenic. He does not consider himself, however, as a sick man yet, and only goes to his physician some time later, when a whole series of secondary symptoms have appeared, of which the relation of cause and effect with the patient's emotional state is often not at all clear either to the physician or the patient. The whole difficulty then consists in finding out exactly the moment of the onset of the affection which has caused it. Before frankly becoming a neurasthenic with all the classical symptoms of a psychoneurosis, a subject may have been, perhaps for a considerable length of time, in a state of unstable equilibrium, so much so that often he does not date his disease back further than a few months, when sometimes, as a matter of fact, if he had included the whole series of phenomena, he would have gone back several years.

If one wants to classify the various manifestations presented by neurasthenics, then, one might say that they could be considered thus:

(1) Phenomena of simple emotional fatigue and psychic and physical disturbances in direct and immediate relation to emotional excitation.

(2) By reason of these disturbances, manifestations due to auto- and hetero-suggestion by deficient and disharmonic attitudes.

(3) After a greater or less length of time, symptoms of all kinds which are the immediate or remote results of functional troubles previously created.

In other words, we will say plainly that every neurasthenic goes through three phases,—a first phase of simple emotional disturbance, a second phase of functional disturbances, and a third phase where the various consequences of the general invasion of the organism by previous functional disturbances finally appear. It is very evident that such a division is somewhat schematic, and that in this succession of phenomena there is for any given period of time neither the coexistence nor necessary exclusion of disturbances presented during the preceding period, and it is just on this account that we find the extreme variability of the symptomatology presented by these patients.

Between the neurasthenic at the start of his disease, and the neurasthenic who has arrived, and the individual who only shows certain traces of some old neurasthenic condition, there may be every possible type of transition.

We lay it down, then, as a general rule, that, when one finds that one has a neurasthenic to treat and is trying to interpret his symptoms, it is always necessary to go back to the emotional cause, whether one has to seek it ten, fifteen, or twenty years before, because it is the thing which has brought about the whole series of consecutive manifestations presented by the patient, and, although the time of their development may sometimes be very short, it may also sometimes be very long.

Here, for example, is a lady fifty years of age, a false gastropath, considerably emaciated, who says that she has been sick for two years. If one tries to find some emotional cause during that period of her existence, one will discover nothing. In her case one has to go back twenty years. As a matter of fact, when she was about thirty she lost her husband, whom she had loved very much. At that time she was greatly overcome with grief. She had a whole series of functional disturbances, particularly emotional anorexia (this was the immediate emotional phenomenon). From that time she has never grown accustomed to the idea of her husband's death. Her emotionalism has become considerably greater. She has become very suggestible, and under some accidental influence she became in this way a false gastropath (a phase of secondary disturbance). Finally, by not eating enough, she grew very thin and weak (the later phase). Here is a patient who, presenting formerly a whole series of other troubles, appeared at first sight as a comparatively recent neurasthenic. In reality, psychologically speaking, she was neurasthenic from the day when under the influence of her great emotion she lost the full control of her will. According to our way of thinking, and we cannot repeat it too often, one is neurasthenic from the moment and during the time that the reason is carried away by emotion. One may or may not have symptoms: it is a question of surroundings, previous organization of life, etc. But in neurasthenia, apart from the initial psychological disturbances which are essential, almost everything, if not everything, is accidental.

Having said so much, let us take a patient corresponding to the type of the neurasthenic who has "arrived," of which we have just been speaking,—a physical or psychic major asthenic, presenting functional troubles of every kind, very thin, suffering from insomnia, having headache and pains in the back, in brief an ideal patient, presenting a complete picture of the excessive symptomatology of severe neurasthenia,—and let us see, in his case, how and by what mechanism all these phenomena which he presents have succeeded one another.

Question him. You will learn, first of all, that he has always been emotional and impressionable, and that he has always taken things too much to heart. His condition dates back at least eighteen months or two years. This, as a fact, is the time usually required for such a diffuse symptomatology to be developed. At that time a great preoccupation came into his life. Let us put it that, having no private means and being burdened with a family, he was threatened with the loss of the situation by which he supported himself and those depending upon him. His wife was a woman of rather weak character, and he could find no one on whom he could lean or from whom he could hope for any moral support. He kept his worry to himself. For a certain length of time nothing in particular happened, he was able to continue his work, but he already found that it required a greater effort on his part. From time to time he had a mental panic. He lost sight of his actual duties, and dreamed of the danger which was threatening him. His sleep became broken, often disturbed and interspersed with nightmares which would express at night the anxiety he felt during the day. By degrees his emotional condition increased. His mental panics were more frequent. His work became extremely difficult and fatiguing, because he thought more and more of the subject of his preoccupation and because he found it more and more difficult to keep control of himself. The least noise exasperated him; if any one asked him a question he jumped. His insomnia became very troublesome, and he would sometimes pass whole nights without sleeping.

Physical emotional phenomena of every kind appeared. Each time that he thought of his situation he felt nauseated. He would grow pale, or else would have a feeling of congestion and break out into perspiration. Sometimes he would have an attack of polyuria. At the table he felt no appetite and had to force himself to eat. He would only eat because he knew he must.

It is hardly necessary to say that such a struggle against an invading emotion cannot go on without causing a very appreciable physical and intellectual fatigue, expressing itself at this time by an impression that physical and intellectual fatigue is much more rapidly tiring than it should be normally. At this epoch brain fatigue may appear, which is expressed by a feeling of tension or, on the contrary, of cerebral emptiness. These are the very impressions that a healthy subject experiences after a too prolonged intellectual work.

Such are, very briefly outlined, the disturbances that our patient will show in the first phase. They may be summed up in a few words: physical and psychic phenomena directly due to emotional stimulation; phenomena of emotional fatigue and real fatigue, due to the excess of work which the constant struggle against the emotional cause imposes.

This situation will be prolonged; our patient is going to go on struggling; he will put forth every energy to keep his emotion from completely overwhelming him. Nevertheless, he has perceived that in spite of all his efforts his work is not so well done. If he were an accountant, he has made mistakes in his figures; if he had clerical work, he has forgotten part of a phrase in copying a letter. He has become restless. He has felt as though he were going mad, and has pictured himself incapable of work, not because he will have been dismissed, but because he really feels himself incapable on account of illness. When this happens, the last straw, if one might so call it, has fallen upon our patient, who, incapable of doing anything to help himself, sinks into the second phase of his illness. It is quite natural that none of these phenomena which have hitherto appeared should disappear on this account; quite the contrary. But new manifestations are going to appear. They will result from a double mechanism: auto-observation and auto- and hetero-suggestion. Our patient, whose intellectual control is now affected, becomes incapable of judging his impressions and of appreciating his various sensations in their true nature and origin.

All the ideas, which his cerebral automatism introduces into the field of consciousness, are preserved and ranked on the same plane. The filter of his voluntary consciousness is out of order, and our patient takes for a fact what is often only a memory which has been in some way mechanically evoked. By this process he may soon acquire phobias. The idea of sudden death or the thought of suicide will flit through his mind. These ideas seem as real to him as if he were entertaining them in earnest. He has a fear of sudden death, and a dread that he will want to commit suicide. He is afraid of doing harm to somebody. There are no ideas of this kind that one may not find, and which though normally fugitive may become fixed in the neurasthenic because they are not submitted to judgment. These phobic manifestations in themselves become factors of superadded emotional stimulation.

All intellectual work tires him, and soon it is impossible for him to do any work. His memory seems to be failing, because to call it forth from such a disorganized brain is evidently very difficult. Our patient even pretends that his intelligence is affected, and that he cannot understand things perfectly, that he can no longer follow the line of thought of the person who is speaking or the author he is reading. This may be quite possible: for he is perpetually somewhere else, perpetually distracted from everything that is going on around him by what is going on within him. He is continually absorbed in his own condition.

Does he attribute all the symptoms which he feels to their true cause,—viz., his emotional preoccupation? Very rarely. But this seems quite natural, because in such a patient his causal emotional preoccupation has already become merged in a large group of superadded phenomena. Physically and intellectually he grows weak; and it is then that he will say that he is sick. Now our patient will begin to watch and examine himself. Naturally he will experience various sensations which will be those resulting directly from emotional stimulation.

We have already spoken above of the peculiar orientation taken by emotional stimuli according to the particular case. We have said that normal individuals react somatically in various ways to emotion. In some it is the stomach which is upset; among others there is a certain disagreeable sensation which appears in the perineum or bladder. In still others emotion brings on palpitation of the heart, diarrhœa, or polyuria, and another will feel his legs give way beneath him. Whatever the subject may have felt, the memory of these sensations will remain. If he does not experience them again, he will have auto-suggestions about the sensations which he is going to experience, and, as a matter of fact, it is the particular fixation which he is most apt to have which will bring about physical reaction consecutive to the emotion on which our patient's auto-observation will become centred. He will have auto-suggestions about his stomach, or his intestines, or his heart, or his lungs, or his urinary duct. He will imagine himself afflicted with some mental or spinal disease. He will picture himself having heart trouble, or tuberculosis, or dyspepsia, or enterocolitis, etc. He may believe that he can have all of these at the same time. Now, if he begins to read and converse upon the subject and gather that little knowledge which is a dangerous thing, or, above all, if some physician turns his thoughts in an unhealthy direction, our subject, who often has at first had a little fear of everything, will now definitely fix his fears upon such or such an organ, which will become for him the centre of divergence for all the troubles he feels.

Thus by auto-observation and auto- and hetero-suggestion our patient will manage to have one or several somatic fixations. But here we must understand exactly what we mean by functional trouble. We have designated under this name the group of phenomena which may occur from the intervention of the psychism interfering with automatic normal functions. But does this mean that the troubles which are felt by our patient have no objective reality, that in a word they may be imaginary troubles? By no means, for our patient suffers exactly as much as if he had real organic troubles. The difference between what he experiences subjectively and what an individual who has real lesions experiences is purely a question of pathology. The tachycardia, or dysuria, or impotence, or gastro-intestinal atony which psychic impressions have created is by no means imaginary on that account. The subject really has palpitations and difficulty in urinating, or more or less complete genital insufficiency, or digestive troubles, just exactly as if he had exophthalmic goitre, or a stricture, or a castration,—just as if he had a cancer of the stomach, for example. The disturbance is no less real for being of psychic, suggestive, or emotional origin.

But outside of the direct action exercised by a psychical stimulus, which may itself be either exciting or inhibitory, on the function, other troubles occur which spring from a very peculiar mechanism which we have already described in the first part of this work. We allude to the disturbances due to disharmony. These are all troubles which result directly by the intervention of attention in the production of acts which are customarily automatic. We have seen this mechanism come in in the production of respiratory troubles, and in the disturbances of digestion and sleep. We have seen it play a considerable rôle in the production of the physical asthenia of the neurasthenic and of all those distressing fatigue symptoms of which they so often complain. We need not refer to them again.

There still remains a whole series of morbid manifestations of a more exclusively psychic nature. We mean "fixed memories." It may be an impression of anguish which sometimes has been fixed for a very long time under the form of a pain. It may be the memory of fatigue, which prolongs an impression of helplessness which the subject cannot make up his mind to throw off. This is the process which often encourages neurasthenics to retain symptoms which at a given time might have remained isolated without any other added phenomenon.

In short, our patient, by the various mechanisms which we have examined, has become, let us say, a major neurasthenic, presenting a whole series of functional troubles. He has now reached the second stage of his affection.

He may pass on to a third phase, to that in which he begins to feel all the consequences of the functional disturbances which he has hitherto presented. If anorexic or dyspeptic, he has probably cut down his food so much that a considerable loss of weight will have followed, bringing with it general depression and having a very great effect upon his bodily health. Let this condition persist for a long time, and he will very naturally become less resistant to and more liable to contract an infection; particularly will he be liable to acquire a tuberculosis.

It does not seem to us, on the other hand, to be anywhere proven that a functional trouble, though it be of purely psychic origin, may not in the long run create true organic lesions. And when the authors of former days included emotional causes in the etiology of a certain number of chronic affections, they perhaps expressed a truth which our too material age has done wrong to scorn. The saying "It was grief or his troubles which killed him" seems to us to have something more in it than a simple popular fiction.

At this period our patient might sometimes be a "mixed case," presenting still a whole series of functional manifestations, but also offering for our consideration certain symptoms which had slowly come to pass from organic modifications which the functional troubles had created. But if this were so, it would, as a rule, be rather rare.

Let us sum up, and we shall see that our patient by a rigorous chain of events, and starting from the single point of departure,—an overwhelming emotional preoccupation, with the loss of intellectual control,—must necessarily present all the phenomena which form the classical symptoms of neurasthenia.

Is there in this affection a single manifestation—we say, a single one only—which can seem to escape from the pathogenic mechanism which we have just developed? We do not believe so. It will be enough, however, to refer to the first part of this work, where as we described each of the functional manifestations we have attempted to bring out its particular pathogeny. Emotion, auto-observation, and auto- and hetero-suggestion, the production of functional troubles, sometimes the possibility of a later organic association—this is the whole history of a neurasthenic; and, if neurasthenia appears to be such a polymorphous affection, it is partly because one may see it in every period of its evolution, and also because the diversity of symptoms presented is due to the multiplicity of possible psychic orientations.

It is also true, that, although the symptomatology of a neurasthenic may sometimes be extremely complex, it may also in certain cases be relatively simple, and be limited to functional troubles in a given organic system. In this latter case it is generally a question less of neurasthenia, properly so called, than of lingering neurasthenic conditions. These are manifestations which have continued to develop on their own account when, the emotional cause having disappeared, and the subject having regained his intellectual control, there still persists, concerning some organ or function, such a conviction of helplessness, strengthened by the accumulation of auto- and hetero-suggestions, that the disturbances persist, even when the cause which originally created them has disappeared.

Thus, we may see people who continue to be false gastropaths, false urinaries, false cardiacs, and false genitals, etc., for a considerable length of time after the occurrence of emotional cause. Their minds are sound, their emotionalism is not really exaggerated, their intellectual control is normal for all that does not concern the functional trouble in question; but it is only necessary to question them to discover the emotional cause, and to realize that at a certain time they had lost their self-control, and it was on that account that a purely functional affection had the chance to develop in them.

However precise and localized the actual symptomatology of all such patients may be, they deserve just as much to be included in the picture of neurasthenia. Although it is with great difficulty, on account of the variability of its symptoms and symptomatic entity, that we can define this disease, nevertheless, it seems to us to have an absolute pathogenic autonomy. There is not one of the phenomena which neurasthenics may present which, either directly or by the intermediary stages which we have described, does not spring from the insufficient adaptation of the individual to some emotional cause, and from his struggle to adapt himself to it. Insufficient adaptation of an individual to an emotion gives us all the phenomena which result from loss of intellectual control which is the specific basis of neurasthenia; and the struggle for this adaptation gives us all the symptoms bearing upon the disordered attempts made by the subject to get hold of himself and to prevent the various functional manifestations which he presents. We cannot, therefore, speak of neurasthenic conditions. There is no such thing as digestive, sexual, or urinary neurasthenia, etc. Neurasthenia is an entity, and if, like any other disease, by disturbances which are more limited in a given region, it may take on certain aspects and peculiar forms, it has preserved none the less its full and complete autonomy.

CHAPTER XVII.

GENERAL CONCEPTIONS OF HYSTERICAL SYMPTOMS.

When, in the preceding pages, we set forth our general conception of neurasthenia and its symptoms, we were led to see that neurasthenia hardly ever develops except in one who is predisposed to it. Is the same thing true of hysteria and its symptoms?—do they only appear in subjects who have a peculiar mental constitution, or what we might call a specific constitution? Before we answer this it seems to us that we must first make a certain number of distinctions.

We have already said that we do not in any way consider that mythomaniacs are hysterics. The very peculiar mental condition of these patients should not, we feel, be regarded as forming a constitutional predisposition to hysteria and its symptoms. What, as a fact, is much more constitutional in the hysteric, is his excessive physical emotionalism, and again the very peculiar action of that emotion upon his psychism. Hysteria may be separated into two broad classes of symptoms. On the one hand there are all those which belong to hysterical attacks and emotional discharge, while on the other hand there are all those which either abruptly or slowly, but always following some emotion, become established in a way which is generally lasting, and unconnected with any attacks properly so called.

This distinction seems to us to be of importance, because, although certain authors consider that all hysteria expresses itself in attacks, we are far from accepting this point of view. We frankly say, on the other hand, that the attack is the least specific thing in hysteria. Between an emotional syncope, or a motor agitation, which the most self-contained individual is liable to feel under the influence of some great emotional shock, and the most characteristic hysterical attacks there exists every gradation. There are some subjects who have a single hysterical attack during their life resulting from the shock of some great emotional excitement. Neither before this attack nor ever afterward have they presented, nor will they present, any hysterical manifestation whatsoever. In short, an hysterical attack is only an emotional discharge. Under the influence of emotion there would evidently be all the more chance of its recurring, because the subject in question would be more emotional than usual. But, in matters of nervous attacks, we are not at all convinced that there is anybody who is absolutely proof against them. There are some people for whom a very slight emotion is enough to start off an attack. There are others who only react in the form of an attack when they are under excessive emotional stress.

In fact, it would seem that from this point of view there is no qualitative difference in the subjects, but that it is simply a question of emotional degree which varies according to the individual. So far, and so far only, can one admit, as far as hysterical attacks are concerned, the existence of individual predispositions which characterizes the more intense reaction to slight emotional excitement. Naturally it must be understood that we are not thinking now of people who like theatrical effects, and who at the slightest annoyance go off into an attack of hysterics, which they themselves know is more than half put on. These patients, as we have already said, are mythomaniacs, if you will, but not hysterics in the very special sense which we attach to this term.

The same thing is by no means true as far as hysterical accidents, properly so called, are concerned. For here, on the other hand, we are very much inclined to attribute considerable influence to the peculiar mental make-up of the subject.

First of all, the candidate for hysterical symptoms possesses a specificity in his physical emotional reaction to a greater degree than the eventual neurasthenic. In addition to the fact that he reacts much more intensely to an emotional stimulus, which is sometimes very trivial, he reacts again and more often in a given physical region, in a way that is almost constant for a given subject, whatever may be the emotion that is at work. That hysteric who later will show functional paraplegia has always felt, no matter what may be the emotion that she is experiencing, that her legs were giving way beneath her. This other has always felt her emotional reactions expressed by a sensation of weakness in the left side. Let some emotion that is stronger than usual overwhelm her, and she will become an hysterical hemiplegic. This is a very frequent phenomenon, and one which we have had the opportunity of seeing a great many times in patients having hysterical symptoms.

What is even much more characteristic is the dissociating action of emotion in the hysteric. In the neurasthenic an emotional stimulus with the physical reaction which it provokes serves as a starting-point for some psychic fixation. All the phenomena which follow spring from this psychic fixation and from the intervention in the functioning of the organs of such phenomena as observation and attention. In the hysteric it is just the opposite thing which occurs. It would seem as though the psychism were composed of badly grouped elements, which emotional excitement is capable of dissociating, surrendering an organ or a functional group to the whim of the will. This is the peculiar feature in the general mentality of hysterics. They are unstable, incoördinated, psychically speaking, in a degree which evidently differs according to subjects, but is always quite distinctly marked. Their mentality has been compared, and not without reason, to that of a child. Their ideas follow one another but never take root. The psychological mechanism of coördination, ideas of time, sequence, and causality, are almost foreign to them. They are, if we might use the expression, "badly put together." As a matter of fact, their centres of mental representation of the various organic functions behave, under the stress of emotion, as if they were quite independent of one another. From this, moreover, arises in these patients the very great specificity of emotional reactions, and, outside of all symptoms which have to do with attacks, the slight degree of diffusion and localization of their symptoms.

All these symptoms have a common characteristic. They are phenomena of immobilization, of psychic forgetfulness, if one might so call them. An hysteric who becomes paraplegic acts as though he has forgotten that he has limbs. In the same way an hysterical hemiplegic has lost the mental representations which correspond to a whole half of her body. This is the rule. It is, however, far from being absolute, and it may happen, on the contrary, that a new representation brought about by some emotional excitement may be added and superposed upon the previous mental representations. Such a representation, without any struggle on the part of the subject, without his having even been aware of it, becomes an integral part of his mentality, and tends to take definite part in it. The thing, therefore, that characterizes the constitutional mentality of the hysteric is his absolute passivity concerning his more or less marked defect of coördination.

This passivity is found in the hysteric once the symptom has been created. While the neurasthenic is restless and preoccupied, while he becomes obsessed concerning his symptoms and is wholly uneasy about them, nothing of the sort may be observed in the hysteric. Were he quadriplegic, it would make no difference to him. This indifference of the hysteric concerning his symptoms constitutes a very peculiar element in this class of patients. But this very special mentality is a natural result of the mechanism of dissociation or passive disintegration which was present when his symptom arose. The paraplegic hysteric has forgotten in some fashion that he ever had limbs. He no longer seems to be aware that he has any. In fact, he acts as if he never had had any, and as if he had never known what it was to walk. The same observations could be made in regard to hysterical deafness, amaurosis, dumbness, and contractures.

Before as well as after his infirmity, the hysteric is in no way preoccupied or liable to obsessions. In that again he differs profoundly from the neurasthenic.

This mental fragility, this lack of psychic coherence, this passivity of the hysteric make it evident that he may be suggestible. He has no power to keep out any ideas which, by the mechanism of the association of ideas and memory, his psychological automatism introduces into his consciousness. In the same way he would consider as real the ideas which had been introduced to him by some hetero-suggestion. But we must make some reserves on this point. The psychological automatons who have served as objects of study for a great many physicians and some psychologists are, almost without exception, perfectly *au courant* with medical observations, and naturally are subjects who have had a long and careful education. These individuals of double personality who are turn-about automatons or conscious beings are but very seldom met by the most experienced physician in his career.

Concerning suggestibility during hypnotic sleep we have nothing to say. We belong to those who think that hypnotism in itself is a method that ought not to be employed. Moreover, does not hypnotic sleep contain, according to our way of thinking, something specifically hysterical? For, looking at it in this way everybody would be more or less hysterical in different degrees. We, therefore, only wish here to take up suggestibility in a waking condition. It must be sufficiently widespread for certain authors to try to base their doctrinal theories of hysteria on extreme suggestibility. One cannot, however, make any nosological distinctions among neuropaths on the ground of suggestibility. Every being is more or less suggestible while in a waking condition, and that is why we have just said that everybody would be more or less hysterical. The neurasthenic himself is still much more auto- and hetero-suggestible than the hysteric, but the mentality is wholly different in these two cases. The first is too much preoccupied with the symptoms with which he is afflicted, while the second, on the contrary, does not pay enough attention to them.

But, on the other hand, one cannot by suggestion bring up at will symptoms in hysterics, any more than one can at will cure these same symptoms. Emotion alone, which is much more powerful than any suggestion, is capable in these subjects, predisposed by their mentality, of creating symptoms by dissociation or by addition and almost certainly in the domain previously determined by the emotional specificity of the subject. But the idea that one can create such symptoms as contractures and paralyses, without provoking emotional states, merely by mental suggestion, in a domain where an hysteric has never been previously afflicted, seems to us far from being easy to grasp, with the exception—it must be understood—of the mythomaniacs and the specially educated.

It is no less true that in the persistence of certain hysterical symptoms, in the continuity of dissociation which emotion has primitively produced, we would very willingly admit the intervention of auto-suggestion, which although certainly not constant is nevertheless frequent. Already this auto-suggestion would be more or less directly created by the memory of the emotional cause and of the phenomena felt during the action of the emotional shock. If the hysteric is indifferent to the symptoms which he presents, it must also be true that he is insensible to the very cause which has determined them, and it is by this intermediary that a suggestive reinforcement of the symptoms may sometimes be produced.

In the great majority of cases the hysterical symptom succeeds the emotional shock. This emotion may act in two different ways: it may directly create a symptom, but it may also act by exaggerating the constitutional mental predisposition of the subject. There is no doubt that an extremely lively emotion may exercise a dissociating action on the mentality, and that in a very large measure it may create this peculiar psychic soil on which the hysterical symptom may be developed. We do not think, however, that this would be so in the majority of cases, and we recognize, as a matter of fact, that the mental predisposition is more often constitutional than acquired.

The very exaggeration, in comparison with the normal state of emotional susceptibility, or the emotional soil if one prefers it, which constitutes one of the conditions of the production of hysterical symptoms, may in itself also be an accidental acquisition, for which the action of lively and repeated emotion, or even simply a continued emotional preoccupation, is responsible. But these are very rare cases, and it is just because, by reason of his habitual mentality, although the hysteric reacts sharply to external emotional shocks, yet he hardly ever becomes emotionally preoccupied or has internal emotions. Cases of this kind, nevertheless, exist, but belong rather to hysteroneurasthenics than to pure hysteria.

If we sum up what has gone before, we would say then: there are subjects who are more readily liable to become hysteric than others by virtue of their emotional as well as their mental constitution, which is more often congenital, but which may also often be acquired. This mental constitution is not to be confounded with suggestibility if, however, one excludes the suggested idea which is strongly reinforced by emotion. Finally, the individual predisposition by the particular kind of emotional orientation of the subject may in a great degree fix the seat of the eventful hysterical symptom.

But in the genesis of an hysterical symptom one must not only take into account the personal factors of the subject who is afflicted with the symptoms. The rôle of emotional shock in the localization of the hysterical symptom is none the less considerable. A woman learns suddenly of the death of one of her family, and experiences some unpleasant sensation. This is one of those cases where in the simple localization of symptoms there will be brought into play specific individual emotional reactions. If the emotional shocks are expressed at that time by a giving way of the limbs, or by difficulty in speech, or by a sensation of numbness on the left side, the subject may have a paraplegia or mutism or hemianæsthesia. Here, on the other hand, is a woman who shows a contracture of the right arm, which came on suddenly when in a moment of anger she wanted to strike her husband. Here, on the other hand, is a young girl the adductors of whose lower limbs are contracted. This contracture followed an attempted rape. It is evident that in these two cases it was the very nature of the emotional traumatism which determined the seat of the symptoms, and the patient became immobilized, in the latter case in a position of defence and in the former in a position of attack. When under other circumstances an hysterical paralysis is located in the limb which was hurt during the traumatism, we would again have a case where the very nature of the shock which was experienced would have determined the seat of the hysterical symptom. There is then a second factor of localization of hysterical symptoms which has its very great importance.

Although we may be quite unprepared to understand the why and wherefore of the specificity of individual emotional reactions, we can better grasp the general mode of action of the emotional cause. It is not a simple thing to do. It is, nevertheless, a feasible thing, while remaining always within the domain of hypothesis.

It seems to us it is by bringing together a sufficient number of cases where the hysterical symptom immediately succeeds the emotional shock, that one can most easily gain an idea of the mechanism which has been present at the establishment of the difficulties which our patients show. We have already said that we consider hysterical accidents as being more often phenomena of dissociation. Now, things happen exactly as if the ensemble which is formed by the psychic centre and the member or the organ which depends upon it, and which the emotional shock has dissociated from general consciousness, continued to functionate autonomously, according to the impulsion felt at the moment when the dissociation was established.

This is a rule which seems to us to be applicable not only to symptoms whose localization is due to some peculiar emotional stimulus, but as well to those which owe their localization to individual emotional specificity. This latter is a still more mysterious mechanism.

Let us take the subject who, under the influence of some emotion, feels his limbs give way under him and who develops a paraplegia. Here dissociation has taken place; the lower limbs have in some way escaped from the voluntary control of our patient when they were under an inhibiting influence. Thus there is established a flaccid paraplegia.

Let us, on the other hand, consider the patient who has had an adduction contracture as a result of an attempted rape. Her limbs were drawn up the moment they experienced the motor stimulus of defence. It is no longer a paraplegia, but a contracture which one then observes.

The same process of reasoning, it seems to us, might be applied to the great majority of hysterical symptoms. It is not strictly applicable to trophic or cutaneous disturbances. These can be explained by the continuity of vasomotor or trophoneurotic action.

It is, however, very true that this is really merely a theory, and we do not pretend to lay it down as anything else but an hypothesis which satisfies the mind.

We have already said elsewhere what we think concerning the period of incubation of hysterical symptoms. We have shown that in reality it was chiefly a period of emotional incubation, and that the time between did not represent the necessary time for the subject to adapt himself to a given hysterical symptom, but rather the time which would permit the emotion to develop and extend and accentuate its action.

As to the systematization even of hysterical symptoms, we have already indicated elsewhere that it took place according to the scheme of mental representations, and it follows that, long before having been a bulbar phenomenon, emotion is a phenomenon of psychic localization. The great majority of hysterical symptoms, particularly the anæsthesiæ, contractures, and paralyses, conform to a topography which corresponds to intellectual acquisitions, and not according to anatomical or functional localization. It is not the region of the nerve or a spinal-cord segment or a region of the psychomotor cortex which is afflicted; it is the territory of one or several of a great number of mental representations. These are, for example, all the conscious or subconscious ideas which preside over the movement or the sensibility of a part of a limb, or a member, or half of the body, which are no longer capable of being called forth, or which no longer reach the field of general consciousness, because, as we have just said, there has been, under the influence of emotional shock, a dissociation or exclusion in some way of the psychism of the subject of all the ideas leading to the zone which is thus afflicted. Emotion acts, in fact, as suggestion would act by dissociation, by retrenchment, and by exclusion. There is nothing extraordinary in stating that the hysterical manifestations may act objectively, as do phenomena of suggestion. It is such an appearance which, we feel, has permitted the suggestion theory of hysteria to be established with some appearance of truth. But, although the effects may be identical, it is by no means legitimate to infer that they spring from the same cause.

It may happen that under certain circumstances a different mechanism intervenes, and that, by reason of an emotional traumatism, ideas springing from subconsciousness and the psychological automatism, and brought about themselves more or less directly by emotional shock, will penetrate and invade the field of consciousness, where, not being critically judged (as the subject is, at the time, incapable of all intellectual control); they are admitted. The symptom is thus born by the addition to the previous mentality of the individual of a new idea which has not been judged, and will follow the scheme of mental representations. Here again we find parallelism with certain phenomena of suggestion.

But in one case or the other the hysterical symptom always appears as being a residue, or an emotional relic.

However this may be, it seems to us that the domain of hysteria may in fact be limited to the very domain of physical and psychic emotional reactions. Everything that an emotion may create in an accidental and transient way hysteria may accomplish in a lasting way. This is a doctrine which we already have had occasion to formulate during the course of this work, and, in the different functional manifestations of an hysterical nature that we have had occasion to take up, we have tried to bring out the value of such a delimitation of hysterical symptoms.

We shall not linger any longer on this necessarily rather theoretic chapter of the general conceptions of hysteric symptoms. Once having laid down our method, we have already had a great many opportunities to develop our way of looking at it. We have shown that, although we admit the secondary intervention of suggestion in the persistence of hysteric symptoms, it does not play, according to our way of thinking, anything more than an infinitely small rôle, if any, in the genesis of these symptoms.

We have said, and repeated, that at the basis of hysteria we must place emotional shock as the capital and almost exclusive pathogenic factor. We have shown how much confusion results from classifying as hysterics those patients who have been completely changed by a long-continued education or training, or else from classifying them with mythomaniacs whose relationship with hysterics seems to us to be quite effaced.

It now remains for us to complete this study by etiological considerations on the relative frequency of hysteria in men and women, by the nature and frequency of emotional causes capable of creating the symptoms with which we have been interested. All these questions have been so frequently and completely treated by so many authors that it seems useless to dwell on them anew. Being somewhat in haste to arrive at the practical and therapeutic part of this work, we think we can sum up all that has gone before by saying, that, just as in general pathology one groups under a single term all the troubles which spring from the same pathogenic cause, in the same way in neurology it seems to us quite as legitimate to study under the common term psychoneurosis the symptomatic mechanisms which recognize emotion as a general and immediate pathogenic factor.

According to the ground on which the seed falls emotion will exercise its action. Sometimes it is neurasthenia which will be developed, and sometimes it will be hysteria with all its symptoms which will manifest itself.

The psychoneuroses thus have a common pathogeny, emotion. But with the same cause very different effects may follow, according to individual predisposition, and, although there may be an autonomy of the psychoneuroses, there is also an autonomy of two types which they may present: neurasthenia and hysteria have each their pathologic entity. The neurasthenic and the hysteric are distinct individuals with an utterly different development, who nevertheless belong to the same family.

CHAPTER XVIII.

GENERAL CONCEPTION OF FUNCTIONAL MANIFESTATIONS.

BEFORE finishing the second part of our work, it seems to us that it would be useful to define clearly our conception of functional manifestations. In general medicine they describe as functional symptoms —and one studies them in nearly every affection along with local and general symptoms—all the disturbances, taken as a whole, which any lesion whatsoever may occasion in the functions of an organ. If, for example, we were considering a pyloric stenosis of organic nature, the gastric stasis and vomiting which would follow would be called functional symptoms.

From all that we have said before, it is very plainly to be seen that the functional manifestation of the neuropath has no single point of contact—apart from the involvement of the same function—with the functional symptom of a patient who has some organic disease.

To express it in a provisional definition which is intended to be limited simply to the subject of our work, we have considered as functional manifestations the ensemble of disturbances and persistent symptoms of which neuropaths complain and which are created in these patients outside of all antecedent somatic lesion.

It seems to us that we are now sufficiently prepared to define functional manifestations in a shorter, fuller, and more concise manner. They consist of all disturbances of psychic origin which are liable to affect the functions. They represent all psychic actions on the bodily organs.

It is this action of the psychism on the physical which is generally very badly understood. There are some ideas which to the present medical generation, accustomed to organic interpretations, form a sort of dead line.

One will readily admit that in certain cases a symptomatology may be purely subjective; that it will have no objective foundation, nor any organic reality. But in such cases one will take it for granted that the subjects who present this symptomatology are imaginary invalids, or hypochondriacs.

One will readily recognize, on the other hand, that there are such things as neuropathic disturbances in an organ which have created no organic change in the organ in question. But one will then refer the symptoms in question to some disturbance of innervation. The spinal ganglia, the major sympathetic nervous system will be brought into play; one will explain such and such a symptom by neuralgia of the solar plexus, or of the cœliac ganglion. One will use it to support some doctrine of the existence of painful zones, more or less distinctly superposed on the sympathetic regions which they hold to be afflicted. And they pay no attention to the fact that by the intercalation of a greater or less number of neurons there is at the extremity of each nerve-fibre a psychic cell; that this may be modified in its dynamism—though this is merely a word—or that it may be subjected to some alteration, whatever it may be, is no less constant than the fact that the whole nervous mechanism on which it depends, but which is also dependent on it, will suffer in its functioning and with it the organ to which it goes.

Let us take a simple phenomenon like pain. It is noteworthy that attention increases it and distraction diminishes it, even while the organic cause of the suffering remains constant. The subjective pain phenomenon thus appears to be only a relation between the degree of physical stimulus and the degree of psychic receptivity. But physical stimulus is not even necessary to produce pain. A psychic stimulus is all that is needed by the common mechanism of memory and by the mediation of emotional anguish, which is responsible for so many localized pains, for an impression of pain to be produced in the psychic centre, and for the periphery to become hyperæsthetic, because then normal sensation is perceived as pain.

That, on the other hand, there exist a whole series of psychosecretory, psychomotor, and psychotrophic functional disturbances is not even open to question. Such are admitted to be facts, especially as far as the digestive functions are concerned. What necessity is there, then, to interpose, between a peripheral disturbance of an organ and a disturbance of its psychic centre, which was the cause, any change or modification of the nervous pathway which unites the centre to the peripheral organ?

In nervous pathology the idea is the same as the thing itself, from the subjective point of view, and in a very large degree it is capable of creating it objectively.

In the same way, for example, when we set forth our conception of false gastropathies it would have been quite inexact for us to say that there is no such thing as dilatation of the stomach or hyperchlorhydria, nor hypochlorhydria, etc.; but we admit that an individual whose mind is psychically fixed upon his stomach after he has experienced some inhibitions, which is more frequently the case, or becomes very excitable, is liable, as a result of his psychical impressions, to have a gastro-intestinal atony, with great dilatation and hypochlorhydria, or, on the other hand, symptoms of secretory stimulation leaning to hyperchlorhydria. Study the false intestinals, the false cardiacs, the false pulmonaries, etc., and phenomena of the same kind will be found. It is not the objective reality of the symptoms presented by the patient that we are contesting; it is the belief in their peripheral origin.

We have seen elsewhere, that, in certain cases following functional troubles, organic affections would start up which were directly caused by them. In this we have the very proof that we cannot in any degree confound a functional manifestation with a purely and simply imaginary phenomenon. We think, in other words, that, in the harmony which tends to establish itself between the mental representation and the peripheral condition, if the mental representation is primary the peripheral disturbance will be secondary.

Such a conception is by no means a pure figment of the mind. It is admitted by everybody as far as the gastric secretion, for example, is concerned. It is the very basis of the normal functioning of the sexual organs. The extension which we have given to it seems to us to be entirely legitimate. As the facts oblige us to admit that a psychic modification is capable of modifying the functioning of given organs, we really do not see, then, how in the relations between the psychism and the organic functions one could strictly limit to certain functions what from all evidence must be a general law.

Therefore, a functional manifestation is characterized by an antecedent psychic disturbance, but also by consecutive peripheral disturbances.

This idea is of the greatest therapeutic importance. But here, even those authors who admit the primary psychical nature of functional manifestations are divided into two schools. One wishes the patients to be treated in a bilateral manner,—that is to say, for the peripheral disturbances which they present and for the psychical condition which is the cause of them. The other, for very definite reasons, thinks that a psychic pathogeny requires an equally psychic therapy. And this brings us directly to the third and last part of our work, where we shall take up the question of treatment, and in particular the psychotherapy of the psychoneuroses.

THIRD PART

The Treatment of the Psychoneuroses.

Psychotherapy and its Adjuvant Processes.

CHAPTER XIX.

CRITICAL STUDY OF THE TREATMENT OF THE PSYCHONEUROSES.

There has been a marvellous evolution in therapeutics during the last few years. From being symptomatic, as it used to be, there is a greater and greater tendency for it to become pathogenic. Medicine no longer attacks the symptom, which, considered in itself, has only a slight indicative value. It concerns itself only with the actual causes of the disturbances which it has to treat. Specific treatments, like that for syphilis or malaria, by mercury or quinine; specific treatments such as serotherapy, and specific treatments such as psychotherapy, which in the presence of affections of psychic origin essays to cure them by psychic action. In short, as medicine progresses, one sees more and more that very little of the old therapeutic arsenal remains, except those remedies which were specific without the fact having been known. This is still the case for mercury and quinine.

That is to say, that in our conception of the psychoneuroses we see no place for drug therapy. That it may from time to time find some indication in an added phenomenon not depending on psychical causes is possible; that sometimes one may help a patient, or at least be able to palliate his symptoms, by means of medication may also happen; but the time has passed when one could pretend to do a good piece of medical work by saturating an hysteric or neurasthenic with bromide or phosphorus. This therapy has lived its day, and we feel that it is time to condemn it, without any circumlocution or restriction.

Naturally, it will always be more easy for a physician to give a patient a prescription, with the therapeutic conclusions which such practices lead to, than to draw forth clearly the psychic or moral cause of the disturbances presented by him. Of course there are patients who, if they leave a physician without having managed to get a prescription or a new régime out of him, will imagine that their consultation has been worth nothing. But if we are not mistaken, a very distinct evolution has begun which has reached even the great public who are sick. They are beginning everywhere to grasp the idea that functional diseases may be treated psychically. If there are really still a great number of neuropaths whose tendency is to run after the honeyed words of a mesmerizer, or even the conjurer of the neighborhood or of their city, we are convinced that it will not be very long before all nervous patients will demand from every physician whether he knows how to treat them by psychotherapy.

It is understood that drug therapy may, in a certain measure, be considered as psychic therapy, but in the wrong sense of the word; and many physicians, even among those who are persuaded of the real psychic origin of the psychoneuroses, lend themselves to this practice.

It will help, they say, if only through suggestion. Whether you order bromides or glycerophosphates, or whether, graced by a more or less high-sounding Greek or Latin name, you prescribe pills of bread crumbs or dandelion, you are acting exactly the same way. If you manage to convince your patient that the medicine prescribed will do him good, there is a very good chance that this will be the fact, and, although you have chosen an indirect method of medication, you will succeed in improving his condition.

Nevertheless, such practices seem to us to be wholly without value. First of all, we hold that one has no right to deceive patients and abuse their credulity. On the other hand, although the medicines may be sufficiently suggestive, they cannot help but cost money. This inconvenience is trifling, one will say. Perhaps so; still, one should not forget that there are certain neuroses among the poorer classes as well as among the rich, and, when by the aid of a great many medicines and of repeated prescriptions you have successively "ameliorated" all the symptoms presented by your patient, you will find him more profoundly neurasthenic than ever, because, being incapable of work, he will have practised the strictest economy in order to buy food. We see too many of these heart-breaking examples in the hospital clientele. But even with the rich patients the method is equally dangerous and quite as inefficacious.

By medication you may ameliorate the gastric or intestinal conditions. Your patient will complain less of his head, or of his kidneys, or his legs, or his asthenia; he will carry about with him a whole series of little vials for some specific suggestive action. He will keep, carefully locked in a cabinet, powders which will cure headache, others that will help his digestion, others that will make him sleep sooner, and often he will not hesitate to have himself subcutaneously injected every month with various tonics that will have the same effect upon him as a whip upon a tired horse.

The suggestive action of medication is, however, supposed to be going on all this time; and the physician will feel triumphant when, on asking his patient, "Well, how is your stomach acting now? how are your kidneys? are you sleeping any better?" etc., and the latter will reply, "Doctor, it seems to me that I am a little better in that way."

Things will go on better, in fact, until some day the patient will perceive that, although he is a little better in each successive point, he nevertheless, taking all in all, feels just as ill as he did before. On that day he will become desperate, and, more likely than not, he will turn against his physician who will have "humored" him, or "occupied" him in such a way as to stop all his activity by the multiplicity of his daily prescriptions. We have seen patients whose whole day was taken up by the treatments to which they were supposed to devote themselves. We have met others who weighed their food, who measured their drinks down to a teaspoonful, because some insidious analysis of urine had shown an excess of such and such a product and an insufficient quantity of some other, which was to be compensated for either by increase or diminution in the matter of food. Certainly during the time that they gave themselves up to all these little ceremonies the patients were distracted, and in their care forgot the very cause which necessitated them.

But all the same, in the end, when the weary and discouraged patient has thrown over his physic and his physician, he will not be able to give up all at once the habits of over-observation which he will have contracted, nor will he renounce that conviction which has been implanted in him that it is outside of himself and in the therapeutic resources which chemistry and physics furnish to the physician that he ought to find his cure. He will repudiate his medications and his doctor, but it will only be to turn to some other physician and to get some other medicine.

It would be hard to say how much time may be lost in this way by patients. We have seen some who have been in miserable health for five, ten, or twenty years. There are some who have drugged themselves during their whole life. There are some people who, without any question, have devoured what would amount to the contents of a whole pharmacy in some small country town, and who have on this account a worn-out stomach and suffer from what is justly entitled medicinal gastritis. Do not let any one imagine that by such processes the physician gains the confidence of his patient, and that, merely by varying his prescription and changing his medications, whose action is useless, he will be assured of his patient's fidelity. Nothing is more false. We have known neuropaths who have consulted ten, twenty, thirty physicians. That is nothing. We have seen a list of fifty-six physicians consulted by a false gastropath in the space of a few years, and a certain patient whom we know, who is unquestionably neurasthenic and not hypochondriacal, changes his physician every two months on an average. He has been sick sixteen years. Imagine his bills.

Therefore, no medication for neuropaths. The method is dangerous and inefficacious, and its greatest inconvenience is the fact that it gives the patient's psychism an orientation which is directly opposed to that which one wants to see him take. No medicine, we say, except what may be quite incidental, for it is perfectly evident that one would be justified in giving a few grains of quinine to a neurasthenic who has a touch of the grippe. But the medication of the wonder-working doctor who wants to exercise suggestion, and the medication of the organicist physician who pretends to reduce a theoretic nervous exhaustion or an external irritability, are equally dangerous, and ought to be equally proscribed.

As for physiotherapy, which is bad if it pretends to be pathogenic therapy, it may, on the contrary, be indicated, and give good results if it consents to be nothing more than the practice of general hygiene appropriate to certain given constitutions.

The only proper treatment for the psychoneuroses, therefore, is psychic treatment. Although by no means all, yet a very great number of neurologists have come to agree upon this point. But there are a great many differences of opinion concerning the psychotherapeutic methods to be employed.

We shall not dwell upon methods of indirect suggestion. They are those which act in exactly the same way as a medicine or any therapeutic proceeding whatsoever to produce upon the subject, without consulting his reason or his will and without any direct action of the physician, a suggestion which might be favorable. These are medical tricks. One should never forget that it is not enough to make the symptoms disappear in order to have accomplished a real therapeutic result in the neuropath. It is necessary to change his mental state, to explain to him how and why he has fallen ill, and how and why if once cured he cannot slip back again because he will have regained the mastery over himself. With miraculous proceedings it is only the symptom which is treated, which, in our opinion, is absolutely insufficient. From our point of view, there is only one series of cases where a physician should have the right to use any proceedings of this kind, and that is where certain sexual neuropaths are concerned. We shall see why further on.

In a general way psychotherapeutic methods are divided into two large classes,—namely, on the one hand methods of direct suggestion, and on the other methods of persuasion. The difference which exists between these two methods is very important. The former pretend to introduce into the consciousness of the subject new ideas, or to destroy existing ideas, without his consent and judgment. The latter want the new ideas to be introduced with the consent of the subject, and if he abandons a conception by means of his treatment this abandonment must be made voluntarily after reflection and with full knowledge of the cause.

Direct Suggestion.—Direct suggestion is only addressed to the psychological automatism, and theoretically it would be all the more perfect and easy if the subject to whom it is addressed would permit very few phenomena of consciousness to intervene during the course of the suggestive act.

The partisans of direct suggestion are, therefore, logical, within their own lines, when they demand that their therapeutic action should be exercised during hypnotic sleep. During these states what is called forth, as well as what is acquired, is done independently of all conscious will on the part of the patient. The action of the physician is all-powerful, and he may at his pleasure add to or withdraw from the psychism of the patient ideas which seem to him useless or dangerous. The suggestive action is not limited to the suppression of various somatic symptoms presented by the patients, but may also be pedagogic in its nature. One may in an hypnotic sleep undertake the education of emotional states, and the education of the will, and analyze and modify the specific psychological reaction of each individual. Such is at least the conception of physicians who are hypnotists. This point of view demands discussion.

Hypnotism raises, first of all, serious questions of a moral and social nature. It is no small problem, in fact, for a physician to ask himself whether he has the right to suppress the free will of a subject, and make it act according to his ideas, even though he have a therapeutic end in view. But this is not the chief question. It resides chiefly in the education of the automatism which, to our way of thinking, is, if not the constant, at least the very frequent result of repeated hypnotic practices. To be convinced of this one has only to see what has become of the educated hysterics of former times. They are for the most part very helpless people, incapable of guiding themselves alone through life. Since the period when they were used as experimental mediums there is only a very small number of them who have been able to go back to normal life. One cannot with impunity accustom a subject to accept suggestions from others. It is a direct and negative attack on the individual personality which is thus put into practice, and, although the personality may be modified by hypnotism, it is most assuredly not along the line of its development, but rather in the line of deterioration and weakness. The reason that for a certain number of years no one perceived the dangers of hypnotism was because one could not see its remote results. In our days, further removed from the starting of the method, we are able to state that it presents a great many dangers which more than overbalance the advantages which may arise from it. It is true that one cannot always make certain neuropathic symptoms disappear as rapidly with persuasion as by hypnotic suggestion. But what advantage is there in suppressing the symptoms if the underlying foundation remains, and all the more if this foundation is modified in such a way that new symptoms will have a better chance of developing upon it?

Hypnotism also raises another social question, for the automatism of major hypnosis may be pushed so far that such subjects might become a real danger to society, if they met anybody in their life, who was ready to take advantage of their automatism to use it for his own ends. One remembers the discussions in which, apropos of a celebrated case, the neurologists of the two opposite schools of Salpêtrière and Nancy took part. It certainly seems that, for certain subjects at least, it was the school of Nancy which was in the right, and that a deeply hypnotized individual might, by the will of others, be urged to perform any act, including crime. For our part we are convinced of this. The judicial chronicle reminds us that hypnotism offers, on the other hand, certain dangers to physicians. A great many women who have been put to sleep have pretended that it was not only their psychological freedom which the physician had forced them to yield. Along this line of ideas there are numerous dangers, not only for the physician but also for the patient, who, by reason of accepting foreign suggestions, finally will admit, by reason of secondary conviction, the most impossible auto-suggestions. This is, moreover, one of the things which prove the psychological danger of hypnotism, because, if the physician really had simply as a therapeutic means given a narcotic to his patient, he would be open to the same accusations. But what he has done in practising hypnotism is to develop the power of the psychological automatism and to diminish the value and intensity of intellectual control, and, in a very great measure, the physician is responsible for the faculty of auto-suggestion which his patient has thus acquired. The most ridiculous ideas which in a perfectly involuntary way cross the field of consciousness, in a subject thus educated, will tend to be admitted without discussion by him as real and demonstrable phenomena. After his mental mechanism has acquired, under the influence of repeated hetero-suggestions, the habit of admitting without criticism, the ideas that a foreign will has tried to introduce into it, it would seem plausible after this that the ideas which spring from the psychological automatism across the field of consciousness should tend to come back into this automatism in the form of facts of memory admitted just as if they had been examined and exactly as may have been in the case of hypnotic suggestion. Although they say that the hypnotic memory in its definition is only addressed to the psychological automatism, yet it tends to develop it at the expense of the functions of consciousness and judgment. Hypnotism is only a logical method for those who believe in a very narrow determinism of the psychic functions, and who, denying the existence of superior psychic phenomena, consider the human mechanism as a tool which one can regulate or put out of order at will. We do not belong to this class. Hypnotism, it seems to us, may do for the psychoneuroses what certain symptomatic therapeutics may do, for example, for an infectious disease. What would one think of a physician who, in order to diminish some symptom,—such as fever, for example,—would order such medicine as would, at the same time that it was lowering the temperature, diminish the resistance of the patient to the infection?

But that is not all. First of all, the hypnotic method should be employed differently for each kind of patient. There are very many subjects who are not hypnotizable. There are others, who are still more numerous, to whom the idea of entrusting their free will into the hands of a physician, even of one in whom they would have the greatest confidence, is peculiarly depressing. One does not give up his will and his personality so easily, and we have known subjects in whom the very emotion which had been caused by certain attempts at hypnosis had brought about new and very serious neuropathic manifestations.

On the other hand, we must understand the exact value of hypnotic suggestion. Here is an individual to whom in hypnotic sleep you make some suggestion for a future time. You order him, for example, to write a letter or to make a visit several weeks, or perhaps several months, later. The suggested date arrives, and our subject achieves the suggestion satisfactorily; but he achieves it in a secondary condition, —that is to say, in a purely automatic state. Once the act is accomplished he retains no memory of it. At no moment has he had, either at the time of the suggestion or during the execution of the suggested act, any phenomenon of consciousness. The suggestion, in other words, was only able to act when the faculties of consciousness were lost. At these two periods, during the order and the execution, the suppression of consciousness is the essential condition of suggestion. In what measure has the hypnotic suggestion, therefore, any persistent action upon the individual when he has regained his state of consciousness? This is a question that one has the right to ask, and of which the negative solution shows how illusory is the pedagogic action of hypnotic suggestion. On the other hand, as a matter of fact, the real action of hypnosis has always appeared to us to be limited to neuropathic symptoms depending more or less directly upon psychic automatism. Hysterical manifestations, in so far as they are accidental, may sometimes disappear rapidly under the influence of hypnotic suggestion. We have seen, on the contrary, many neurasthenics who have never found that such therapy has been of any benefit whatsoever for the functional symptoms presented by them. This is because in such cases it is a question of troubles engendered by preoccupation, and in which the intervention of the psychological automatism is only secondary.

Along this same line of ideas bearing on pedagogic influence,—or, if one so prefers it, of the possible modification of the soil,—a very important thing in matters of psychotherapy—which hypnotic suggestion may bring to pass, one must always take into consideration the patient's usual habit of thought. It is very evident that the value of a psychic acquisition is measured by the number and importance of the ideas with which it is associated. For a religious subject it is certain that any idea which has to do with his convictions will have an enormous value in directing his thoughts. To a cowardly subject any idea bearing on the subject of sickness or death will have considerable weight. On the other hand, by the action of repetition, any idea which is associated with a great number of facts in life will gradually assume a greater and greater importance in the psychism of the subject. But the value of hypnotic suggestion is to express itself, as it were, on a blank page, to associate itself with nothing and to be dependent on nothing. But what effect can it have, under these conditions, on the psychical or moral orientation of a patient?

On the other hand, it has seemed to us, in some cases, that hypnotic suggestion may overshoot the mark, and tend continually to put the subjects into subconscious states approaching those secondary conditions where suggestive action then becomes preponderant.

However it may be, hypnosis is none the less extremely interesting from the point of view of psychological analysis. Were it only that it has permitted the dissociation of the automatic functions and the functions of consciousness, it should, for this reason alone, receive the thanks of physicians. For, by this very act, it permits one to see that all psychotherapy should first and foremost be addressed to the functions of consciousness, and that a method such as hypnotic suggestion which is addressed to the functions of the automatonism can no longer be practised at the present time. In other words, the results of the psychological analyses which are made possible by means of hypnotic sleep condemn its use as a therapeutic method.

A very different thing from hypnotic suggestion is suggestion during the waking state. This is practised under peculiar conditions. In a semi-obscure room removed from the noise of the street, the doctor settles his patient comfortably. It is necessary that there should be no physical discomfort and that his attention should not be attracted by any outside phenomenon. Then the physician tells him to close his eyes and to put himself into such a condition that no thought or sensation may come in between the psychism of the subject and the suggestion which the physician is going to make. It is understood that the patient, when thus placed in this condition of receptivity, which under these circumstances is voluntary, is not supposed to discuss anything. He must, without reasoning, and without any psychic reaction whatever, accept the suggestion. This will chiefly be put in the form of repeated affirmations. It could not, naturally, be in any degree an argument or a demonstration, of which the first result would be to awaken the psychism of the patient. One could, if absolutely necessary, multiply his statements by dividing them into short sentences. One might subdivide the symptom picture presented by the patient into a series of elementary symptoms, and oppose a suggestive statement against each one of these. Surrounded with a little sense of mystery, and by the very force of things complicated by phenomena of auto-suggestion, and having its results perhaps only through the intermediary of this auto-suggestion, there is no doubt that this practice may lead to a great number of good results in the therapy of neuropathic symptoms.

It is very evident that this method has none of the preliminary inconveniences of hypnotic suggestion. It does not make a disagreeable impression upon the patient, who has no fear, as in hypnosis, of feeling himself both psychically and physically abandoned to the mercy of his physician. The latter, moreover, always takes pains to reassure his patient on this point, and promises to awaken him if he should happen to fall into an hypnotic sleep.

As a matter of fact, it often does happen that during this practice the patient goes to sleep and falls into an hypnotic condition. Also, there are a great many physicians to be found who do not see that suggestion in the waking state differs from hypnotic suggestion in any way except in degree, and who consider the peculiar condition in which the patient must be placed to submit to suggestions as merely a less marked state of hypnosis.

However this may be, although we regard this method as in all respects less dangerous than hypnotic suggestion, yet we wish to point out a great many objections which it seems to raise. Evidently the most important objection is that in this treatment one deliberately directs one's attention to the symptom, and completely neglects the underlying mental stratum. By direct suggestion one weakens instead of strengthening the patient's critical power. It does not in any way accustom him to judge his impressions and to recognize the value of his sensations. Here again the attempt to help improve the symptoms or to cure by outside suggestion only tends to reinforce the patient's auto- and hetero-suggestibility, which form the very source of his symptoms.

In an intermediary position between indirect suggestion and persuasion there are some rather specialized therapeutic processes which tend to arouse, either by direct or mediatory action, curative autosuggestions in patients. In this way, by starting from the suggestive power of a saying, either written, read, or repeated mentally or aloud, one can make the patient who is afflicted with neurasthenic headache or hysterical paralysis either write, or read, or say, "I have no headache; I can walk." Such a method may be varied infinitely, and depends chiefly on the fact that the word, or the gesture, constitutes by its relation to the psychism of the patient the reality of the idea or action.

Here, as the intrinsic suggestion is worthless, it is likely that the unfavorable effect produced on the mental make-up is not so great. It must be added, that from the therapeutic point of view the results are not very brilliant, and that, in spite of all, a method which accustoms one to interpose psychic operation cannot but be inconvenient to the mental constitution of the subject in question. We have seen patients of this kind who could not bring themselves to decide upon any action whatsoever without repeating to themselves a great many times: "I will do such and such a thing." The word, for them, had become the means of action, and the necessary intermediary between the action and its conception. This is the ultimate outcome of such therapeutic practices as we have just described.

We have now briefly analyzed[1] the different psychotherapeutic processes which taken as a whole—although varying in the degree in which they suppress consciousness—are addressed to the cerebral automatism and practically lead to relapse.

PERSUASION.—We come now to psychotherapy by persuasion. Here there is no more stage setting, no more drawn curtains, no more closed shutters—nothing which would be calculated to impress the patient. The conversational attitude, the familiar manner of talking things over, the heart-to-heart discussion, where the physician must exert his good sense and feelings, and the patient be willing to be confidential,—this is what is meant by psychotherapy by persuasion. It consists in explaining to the patient the true reasons for his condition, and the different functional manifestations which he presents. It consists, on the other hand, moreover, and you would say almost wholly, in establishing the patient's confidence in himself and awakening the different elements of his personality capable of becoming the starting-point of the effort which will enable him to regain his self-control. The exact comprehension of phenomena which he presents must be grasped by the patient by means of its own reasoning. The general elements which may in some way build up his mental synthesis must be drawn upon by his own volition. The part that the physician plays is to recall, awaken, and direct. He has nothing to do with suggestions. All conceptions and ideas which the physician puts forth should be such as would appeal to the patient's reason, and should not come into collision with either his convictions or his feelings. When the physician shows a patient in what way he has erred, what are the faults of his character and his moral condition and his reasoning which are the cause of the genesis of his affection, he does not demand that he shall accept what he has told him as an article of faith: he asks only one thing,—that he should force himself to reflect and to understand.

Far from acting, as do direct suggestions, by restricting the personality, persuasion, on the contrary, tends to permit the personality to develop, in liberating it from all the disordered actions which may have been established by bad moral hygiene or by vicious physical or psychic attitudes. And if, as is the rule, the subject is cured, it ought to seem to him that he has evaded his neuropathic condition through his own efforts, and that it is he himself who has successively cut or disentangled the bonds which had kept him there. One can see how, in this way, the self-confidence of the patient who is cured is augmented. His feeling

[1] For a more complete and definite exposition of different psychotherapic processes we refer the reader to the work, "Isolation and Psychotherapy," by J. Camus and P. Pagniez, published under the direction of one of us (Paris, 1904, Alcan).

of safety is complete if he has been wisely treated,—quite complete enough in all cases for the patient, conscious of the faults which he has committed, and recognizing the dangers which threaten him, to know that he can and must guard himself against one and the other. The risk of relapse to the neurasthenic cured by persuasion is almost nothing. He may have times of weakness, but he will remember and pull himself up and get hold of himself again.

It goes without saying that persuasion can only be applied to individuals whose mental mechanism is virtually sane. If it is brought to bear upon subjects whose psychic functions are either congenitally or accidentally and organically affected, it is certain to meet with defeat. There is no psychotherapy, such as we understand it, for people with major obsessions, for melancholias or circular psychoses, any more than there is psychotherapy for the psychoses. We feel that it only casts discredit upon the method to think of applying it to this class of patients. One cannot give a new orientation to a mentality which is, as it were, crystallized in a definite situation. And although some authors may have had improvements or cures among patients afflicted by some kind of mental affection, it has been owing to a happy chance for their subjects, but an unfortunate one for them, for it has been the starting-point of their errors. They have found themselves confronted by periods of natural and spontaneous remission which occur in the great majority of subjects afflicted with these mental affections.

On the other hand, and even where the psychoneuroses are concerned, there are peculiar cases which we shall have to consider in the course of this study, where persuasion loses its power. Often it is a question of an almost pathological mentality in certain subjects. On the other hand also, it is because, before having had recourse to psychotherapy, peremptory indications—drawn, for example, from the subject's general condition—have obliged one to act first and talk afterward, and sometimes too late.

If, however, psychotherapy is the chosen method to be applied to the great majority of patients, it must also be recognized that there are cases, and very many of them, where it can only be practised under certain given conditions, which are necessary and preliminary to the treatment. The most frequent of these conditions is isolation, and there are nervous people for whom, without isolation, all psychotherapeutic methods would be in vain.

There are, therefore, in the treatment of the psychoneuroses certain psychotherapeutic accessories which we shall have to study. Essentially a psychoneurosis is composed, as we have seen—

1. Of a mental and moral foundation which is either constitutional or acquired, and due to some emotional stimulus.

2. Neuropathic symptoms properly so called, or functional mani-

festations, grafted on to the psychic stock which has hitherto been established.

3. Additional phenomena, expressing the persistence of functional manifestations in the organs.

For convenience in description, and after having devoted several pages to the medical examination of neuropaths, we shall take up successively the treatment of each one of these constituent elements of the psychoneuroses. Naturally, this must be a schematic and purely artificial division, for in the treatment, just as in the disease, symptoms are evidently bound up together. Finally the actions exercised upon the different troubles presented by the patients depend one upon the other.

Having prepared the way, we shall then take up the accessories of psychotherapy. In a final chapter we shall try to see how and to what degree the psychoneuroses are susceptible of preventive treatment, and how the physician who, in a prophylactic manner, has been until the present bound up in his ideas of physical hygiene may also assume the right to interest himself in this question of mental hygiene, which, moreover, is so often an accompanying element of physical hygiene, as it is also a requisite to a very great degree of the general health of society.

CHAPTER XX.

THE EXAMINATION AND QUESTIONING OF THE NEUROPATH.

UPON the first encounter between the physician and the neuropath depends the fate of the combat. If from the first conversations you have not been able to awaken a reciprocal sympathy in your patient, and if you have not succeeded in gaining his confidence, it is useless to go any further. The result that you will obtain will be worthless or mediocre.

But it would be wrong to imagine that it is extremely difficult to gain the confidence of a neuropath. The nervous person is usually extremely susceptible. He is not at all willing to show confidence in any one who has not gained it, but he is also extremely sensitive to kindly treatment, and quite ready to confide in any one whom he sees interested in his fate. Also, if the neuropath in his explanations is often somewhat prolix, and if he bring into his descriptions things which seem to you wholly unimportant, do not become impatient with him. It will sometimes happen that a detail which seems insignificant at first may, as matters develop, be extremely useful to you. It will also happen that when carried away by his own subject the patient will reveal himself much more completely, if you let him go on, than if, with the air of hurrying him on to be rid of him, you try to get him to be concise when it is impossible for him to be so. Not only must you let him speak, but you must listen to him. You must make notes, in your memory at least,—and, if that is not trustworthy, in writing,—of all the ideas which the patient may have concerning the nature and the causes of his condition. These notes you will use later on. They will often serve to convince the patient of his own contradictions, and it is hard to realize how often it is necessary to reply to an argument, which is just beginning, with "But you told me that several days ago."

Before entering into any discussion with your patient, you, as the physician, must yourself have acquired as complete an idea as possible concerning his condition and the mechanism of his symptoms. It is not the time beforehand to launch out upon any systematizations based upon your own reasoning: you will run too much risk of making a mistake, and of calling forth the confidence but not the convictions of the patient.

Then, when you make an appointment with your patient, try to have at least an hour free before you. This is seldom too much. Often it is not enough. If in this hour you have not finished your examination, ask your patient to come back the next day. If possible make your examination in three or four visits, but do not begin any therapeutic measures before having finished it. In the first conversation plan it, if possible, to understand thoroughly the character of your patient. This is really very important, because in neuropaths, however they may be affected, you will nearly always detect by careful questioning some former tendency, which may be more or less marked, to emotionalism; this is what makes it possible to say that with these patients nothing new has been created, and that all the symptoms of which they complain are only an exaggeration, sometimes extreme and sometimes an unhealthy exaggeration, of their former character.

Finally, and chiefly at the beginning of the treatment, the psychotherapeutist must very carefully weigh his words. The neuropath, in fact, is usually endowed with an excellent memory for everything that pertains to his condition and his health, and, paying great attention to the words of his physician, he will seize upon the slightest apparent or real contradiction to anything pertaining to what has been said before. By this fact his confidence in his physician would be injured, and the results of the treatment, if not compromised, would at least be delayed.

As a rule, the patient who reaches the neurologist has already been seen by a certain number of physicians, who will have always, or at least nearly always, expressed the results of their examinations in terms which are purely physical. Thus, your patient, at first, is going to tell you about all the troubles which he supposes has injured the general functioning of his organism, and to which he refers his whole present condition. He will tell you of his asthenia, of his pains, of his headaches, and of his gastric and intestinal troubles. When he has exhausted the series of clinical manifestations, take your turn, and try to find out if he has had any trouble with organs which he has not mentioned in his dissertation. You will then, in this way, avoid having him say, the next time he comes to see you, "Oh, doctor, I forgot that——" In other words, in speaking he will attribute this forgetfulness to himself, but, as a matter of fact, in his inner thoughts he will think that you have examined him very carelessly. Do not, therefore, forget, in this first phase of your questioning, any organ or any function. Whether it happens to be a man or a woman, be sure not to forget to ask a certain number of questions concerning the condition of the sexual functions. These disturbances the patients will be very anxious to hide, and, if they manage to conceal them from you, they will consider that they have scored the first victory over you. They will then have the upper hand, and you will have difficulty in obtaining it again.

After having reached the end of this examination of what one might call physical consciousness, sum up everything that seems to you to have come from it in the form of facts which you have appeared to acquire. "In fact," you will say to your patient, "you complain of suffering from insomnia, characterized by . . . ; coming on regularly (or intermittently) . . . , accompanied by . . . ; you have gastric disturbances, appearing at such a time of day, under such and such conditions, and influenced (or not) by your food . . . etc.'' From this time on, your subject must have the very distinct impression that you are completely *en rapport* with his physical condition. It is necessary, however, that from all this you should have made private notes of the various logical points in the symptomatology described. Finally, this part of your questioning will only come to an end when, before your little exposition, which perhaps may have to be done over several times, your patient will say to you, ''Yes, that is exactly how it is.''

He will immediately propose that you should examine him, but the moment for this examination has not yet come. The major part of your work remains to be accomplished. This means that, from this moment on, you must establish for yourself the chain of development. It is necessary to know, first of all, how all these related disturbances have followed one another; it is of the utmost importance to find out their relations to emotional causes, and to the phenomena of auto- and hetero-suggestion which may have caused them, and the affective and transient symptoms of physical life which may, by the mechanism of the psychic crystallization of memory, have given rise to actual symptoms.

If a woman, for example, presents gastric disturbances, do not forget that her troubles may have really been justified in the beginning by pregnancy. In a man, it may have been a passing attack of alcoholism, dating back some years, which has brought back to him the manifestations which he now presents. In another case, it may be a transient action due to medicines, in still another to some alimentary intoxication, while in another it may have been a conversation or something that the patient read. In this case it may be contact with patients who were really suffering from some functional disorder, while in that one it may be the memory of some heredity which is the cause of it. It is very hard to imagine the great variety of causes which in some form of functional manifestation or other may give rise to very analogous effects.

This analysis, this searching for the psychic origin of the symptom or symptoms, must be pushed until one obtains some result. It is the absolutely essential condition of treatment. It may happen that you will not find it the first time. It sometimes requires three or four conferences, before one can obtain a sufficiently precise idea. Do not be disturbed by this. Your patient will bear you no ill will, for, already finding that you are interested in considering every detail so thoroughly, he will have complete confidence in you.

You will then have to establish the condition influencing the variability—an almost constant factor—in the symptoms of your neuropath. The immediate or more slowly perceived beneficial or harmful influence of distraction, of emotions, and of preoccupations foreign to the symptom in hand,—all this must be brought out by your questioning. Note that from this time on, and without meaning to, you are practising therapeutic measures. When your patient leaves you, he will be always thinking about the questions which you have put to him; he will already have experienced a mental orientation which cannot but be favorable to him. It often happens that after simple questioning we have seen patients come back the next day and tell us, "Doctor, I have been thinking of all the questions that you asked me yesterday, and I have been asking myself whether or not it may be that I am simply nervous, and a little irritable."

Have you now finished with your questionings? Certainly not. You are still far from knowing all. You must now try to find out the general cause of the patient's condition. Often, at the start, he will not have told you it. But led on by his confidence, because he is convinced that you are interested in him, and that you have shown a willingness to devote your time to him which other physicians have never had the courage to do, he will reveal himself to you more readily. And when you ask him, "Now let us see, before all these symptoms appeared, did you not have any special sorrow, or annoyance, or emotion, or some serious preoccupations?" more often he will reply in the affirmative and will tell you what it was. It may happen that the emotional cause was of too intimate a nature, and that sometimes it involves responsibilities of others, as well as those of the patient himself. But it will only be a little time before you will know it, and that will be when you really become his true friend. But at the start you will have been able to know that it exists, even if the patient has chosen to hide it; for if, as a matter of fact, you watch him closely at the time when you put such or such a question, you will see him hesitate a little, or grow pale, or flush slightly, and show some signs of physical emotion at the memory which you have just called up. Sometimes you will see your patient slightly agitated, his words will be abrupt, his face will contract slightly as if he wished to keep back tears which were only too ready to flow. Sometimes all that is necessary at that moment is a kindly word of sympathy which proves to him that you are quite ready to give him a little affection and a little of yourself. He will then let himself go, and will tell you just what the trouble is. Your patient is then three-quarters cured.

You must then learn the whole history of your patient's life,—all the pleasures that he has been able to get out of it, and all the rancor which may have accumulated in it. You must know the smallest detail of his family life and his conjugal life. Through his tastes, his actions and his reactions, you must manage to form a complete and coherent picture of his mental and moral condition. You must find out whether he is inclined to be sentimental or emotional, or, on the other hand, is cold and indifferent. Has he or has he had a strong feeling of self-esteem or of pride? Is he restless, uneasy, or scrupulous? Has he religious or philosophic convictions? If so, what are they? It is of the utmost importance to know everything in order to understand everything. If you know every trick of a patient's mind, you already, if you will pardon the expression, "have got him."

For this last examination there is no need of any profound psychology. The psychology of every-day life, such as that which a good artisan or honest farmer would use, is quite enough. But it is very evident that the terms which you would employ in your questioning would vary according to the mentality, and the education which the subject has received. But whether it is the case of a prince of science, or a leader of finance, or the heir to a throne, or the most modest of his subjects, those feelings which alone are able to stir men are extremely simple and quite alike. It is the business of scientific psychology to separate them into their psychological ions; the practising physician need not trouble himself about them. He has only need to know the simple bodies which, changing their names according to various languages and latitudes, are, nevertheless, always identical.

It would be a great error to imagine that, in order to be able to obtain a complete confession from a patient, it is absolutely indispensable to be mature in years or have great authority. Naturally, by virtue of his respectability, or his age, or his fame, the physician may make more or less impression on his patient; but the youngest physician, practising in any little place in the country, may arrive, and sometimes even in a shorter time, at exactly the same result, with the condition, however, which in this case is absolutely indispensable, that, loving his profession, and looking upon it as something more than a trade, he knows how to make himself beloved.

However it may be, now that your questionings have been achieved, there still remains for you to make a physical examination of your patient. This examination ought to be absolutely thorough. Your subject should be entirely undressed, and preferably lying down. All the organs and all the functions should be scrutinized by every method of examination at your disposal. An analysis of the urine should be made. Briefly speaking, when your patient goes away from this examination, he ought to feel himself laid bare physically as he had been psychically. It will sometimes happen in the course of this examination that you will discover somewhere some organic defect. It will then give you the key to many of the added phenomena for which otherwise you have had no explanation. You must not conceal the existence of this trouble from the patient. Above all, you must not stoutly maintain that there is nothing the matter when there is something the matter. By wishing to cure him completely, you will not cure him at all.

On the other hand, you must conduct this examination in such a way that it does not make any strong impression on your patient. It is a useful way to give the impression that you are making this examination because you wish to do your work conscientiously, and not because you suspect him to have some serious affection. In case of need, as you proceed with this examination, in order to avoid raising any terrifying doubts in your patient's mind, you may assure him of the healthy condition of such an organ or the proper functioning of such a function which you have just examined.

But here, on the part of the examiner as well as for the one questioned, there must be nothing kept back, and nothing passed over in a mysterious way. In other words, once this examination is finished, there must be a complete sense of confidence between yourself and your patient, and, just as he has hidden nothing from you, in the same way you must keep back nothing from him concerning his condition.

You have thus brought yourself into perfect touch with your patient. You know him psychically, morally, and physically as well as if you had lived side by side for years. Then and then only you will have the right to undertake the therapeutic part of your work. This, if you have hitherto followed the line which we have just indicated, will be remarkably simplified.

To approach the subject in this way will evidently take some time. You will perhaps be obliged to take it up on several different occasions, in case your patient, or you yourself, become fatigued. That does not matter; the time is not lost. The key to success in psychotherapy is found in a clear and primitive comprehension of things. And we say absolutely, to those who do not know how or have not the patience to work in this manner, that they have no right to judge the value of psychotherapy by persuasion. If in their hands it shows but very little good result, it is because they have not given time enough to their patients to cure them.

CHAPTER XXI.

THE MORAL AND MENTAL SUBSTRATUM. ITS PSYCHOTHERAPY.

AT THE very start of this study we must make a distinction. Neurasthenia and hysteria, as we have seen, are accompanied by very different mental and moral conditions. Their therapy, therefore, cannot be considered from the same point of view. So we shall take up successively the neurasthenic and the hysteric.

In order thoroughly to understand the real mental and moral condition of the neurasthenic, it seems to us necessary to state a few preliminary ideas. All the phenomena of life may be classified in a certain number of phases which one might sum up as follows: First, stimulus, whether of external origin or called up by internal emotion. Then, the phase of consciousness; where the subject, thanks to his intellectual control, is able to judge the nature of the stimulus which he has felt. Then, the phase of appreciation, if one might so call it, where the impressions, having had no intellectual quality in any absolute way, take on, by reason of their relation to the personality of the subject, a relative value. Finally, the phase of reaction of the personality, which may or may not manifest itself in the form of action. Stimulus and reception, comprehension or judgment constitute passive phenomena in which only those qualities of stimulus submitted to the intellectual faculties of the subject come into play. This, in a word, is the phase of consciousness. In the normal subject, the personality only comes in a secondary way to judge the relative value of the consciousness thus acquired, to adopt it, without any reaction, if one feels practically indifferent to it, or, if not, to proceed to adapt one's self to it.

In learning any fact whatsoever, we look at it first intellectually, under its various aspects, we register it in our memory, merely as a simple phenomenon of consciousness, if it can neither hurt us nor be of use to us. If we find that it is going to be useful to us in some way, we receive it into our personality, whose general direction may be modified by it. If it is harmful to us, and if we have adjudged it intangible, we force ourselves to change our ideas and adapt ourselves to it. If, on the other hand, we judge that we may have some power, if not over the fact, at least over its consequences, we make an effort, by various reactions, to act directly either on the fact or on its consequences.

This is the manner in which a person who is quite morally and mentally sane will act. In such a subject, by reason of his judgment, which has hitherto been purely intellectual, the reactions of the personality are in fact reduced to a minimum, and the adaptation to the case in hand will be, moreover, all the more easy in proportion as the intellectual appreciation will have been more perfect and complete. In order to fight an enemy, according to the common formula, the important thing is, first of all to know him, to know the forces that he has at his disposition, the ground on which he will develop his plans, and the side on which he will probably attack. In fact, the man who is to be victorious, from this complete point of view, is the one who, before performing any action, and before permitting anything to come into his personality, is able to look upon things objectively, to consider them as if they had nothing to do with him, and to forget for the moment that he is to judge them.

As a matter of fact, this ideal individual does not exist in nature, except in a very small number of instances, and the one who is undoubtedly the furthest removed from this ideal is the actual or virtual neurasthenic.

When one speaks of the emotional or constitutional neurasthenic, one does not merely allude to the various reactions which, with a more or less specific individuality, he is likely to show in physical life. The neurasthenic has in addition to that a very great moral emotivity. The latter is measured by the precocious and too interested intervention of the personality, even in the very cases where it would seem *a priori* that it ought to be indifferent. When one says that the neurasthenic takes things too much to heart, that he considers almost everything of almost equal importance, one does not mean by that that he has no perception of intellectual value. The most subtle problem of geometry might be solved by a neurasthenic, or the most charming description be written by him. One only means to say that he does not know how to interpose between the various events which may affect him—even without, as a matter of fact, touching him or having any reaction on his personality—sufficient time to allow for a purely speculative examination of things. His personality comes into play although, intellectually speaking, the phenomena in question are barely subconscious. It is naturally evident that, as he cannot adapt himself to things which he does not know, the reactions of his personality will be diffuse and more or less incoherent. They will be expressed in this way by hesitations in decisions, scruples, and finally by preoccupations. In other words, the degree of the persistence and of the utilization of intellectual control will measure the degree and the absolute value of personal reactions. Under insufficient intellectual control, the reactions must of necessity be non-adapted or non-adaptable, and mental phenomena, and more especially moral phenomena, will result from the consciousness of this non-adaptation. Feelings of insecurity, and incompletion, to employ Janet's expression, slight and diffused phenomena of anxiety, and a feeling of helplessness and failure, will occur. It goes without saying, that, step by step, the neurasthenic, perceiving his inability to react usefully, will derive from this a general conception of psychic and moral depression, and a sort of experimental pessimism. All these feelings of insufficiency that the neurasthenic has are, therefore, not purely illusory, but spring simply from a bad psychical and moral hygiene.

We must now ask ourselves, what are the elements which may contribute thus to weaken the intellectual control of people? We already know the majority of them.

We have seen in connection with this that certain emotional causes, by the very intensity of their action and the suddenness of their onset, could not possibly be immediately or even rapidly adapted. We have also developed elsewhere the idea that, just as certain subjects possess specific, psychic emotivity, so in their personality there are zones that are peculiarly sensitive to the emotional excitation which may affect them.

The fact still remains, however, that there are people who are constitutionally of a restless nature, who are in a condition of subcontinuous emotionalism, and who for this reason weaken by means of their internal activity the value of their intellectual control. All external phenomena become factors of emotion for them, because, living a too exclusively internal life, without any especial religious, moral, philosophical, or practical direction which is sufficiently intense to inhibit stimuli of external origin, these, when they occur, take them by surprise, and trouble them because they are never prepared for them.

Then there are all the vanquished ones of life, who, having struggled against circumstances for months, or perhaps years, have not been able to triumph over them. They are in a defiant state themselves, in a state of subcontinuous restlessness. But this has nothing to do with any constitutional defect. They fail to use their intellectual control, just as they would neglect to use some instrument whose inaccuracy or poor condition had been experimentally proved to them. For these individuals, the lack of intellectual control constitutes a true reaction of abandon, a confession of defeat. Henceforth these subjects will allow themselves to be borne along by events, and the only reactions, or as we have described the non-adaptations, which they will present will come from the onset of external stimuli against their personality, which is here completely subconscious and no longer voluntarily able to act. But these subjects do not, properly speaking, become neurasthenics. They are the wastes of life, and, when the reaction of abandon is absolutely complete, so much so that they no longer make any attempt or any struggle toward adaptation, the various phenomena of the neurasthenic state cannot help but follow, and in the very line along which we have described the psychoneuroses. In order for a subject to present fully the usual complete mental and moral condition of the neurasthenic, he must needs have more or less lost his intellectual control, but he must also be in the position of trying to recover his self-control.

In reality, the etiological factor which seems to us important, and from which results the participation of the intimate personality in a whole series of facts which ought to be foreign to it, such as the intervention of the subconscious in phenomena which ought normally only to depend upon the consciousness, the essential thing is the lack of general direction.

The personality—the subconsciousness, if one prefers it—is continually, so to speak, overflowing the phenomena of consciousness, especially so if the subconscious is not dammed by the power of the general idea, or if the whole personality is not tending toward the accomplishment of some end or the satisfaction of an ideal. The individual who knows what he wants and where he wants to go, the man to whom some religious or philosophical idea serves as a guide, the person who simply directs this or that affective tendency, the subject, in fact, who in order to determine upon some line of life trusts himself absolutely to some leader or director of conscience,—such a man cannot become a neurasthenic. Whether, like a child accompanied by his parents, or like a soldier who trusts in his chief, he merges his personality, or whether the personality is in some way externalized toward an ideal, the result is the same; the individual has moral support.

In this respect two classes of patients should be mentioned. There are those who, by reason of education or by their constitutional insufficiency, have never been able to direct themselves in this way. There are others who, on account of some external cause, have lost this orientation. If the end toward which they are working is suddenly withdrawn or becomes intangible, if the affection in which they were trusting has disappeared, if the ideal which has guided and upheld them is suddenly destroyed, then, but then only when completely broken down, are they susceptible of becoming neurasthenics. Our experience shows us many such examples every day. The priest who has lost his faith, the ambitious man who has been definitely supplanted, the lover who has been dismissed,—all these are in a fair way to become patients. It must also be added that, most undoubtedly, any religious or philosophical ideal, particularly in the shadow of human vicissitudes, gives quite another kind of strength from that which comes with the pursuit of some real or material aim.

However it may be, the characteristic thing about the neurasthenic—whether it is constitutional or, as more often happens, accidental—is his disoriented personality. His intellectual control is singularly weakened by it, and various manifestations of the psychoneuroses follow almost at once, such as restlessness, a feeling of insecurity and pessimism, which, as a fact, is nothing but the expression of absence of direction and lack of any aim.

In former times the emotions were catalogued differently and divided into asthenic or depressing emotions and sthenic or strengthening emotions. This division seems to us to exist still, and at the same time it has great therapeutic interest to us. Nevertheless, we must, first of all, understand just what one means by a depressing emotion or a sthenic emotion. According to our way of thinking, an emotional stimulus has no intrinsic value. One cannot say *a priori* that an emotion of such or such a nature—with certain exceptions, of course—will necessarily exercise a stimulating or a depressing action on every individual. Good news may under certain conditions have a depressing action, and, on the contrary, bad news may be strengthening. We may perhaps at this point of our study explain our meaning on this point more easily. It is evident that one might consider depressing any emotion which would tend to dislocate or disorient the personality, and that one could, on the other hand, regard as sthenic all emotional action which will react in the sense of the reorientation or the most complete orientation of the personality. Therefore, as far as the mental and moral foundation of the neurasthenic is concerned, the therapeutic action of a strengthening emotion seems to us absolutely preponderant,—we might almost say the only one to act.

Quite apart from any therapeutic action, one sometimes sees subjects who are more or less profoundly neurasthenic and who on finding themselves suddenly in the presence of some new situation completely forget, under the influence of emotional excitement, that they are neurasthenic, and almost immediately recover their mental and moral health. Emotional stimulation has, in fact, exercised a synthetic action of orientation on the personality of the subject. Having found an object in life, he has ceased to be neurasthenic. Physicians may not perhaps often have opportunity to observe facts of this kind, but, if one looks around one in daily life, one sees them all the time. We all know people who were on the verge of becoming neurasthenic—who, as a matter of fact, as far as their symptoms were concerned, were already neurasthenic—and whom some emotional excitement had put upon their feet. The rareness of such cases—which is, however, purely apparent—lies in the fact that the physician so seldom sees neurasthenics at the beginning of the development of their disease, and that he seldom comes in contact with these patients until after symptoms of every kind have occurred which modify the aspect of the trouble.

Is it possible that such subjects have realized the benefit of a restorative emotion, or because they have previously gone through some long process of reasoning? Certainly not. Phenomena of this kind take place, as do the phenomena of the upsetting emotion, in the subconscious. The individual is not aware of it. He gets hold of himself first and reasons afterward. It seems to us, speaking from the therapeutic point of view, that it is rather illogical to think that subjects who are known to have lost some of their intellectual control, and who are subject to exaggerated emotional reactions, can be benefited by reason if sthenic emotion can do nothing. It also seems to us that psychotherapy ought, if it wishes to modify the mentality and morale of its patient, to address itself almost solely to the feelings, and very rarely approach the high summits of pure reason. If the neurasthenic condition comes on at the time when emotion has overthrown the reason, it does not seem to us quite logical to infer that a course of reasoning will be the best therapeutic measure to help the patient to re-establish the balance of his reason.

Does that mean to say that we do not consider that reasoning has any value? We do not mean to go so far as that. We think, on the other hand, that, at least as far as all the functional manifestations are concerned,—even in cases which, like certain phobias, are of a purely mental nature,—it is necessary to furnish the patient with such a clear explanation of things that he may himself get an exact idea of them.

But, as far as the moral depth of the neurasthenic is concerned, we frankly do not think that general considerations of an ethical nature have ever directly modified it. On the other hand, the neurasthenic in all that concerns his condition hardly ever rises above his particular case. He is quite able to appreciate the beauty of one's argument, but he does not think of applying it to himself and he does not attribute any immediate therapeutic value to it. In psychotherapy reasoning is indifferent. But what does do good is the confidence which can be inspired in a patient by a physician whom he feels to be morally and intellectually his superior, and the value of the reasoning lies wholly in the impression of confidence and security introduced into the mentality of the patient, who, feeling himself in good hands, finds himself comforted and strengthened. In such cases we are reminded of the words of Pascal, "The heart has reasons which reason never knows."

It would, in fact, be too naïve to believe that the psychotherapist has at his disposition a method of special reasoning, and, unknown to any one but himself, a specially convincing lingo. It is the confidence which he inspires and his manner of saying things which are the cause of his success. More than once we have heard patients make the following remark: "It is very curious, doctor; I have already been told practically the same thing as you have told me, and, although I have understood it, yet I have not been convinced." "And why?" we ask them. The reply is always the same: "I did not feel any confidence in the others, but with you it is quite different." The whole explanation of the results of psychotherapy lies in this reply.[1]

---

[1] An indication of the rôle which confidence plays in the treatment by psychotherapy lies, as one of us has already shown,* in the difference which exists in the length of time required for the treatment according to whether the case is in private practice or in the hospital. The neuropaths whom we treat by the method of isolation at the Salpêtrière, in the Pinel Ward, come to us, for reasons which it is easy to understand, in a much more serious condition—for they have struggled to

---

* J. Dejerine: "Le Traitement des psychoneuroses a l'Hôpital par la methode de isolement," Revue Neurologique, 1902, p. 1145.

It is clear, from what we have just said, that the first work of the psychotherapist should be to reconstruct his patient's personality, and in order to accomplish this reconstruction he will have to depend almost entirely upon the sthenic emotions. How should he begin this undertaking?

A very thorough knowledge of his patient's personality and life is evidently absolutely necessary for him, in order to know with any degree of certainty what chords are likely to respond, and how, starting from this point, he may synthetically build up the disintegrated personality. But, first of all, there is a very general rule which does not require any very profound questioning. As a secondary consideration, but one that is nevertheless very effective, is the very fact of his disease, which has been and which still is a cause of continued emotion to the patient, exaggerating pre-existing phenomena, or at least assuring their continuity. If, as the result of your questioning and physical examination, you feel quite sure of the purely functional nature of all the troubles presented by your subject, you ought to assure him at the start of the certainty of being able to cure him, and to tell him approximately how much time it would take. One could hardly believe how much power there is in a simple statement of this kind, made by a physician who has his patient's confidence, in helping to change rapidly and completely the patient's moral condition. We have seen patients who have been ill for years, and who, at the simple idea that in a few weeks or even a few months they would recover their physical and psychic health and personality, were overcome by intense emotion, which, however, was peculiarly helpful to them. We have known some for whom this conviction of the immediate prospect of a cure was alone sufficient so to change the current of their thought that they were able to begin to plan and make decisions, and were in some respects cured even before their treatment had begun. Is this the result of reasoning? Cer-

---

the end of their power—than the patients of the richer or more comfortable classes. Nevertheless, they are cured more quickly, on the average, than the latter. The reason for this is as follows: These subjects, who are quite as intelligent and often have much better sense than society people, have been, first of all, less spoiled by their physicians, and they have a much more lofty idea of the power of the head physician of the hospital; but that is not the principal reason. It is the surroundings which here, first of all, create the atmosphere of confidence. In the first place, the statement that they will get well is made publicly, before a more or less considerable number of students, thus starting off under such conditions, which are quite different from those which one finds either in the doctor's office or in the private room in a hospital, where the conversation takes place alone, without any witnesses present. Patients in private practice have often said to us after a few weeks of treatment: "Now, doctor, I am convinced; but I must confess to you that at first I could hardly say as much, because I have been told so many times before that I would be cured."

In our hospital practice it has happened more than once to one of us, that, after one or two consultations in public before the visiting consultants of the Salpêtrière, we have been able completely and definitely to cure intense pains of various kinds which dated back several years. When, afterward, we have asked these patients how and why the faith in their cure had come to them, their retainly not. It is the simple introduction into the patient's mind, but this time with a feeling of certainty, of something which until then he had scarcely dared to think of as possible. This idea, independent of all new medical action, continues its strengthening action, because there have appeared with it such elements as faith, hope, and confidence, which, although having almost no intellectual value, yet have considerable emotional power.

The second psychotherapeutic action which the physician will have to exercise will be what we might call a liberating action. Many patients entertain, along with their many other causes of moral depression, feelings of scruple, remorse, and self-reproach. Such a one will be greatly worried because on account of his illness he cannot support his family and provide for the future of his children. Another will have played some responsible part in some great moral or business catastrophe, and lives in the idea that the harm that was done is irreparable. This one will reproach himself because he has deceived his wife, because he has hidden from her the fact that he has a natural child. . . . One could hardly believe how many and how strange are the sorrowful secrets which cause a feeling of moral depression in many patients.

The building up and the redirecting of the personality of the neurasthenic cannot be begun until the patient has got to the point where he is ready to sweep away all these continued emotional causes which are the factors of the persistence of his condition. Now, we do not deny that here reasoning will have considerable effect. Evidently the physician will do right to point out to his patient how much his preoccupations and reproaches and remorses are exaggerated, and in all cases how useless they are. It will be his duty to tell him that the best method in his power to restore his health is to consider the past as behind him, and to start afresh with new courage. But the thing which above all has liberating action, giving a sense of freedom, is the act of con-

---

sponse was invariably the same: "At first I was so stupefied at hearing that there was no lesion in the case and that in order to get rid of my pain I only had to doubt that I had it, that when I went away I said, 'This doctor has not seen through my case at all.' Then, on reflection, I said to myself that it would be impossible for a physician surrounded by such a great number of students to be other than a very able man. It was in this way that there was born in me confidence in the certainty of my cure." We have taken this example of pains because this has to do with one of the neuropathic manifestations which is often the most rebellious and the most difficult to cure; we do not count, as a matter of fact, the numerous false gastropaths, false enteropaths, false cardiacs, false urinaries, etc., which we have cured under the same conditions,—that is to say, after one or two conversations in public.

There is still another reason why so many neuropaths are cured more quickly in the hospital than in private practice, and that is because in the isolation hall there are patients who are more or less advanced in their cure, and whose presence gives confidence to the new-comers. Then, again, patients who have been cured for a greater or less length of time often for several years sometimes come back to pay a visit to the director, and are shown to those in the ward. All these are elements which rapidly bring a feeling of confidence in the cure, and which are naturally lacking in private practice.

fession itself. All the physician's efforts ought to be directed to this when he feels "that there is something there." It is the emotional condition which the confession brings about that exercises its stimulating action in such cases, and they were profound psychologists who instituted confession as an important religious practice. It is commonly said that a sin confessed is half pardoned. We frankly say that one pardons one's own fault when one has confessed it. And it is this liberating action which the physician should first of all seek. It is in some way accomplished independently of him, once he has been able to call forth the confession, and the rôle which reason plays is here, if not wholly negative, at least of purely relative importance.

Here, then, we have a patient believing in the possibility of a normal future as soon as he believes in his cure, and relieved of a great weight upon his conscience by the act of confession. The part that the psychotherapist has to play by no means ends here, although such an important part has already been accomplished. The physician has realized the conditions which will permit his patient's personality to be directed again into healthy channels. It is the idea of this orientation and the general direction which the patient must take that he must now lay down for him. No future can be established in the air. If under some circumstances the personality of the patient has spontaneously taken its former direction, yet in a great many cases, where the disintegrating action has been sufficiently profound, this is not the case; there are also a great many subjects who have become neurasthenic for the very reason that, to a greater or less degree by the tragedy of life, the very things which form the basis of their life's work have disappeared.

It is just here that the tact of the psychotherapist comes into play. We lay it down as a principle that at this period of treatment it is in the very personality which the patient has previously had that one must look for the elements of direction and re-orientation of his personality and of his life. When one has to deal with subjects whose intellectual control is weak, and who, having confidence in their physicians, are as a result often very much disposed to take everything that they say as an article of faith, we do not feel that one has the right to impose one's own way of looking at things and the understanding of existence. The power of reasoning in these patients is much more destructive than creative. By attempting to lay down any philosophical theory or directing action on the patient, one would risk distracting or destroying the elements which when awakened are capable—such as religious faith, for example—of exercising the most marvellous curative action upon him. Such an action would leave the patient more unbalanced and disoriented than ever.

It is only necessary, we feel, to touch the chords which have hitherto been responsive. Thus and thus only, and not by deductive reasoning, but by the simple indication which becomes for the patient the starting-point of sthenic emotion, the old personality, which had actually fallen to pieces, may be built up again. You are, we will suppose, treating a patient whose life has been given over to altruistic deeds, who is devoted to a mother, to a wife, or to children, and whose neurasthenic condition has been caused either by some affective disillusion or by the death of some being who has been the object of all his preoccupation. It is to these general affective tendencies that you must direct yourself. You must know how to make him understand that others will exist for him, and that there will be other work which will claim his activity. If need be, by examining very carefully the life of your patient and the way he acts, you may attempt to go into detail with a little more definite plan. You will in this way, by creating an emotion in him which is sthenic because it conforms to his former tendencies, call forth the most constructing and uplifting sense of action. But your personality and your conception of life and of things must on no account enter into it, because it has no right to do so. Your function will only be to understand your patient.

Here is another who has a strong religious belief. Do not hesitate to tell him to trust to it. Here is another who is an ambitious man, who has failed in his ambition. Try to make him understand the possibility of turning his ambition toward some other end. And even if you find another who is a high liver and a materialist—though such people very rarely become neurasthenic—it is right for you to tell him to take all that life may have still in store for him in the pleasures which he prefers.

Later, when your patient is once cured and returned to his former condition, if you think that he has an unhealthy and dangerous point of view as regards life, you may, and you even ought to enter into a discussion with him, and draw out from him the inconveniences or the lack of logic in his way of looking at things, or of behaving himself. When you get to that point, you will stand shoulder to shoulder with your patient, and you will then need have no fear about adding to his doubts or his depressing uncertainties. You will run no risk of postponing his cure by wanting to make it too complete. When you get to this point, but only then, you may assume the rôle of the moralist.

Even for the individuals whose ideas are directly responsible for the neurasthenia which follows them, this treatment of intervention should be conducted in two stages: First of all, the reconstruction of the former personality, even with its defects and moral inferiorities. It is only much later that one will have the right, or that one should feel it to be one's duty, to attempt to eradicate their defects, and to try to turn their badly directed thoughts into new directions. This springs chiefly from the very conception which we have given of sthenic emotions whose action has always appeared to be preponderant in psychotherapy in the moral depths of the neurasthenic. Emotion, which we try to use therapeutically, is useful only in so far as it acts in the redirection of the patient's personality itself. One can understand how the part which the physician has to play here must be profoundly humane. It is necessary for him to adapt himself wholly to the mentality of his patient, and to be filled with kindness, pity, and indulgence, so that he can understand the most subtle sentimentalities, and sometimes also the most flagrant immorality. His function is to be always that of the consoler, the comforter, the giver of hope, and the director of a possible new life. In order that his work may have any result, he has to put a great deal of himself into it, and he himself must feel something of the emotion which he is seeking to bring forth. His rôle is that of a lay confessor, or a moral director, judging things not at all from the point of view of life itself. He must understand everything, and absolve everything. He must know, moreover, that in the great majority of cases his patients are people who are too grave, and who err through over-conscientiousness, and by reason of their excessive scruples and exalted sentimentality. Their weaknesses are not a subject for satire or irony or ridicule. They deserve pity, one might almost say respect. There is no doubt that such a conception of the function of the physician is peculiarly remote from the usual methods of practice. There is no doubt, however,—although it is so very simple, and demands neither philosophic conception nor strenuous logic, nor even any very great psychological subtlety,—that it does not lie in the power of all those who are anxious to avail themselves of the value of the moral action which they wish to exercise.

May we be permitted to quote a few lines in which Bernardin de St. Pierre has defined, more exactly and better perhaps than we could do, and with a sort of prescience of what is needed, the very rôle that we would like to have our physicians consent to play to our patients?

"I wish that there might be formed in large cities an establishment, somewhat resembling those which charitable physicians and wise jurists have formed in Paris, to remedy the evils both of the body and of one's fortunes; I mean councils for consolation, where an unfortunate, sure of his secret being kept and even of his incognito, might bring up the subject of his troubles. We have, it is true, confessors and preachers to whom the sublime function of offering consolation to the unfortunate seems to be reserved. But the confessors are not always at the disposition of their penitents. As for the preachers, their sermons serve more as nourishment for souls than as a remedy, for they do not preach against boredom, or unhappiness, or scruples, or melancholy, or vexation, or ever so many other evils which affect the soul. It is not easy to find in a timid and depressed personality the exact point about which he is grieving, and to pour balm into his wounds with the hand of the Samaritan. It is an art which is known only to sensitive and sympathetic souls.

"Oh! if only men who knew the science of grief could give unfortunate people the benefit of their experience and sympathy, many a miserable soul would come to seek from them the consolation which they cannot get from preachers, or all the books of philosophy in the world. Often, to comfort the troubles of men all that is necessary is to find out from what they are suffering." (Bernardin de St. Pierre, "Etude de la Nature," 1784.)

One could not express any better, or any more directly, what we never cease to maintain, however lacking in science it may seem at the first, —namely, the real therapeutic action of kindness.

Liberated morally, and having regained consciousness of self, and freed in addition from his functional manifestations by the appropriate processes which we shall study further on, the patient is cured. He is cured from his actual attack. But his mental foundation, his psychological constitution, still remains in the same condition which permitted him under emotional influences to become a neurasthenic. The rôle of the physician is, therefore, not ended. He must still build up his patient's life, still practise prophylaxis, and get the patient into a condition where his character will be established. He has the right to exert this action not only upon a patient, but upon any subject whose moral and mental constitution seems to indicate a predestination to a neurasthenic psychoneurosis. Furthermore, it seems to us that even in the education of a child there is a place for peculiarly prophylactic moral hygiene for all who have any neuropathic tendencies. We shall devote a special chapter to this study. Here, however, the therapy would be quite different, and reason and explanations would become preponderant.

Is there such a thing as general psychotherapy for hysteria, as there is a general psychotherapy for neurasthenia?

We have seen in a preceding chapter (Part II, Chapter XVII), that the hysterical symptoms were much more closely dependent upon the mental constitution than upon any very peculiar moral condition. Undoubtedly there is a therapy of re-education for this especial moral constitution, which we shall glance at when we take up the study of the general prophylaxis of the psychoneuroses.

But, independently of this very particular rôle, and which concerns the future more than the present, the immediate therapeutic action still springs from psychotherapy. We have mentioned in fact the action exercised by the permanent emotional causes on its production, or by the mechanism of memory and evocation on the persistence of hysterical symptoms. Here again, the liberating action of confession ought to be brought into play, for we have seen a great number of hysterical symptoms which had hitherto been rebellious give in, in a very definite way, when the subject who had suffered from them had acknowledged what their origin was. This fact seems to us to be of great doctrinal importance, for it shows how much effect the synthesis of a sthenic emotion may exercise on a personality. It is to just such mechanisms as these that one must attribute the therapeutic influence of certain places to which pilgrimages are made. Sthenic emotion may act just as well upon a mental state as upon a moral state, just as a depressing emotion exercises its disintegrating action as much upon the moral as upon the mental state of the subject which it attacks.

Therefore, as a therapeutic agent its efficacy is not so generally evident in the hysteric as in the neurasthenic, but must not for that reason be neglected. We think, therefore, that it is right to try to arouse in the hysteric almost the same sthenic emotions as in the neurasthenic; that it is wise, as with the neurasthenic patient, to inquire into his moral condition, and to try to find out whether his personality has not been more or less completely disorganized by the emotional stimuli which he has undergone and which his memory so frequently evokes. In the great majority of cases, such inquiry into one's moral condition and the complete liberation by confession are the necessary conditions—the *sine qua non* of the cure of hysterical symptoms.

It is no less true that the thing which at a given time dominates the picture of hysteria is the characteristic symptom. Some peculiar mental make-up has permitted this certain symptom to be produced, and, as the therapy of the patient's mental make-up is necessarily connected with that of the symptom, we shall continue the study in the chapter devoted to the treatment of hysterical symptoms. Let us say, however, at the start, for this is a point to which we shall return a little later, that any therapeutic work would be very incomplete if it confined itself to making the symptom disappear, or, in other words, to treating the symptom without paying any attention to the mental condition, or without offering the patient any refuge, by means of a well-conducted psychotherapy, from new manifestations of his affection. This purely symptomatic therapy is, in fact, comparable to that which consists in treating a syphilitic headache with antipyrine and neglecting to treat the syphilis.

CHAPTER XXII.

A GENERAL PSYCHOTHERAPY OF FUNCTIONAL MANIFESTATIONS.

When a physician has to deal with a subject afflicted with functional manifestations, he is apt to think that he has an easy task before him. But the psychotherapeutic procedure which consists of saying to the patient, "There is nothing the matter with you; you are only nervous; don't pay any attention to it . . ." seems to us a little too simple, and. above all, quite inefficacious. This, however, in the majority of cases is practically the limit of most physicians' psychotherapy. They pay no attention either to the mechanism which has engendered the functional trouble or to the whole series of symptomatic phenomena which have come in to complicate the situation. If the mechanism is not taken apart bit by bit, there is every chance that it will be built up again, and will bring with it all the troubles which the physician's authoritative statement has been for the moment able to disperse. If, on the other hand, as is ordinarily the case, the additional disturbances exist because of the patient's incapability, even though he be convinced of the fundamental neuropathic nature of his case, of completely freeing himself from his troubles, the symptomatic ensemble persists. In matters of functional manifestations the "Know thyself" of the Socratic doctrine is exactly the thing by which the patient realizes his maximum chance of a definite cure.

The first thing, therefore, that the physician has to do is to interpret and explain. It is necessary for him to take into consideration all the constituent elements of the functional manifestation. If there is any organic tumor or growth, it will be wise to refer to its existence and to show the patient what is the usual symptomatology which such subjects present who are affected with any real lesion; by a sort of subtraction, one will thus finally get to the point where one will draw out from the whole array of symptoms of which the patient is complaining those that are legitimate and those that are not.

To our way of thinking, it is a very serious error to undervalue the rôle played in certain cases by the organic defect; and it would also be a great mistake to try to deceive the patient, when there is any such thing, as to the true organic difficulty in his condition. As it would be a material impossibility for him to get rid of all his symptoms, it would be too much to wager that he would not get rid of any of them.

Outside of functional manifestations which have their starting-point in some actual organic defect, there are some that have originated from some passing organic phenomenon. It is necessary to take these into consideration also, and to explain to the patient that originally his symptoms sprang from some real trouble. This is because it often happens that certain functional manifestations bear a relation to some definite or transient organic defect, antecedent even to the neurasthenic condition. The patient who knows what the succession of phenomena has been in his own case will find it very difficult to admit, without any preliminary explanation, that what he is feeling now is purely neuropathic, and when one tries to prove too much to him one will prove nothing at all.

Finally, there exists with the major neurasthenic a whole series of manifestations of which some have to do with emotional fatigue and others are related to later organic weaknesses. It is right for the physician to explain to his subject not only the neuropathic origin of his symptoms, but also the real nature of the troubles of which he complains. What he must then point out to the patient is the direct curability of his troubles, and what he must avoid, while of course making reservations concerning the exaggeration and prolongation of mental origin, is telling the patient of the purely psychic nature of these difficulties.

There is, therefore, a whole series of therapeutic shoals on which the physician may be shipwrecked if he trusts to any too decided systematization, but which with a little tact and good sense it is quite possible for him to avoid.

However, it is not only real phenomena which must be taken into consideration. One must pay the greatest attention to what we have already elsewhere called disharmonic disturbances. Here is an organ or a function which for weeks, months, or even sometimes years, under the influence of neuropathic disturbances has been mobilized in some vicious attitude, or whose functioning has been quite abnormal. It is clear that phenomena arise which are the direct result of the bad habits that are formed and that they must not be associated with purely psychic manifestations. Moreover, a peculiar therapy must be applied to these latter phenomena. This therapy is called re-education, a method which, by various and different processes, according to the functional manifestation in question, progressively corrects the vicious attitude, and frees or releases the patient from the bad habit which he has formed. For every organ and every function that is affected in this way there is some particular form of re-education. But, speaking in a general way, explanations form a very considerable part of it, for one must show the patient how and in what way he has sinned, and what is the exact rôle which in the general group of phenomena experienced by him is played by disharmonic disturbances.

All these eliminations being made, we get to what is properly called the psychic part. This, unquestionably, is very important. But the most dangerous error, also the most frequent, is that of confounding the psychic manifestation with the imaginary manifestation. The hypochondriac is the only one who has imaginary manifestations which are the pure fabrications of his mind, although sometimes due to medical questioning. The symptoms of a neurasthenic are legitimate sufferings, quite as legitimate as if they were due to some affected organ; only, instead of having had a peripherical origin, they have had a central starting-point,—that is, a psychic starting-point. It is quite understood that the neurasthenic is apt to exaggerate his sufferings, and one must always remember this fact, which is true even for patients who are organically afflicted, that the pain which is a purely subjective phenomenon is felt in proportion to the attention that is brought to bear upon it. But to tell a neurasthenic that what he feels is "merely an idea" shows a very poor comprehension of the exact mechanisms of the troubles from which he is suffering. It is, therefore, very wise to make the patient grasp the fact that psychic phenomena and organic phenomena are by no means independent of one another, but that their reciprocal action is felt in a double sense, either by an organic trouble created by a psychic impression, or else, which is true in this particular case, that a previous psychic impression may disturb an organic function. The functional disturbance of psychic origin thus realized is itself susceptible of having a psychic expression, and of strengthening the pathological convictions for the patient, which in their turn become factors of a still more marked disturbance. Thus is formed the vicious circle into which psychotherapy must penetrate. The patient, from the moment that he finds that you are not going to treat him like an invalid who is making believe, is quite disposed to admit the very reassuring mechanism which you explain to him. It will be proper thenceforward to show him just what is the exact and precise origin of his auto- or hetero-suggestions, and what is the influence which emotional causes exert upon him. It will be necessary to demonstrate to him the rôle played by all associations of ideas, and memories which bound by ties of succession or causality to the pathological idea are apt to recall it and with it all the disturbances which depend upon it. In this way you will be able to explain to him the apparent regularity of certain manifestations which always spring up at a given moment, because following the ordinary psychological mechanism, which one can easily understand, it is at the very moment that the psychism of the patient finds itself directed toward the manifestation which it presents.

The rôle of association of ideas and the awakening of the pathological idea through memory has always seemed to us of very great importance. It is in this way we feel that a great number of functional manifestations are prolonged and complicated and exaggerated. It is also by reason of not taking this fact into account that so many therapeutic procedures based on the re-education of a will, which moreover is often by no means deficient, only leads to very uncertain results. The essential thing for a neurasthenic is, first of all, not to struggle, but rather to make himself forget, and, when one advises that certain patients should be isolated for a time, it is precisely in order to reduce to the minimum the chances for recalling the pathological idea. This recall is produced during the course of the treatment by the intervention of psychological associations, of which the objects and familiar things of the environment in which the patient has lived constitute one element while the functional manifestation forms the other. If later one advises the patient who has grown strong and understands his case, to struggle against a new attack, and against all memories which tend to invade his mind again, nothing can be better. But at the beginning of the treatment, as far as the functional manifestation is concerned—except, however, where in certain cases there is more precise indication—the thing that one must pay particular attention to is to preserve silence, at least in the psychological recesses of the patient's mind.

One only forgets—one can only forget—the things which no longer preoccupy and disturb one. To know one's enemy is already to be in a position where one does not fear him. To fear him no longer practically means the same thing as to neglect him. The whole treatment of functional troubles, outside of some particular cases, lies in so disposing the patient's mind that he has a feeling of intelligent security in regard to the symptoms with which he is attacked.

A patient will only feel himself cured when in all good faith he can say to you, when speaking of his troubles, "I never think of them now."

Under some circumstances, and in the presence of convictions which are too deeply rooted in the patient, one might be led to penetrate his systematization by taking him by surprise. The principle of this process consists in making the subject do, without his having paid any attention to it, some particular act which he believed himself incapable of accomplishing, or, again, by warding off, by some happy intervention, the usual returns of the pathological phenomenon. The employment of such proceedings naturally necessitates a certain ingenuity on the part of the physician, for it is very important that he should succeed. He will run the risk, in case of failure, of increasing the disturbances against which he is struggling.

When it has happened, for example, that he has been able to get an asthenic individual to take a little walk with him, or when he has been able by keeping up the conversation to go past the given hour at which such or such a gastric trouble is due to appear, he must take care not to be in too great a hurry to show his triumph. The patient will immediately seek excuses for his lapse from his functional troubles, and there is a very great chance that on the next day he will come back to you completely upset, or more dyspeptic than ever. "Doctor," he will say to you, "you let me do a very imprudent thing," or else, "I began to feel a pain in my stomach when I went away from your house, and it has never left me the whole day." Keep your triumph, then, for a time at least, a secret, and if, on the next day and the day after, nothing new has happened, then—and then only—show your patient the illogical character of troubles which may be made to disappear by distraction.

But do not be deceived. This "trick," if one might use that expression, is only very rarely necessary and is not always without danger. One can hardly employ it systematically without regret. There are a great many very precise indications which it will run up against, as we shall see further on in the peculiar manifestations of sexual disturbances.

Does this mean that in the treatment of functional manifestations the emotional elements, whose action we have seen to be preponderant in psychotherapy on the moral condition of the neurasthenic, have completely lost their sway? By no means. In the first place, no explanation whatever will be accepted by the patient until he has confidence in his physician, but, even if the patient's reason may progressively respond to convincing arguments, it may happen that his feelings do not keep up with the march. He will be quite aware that he is unreasonable, and that he is behaving in such or such a manner; but he would much rather be considered unreasonable than to change his ways, if the emotional elements, which at bottom are the only ones with any determining power, do not come into play. He may know that he is wrong in suffering, but he will continue to suffer, and that will not change his situation in the slightest. If, on the other hand, you have, to use a slang expression, "got him," if he feels perfect confidence in his physician, he will feel perfect faith that his symptoms will by and by disappear, and then you can get him to do almost anything that you want. Anything that you wish him to do or any effort necessary to break up the vicious circle connected with all his functional troubles he will do, even though he may for the time being suffer considerably. His cure will then take place rapidly, because not only will he have taken a new direction through his reason but will be urged along in it by his feelings.

As a matter of fact, in the therapy of functional manifestations, the physician has not only to struggle against pathological convictions and against errors of interpretation, but he has also to combat apprehensions. The latter naturally result from the former. But when functional manifestations have been prolonged for a sufficient length of time the apprehension becomes involuntary and subconscious, and tends to persist even when in the mind or the pure reason of the patient the convictions have been destroyed and the errors repaired. And it is only under the influence of the action of sthenic emotions that the patient can get control of his apprehensions and manage, after a greater or less length of time, to forget them.

The treatment of functional manifestations demands more explanations and more reasoning than the treatment of the moral depths of the neurasthenic. But in one case as well as in the other we cannot say too often that there is no such thing as cold-blooded psychotherapy.

And if this is true for the treatment of the functional manifestation considered in itself, it is still more true if one considers the mental depths themselves which have permitted these manifestations to become established and which contribute to make them persistent. The general conviction of helplessness, the habit of auto-analysis and auto-observation, the search for the symptom and its magnification,—elements which are, moreover, rather of the moral than of the psychic order,—have participated in the genesis of all the symptoms which the neurasthenic offers. It is very certain that, by explanation and reasoning which permits the patient to become reassured concerning the origin of all his troubles, all these psychological phenomena will have a great chance of becoming diminished.

But there will, nevertheless, always be something left behind,—a sensation of vague insecurity, a feeling of anxiety about the return of the troubles which have disappeared. This is something which can only be completely abolished under the influence of strong emotional growth. This is the same thing as saying that one cannot treat a functional trouble alone, even by the most persuasive or the most incisive psychotherapy, without at the same time being concerned with the general moral condition of the patient and without trying to modify it, and that only can be brought about through feeling and sympathy.

CHAPTER XXIII.

THE ADJUVANTS OF PSYCHOTHERAPY.

BEFORE taking up the study of the detailed treatment of the functional manifestations, it seems to us advisable to glance at the rôle which certain therapeutic agents, such as isolation, rest, and overfeeding, play in the treatment, and state a little more definitely just when they are indicated, for one will often have occasion to utilize them, and under certain circumstances they are necessary adjuncts of the psychotherapy of persuasion.

There was a time when, associated with rest and overfeeding, isolation formed the basis of all therapy connected with the psychoneuroses. According to our way of thinking, isolation, even accompanied by rest and overfeeding, is never enough. Neither is it any more considered to be always absolutely necessary. Just as there can be no such thing as any "sure cure" for the psychoneuroses, so it would be irrational to look upon the isolation of neuropaths as a therapeutic necessity from which one might never depart. It only applies to particular cases and is subjected to a few general rules.

But, first of all, what must one understand by *isolation?* The usual thing is to consider isolation as, first and foremost, consisting of the almost absolute seclusion of the patient, which can only be accomplished in a sanitarium or a hospital. A patient is shut up in a room, into which no one but the physician and the nurse may enter. He receives no letters, is allowed no visitors, and is permitted no relations with anybody except those people who are in care of his treatment.

One step further in isolation, which is really rather one step further in the rest treatment, may be obtained when one keeps the patient's room in a state of semi-darkness, and when one does not allow him to have the slightest knowledge outside of the very narrow environment in which he finds himself.

One degree less consists of permitting the patient, although he may not take any part in it, to know what is going on outside, and to watch and be interested in the life around him. This is already the beginning of outside interests for the patient.

Provided that one approaches this by regular gradations, or, on the contrary, that one is satisfied that it can be introduced at the start, one may go quite far in this method of modified isolation, even so much so as simply to ask the patient to withdraw from his daily duties and his customary surroundings.

This is because, as a matter of fact, isolation is not a simple therapeutic agent. It is not an end; it is only a means which is absolutely necessary in a great number of cases, in order to be able to apply psychotherapy with success.

Reasons of an extremely varied nature, which sometimes are completely foreign to the patient considered by himself, may make it necessary.

Here, for example, is a subject who has a very bad family environment, and who has often found the cause of his neurasthenia in this environment itself. There, on the other hand, is a family who treats a neurasthenic like a make-believe invalid, and who consequently exaggerates the sufferings of a poor wretch, who often "wants to do things, but really cannot," or else, on the other hand,—and this is more apt to be the case,—it is a family who by its too fussy care and perpetual anxiety encourages the patient in his depressing ideas and in his unhealthy point of view. Thus, we see that the psychotherapeutist has many reasons which point out very definitely the need of isolation from one's environment.

Let us take the mother of a family who although neurasthenic still keeps up her pride in the appearance of her home. Just as long as she lives there she cannot help but play the part of wife, and attend to her duties as mistress of her home. The education and the health of her children are continually on her mind. What really serious psychotherapeutic action could one practise upon her under these conditions? It is very evident that there will always be a continual tendency for her thoughts to turn toward her home and her loved ones. Here isolation and separation from her environment are absolutely indicated. It would not be the gravity of the patient's condition that would be the principal reason for her isolation.

Let us suppose, on the other hand, that a subject who has been neurasthenic for some years, and more or less phobic, and afflicted with numerous functional manifestations, has always lived in one spot. Cannot one understand that under these conditions his sickness, as it were, hangs on the very walls which surround him? Each piece of furniture and every little object under his hand has been, as a matter of fact, associated with some distressing moment of his life. It is perfectly clear that, by the common mechanism of the association of ideas, his surroundings will continually recall to the patient his sickness and all his symptoms. Go, under these conditions, and tell him to *forget,* for that is the last word of psychotherapy concerning functional manifestations, as we shall see later on. Here, again, you will see that isolation, which means isolation from his environment, is obligatory.

Take an individual who has become neurasthenic because he has lost one of his family, a wife or a child. Cannot one see that, if he remains in the same environment in which he experienced these sorrows, the emotional cause will have every chance of prolonging its disintegrating action in a way that will be almost indefinite? Until he has completely gotten hold of himself the patient ought to be wholly separated from his former environment.

Here is an hysterical patient who is subject to attacks of paralysis and contracture. How can one hope for any improvement in his symptoms if he is left with his family?

Here, again, is a case of mental anorexia, showing the results of excessive lack of nutrition. How can one obtain any favorable result if the patient remain in the family circle? Here, as in the preceding case, absolute isolation is necessary.

In all these cases isolation from one's environment and from one's daily routine is the underlying condition of psychotherapeutic treatment, whose action otherwise would be rendered completely useless.

There are, on the other hand, subjects who are in the very midst of some moral upheaval, in a condition that one might describe as extreme emotional hypertension. The slightest thing depresses them; they are extremely irritable. Here isolation is indicated, and not merely isolation from one's family circle and from one's daily surroundings, but, still further, complete isolation which shall be almost absolutely free from any external excitation. With such subjects we enter upon a series of cases where isolation is not merely a condition of psychotherapy, but where it becomes the condition of absolute rest, which is necessary for certain patients. Such is the case, for example, with people who suffer from extreme exhaustion. The statement of this formula, that complete rest can only be obtained in isolation, gives us the key to all the cases where strict isolation is indicated.

This same strict isolation may be utilized under certain circumstances as a true psychotherapeutic measure. Certain subjects with a weak will, many hysterics, and children, as a general rule, in order to be freed from an isolation which weighs heavily upon them, will find themselves capable of getting their ideas to work, a thing which could not have been accomplished otherwise without great difficulty. But, they will tell us, in this cloistral isolation the patients will be apt to become very uneasy and disturbed concerning the health of their families. How can one deprive a mother of a family of news of her children? Your subjects' minds cannot be at rest and in a tranquil state, and therefore they will be in very poor condition to get well. If things happen in this way the objection would be wisely taken, but this is not the case. Every subject who is obliged to go into strict isolation, and who is consequently deprived of letters and of visits, will receive every day absolutely exact news of what has happened in his family. Furthermore, he knows, for he is told at the start, that if one of his family should fall sick he would be immediately told of the fact, and would be allowed to interrupt his treatment and go home. This is the only way in which strict isolation can be undertaken without disturbing the moral tranquillity of those who are obliged to submit to it.

We only insist on isolation either in a sanitarium or in a hospital because, by reason of the great number of patients being brought together in different periods of their disease, there is necessity for a special discipline.[1]

Let us say, however, that each time that strict isolation is indicated, it can only be practised at a hospital or a sanitarium, because there, and there only, the patients will find the proper personal attendance adapted to the various cares which their condition demands. In short, in order to have the psychotherapeutic action which the physician lays out practised continually, it is of great importance that it should not be interrupted by maladroit interventions of some second person. By breaking the disciplinary rules of strict isolation, by ill-chosen conversations, or simply by those that last too long, the nurse or attendant may be as dangerous to the neuropathic patient as he would be if he handed around iced drinks to pneumonia patients or if he gave a typhoid patient all that he wanted to eat. The choice of the persons who assist the physician is, therefore, of very great importance.

To sum up, we would say that isolation may be prescribed in three different degrees,—namely:

(1) Strict isolation.

(2) Absolute isolation from one's family circle and environment.

(3) Isolation from one's family circle alone, or from one's environment alone. In this latter case one either takes the patient away from his home but allows one of his family to accompany him, or else lets him stay in his home but separates him from the people who usually surround him.

It is evident that the third degree differs only quantitatively from the second, as, as a matter of fact, one's environment forms a constituent part of one's circle, and that there are particular cases which, according to the causes which have brought about the patient's condition and the symptoms which he shows, and also according to the positive or negative therapeutic value of his surroundings, indicate that there is a necessity of absolute isolation from one's family circle and from one's environment, or from only one of these two elements.

Cloistral isolation cannot be realized except at a sanitarium or at a hospital. This is because the hospital or sanitarium offers the best opportunity of isolation of the second degree. One could also under certain circumstances send a patient to a hydrotherapeutic or thermal establishment, or to stay in the country, anywhere, in fact—but this is the imperative condition—where he could find proper psychothera-

[1] One will find in the work of Camus et Pagniez, l.c., very complete details concerning the organization of hospital isolation such as has been practised by one of us for fifteen years during his service in the Pinel Ward at the Salpêtrière.

peutic treatment. Isolation from one's family alone can also be accomplished under the same conditions by permitting a patient to be accompanied by one of the members of his family.

As to isolation from one's social environment, it does not have to take place so very often, and it is rendered necessary for very special reasons. As a general rule, it will be much simpler to separate the patient from both his environment and his family circle at the same time by proceeding as we have just indicated.

The reader may ask whether it is possible for us to indicate approximately, among patients afflicted with a great variety of neuropathic symptoms, what is the proportion of those for whom isolation, in its various degrees, is necessary? Here it is evidently a question of kinds. Nevertheless, in order to get some idea of it and to show how slightly our experience has inclined us toward any systematic treatment of the psychoneuroses by isolation, we might say that for at least a third of the neuropathic women who have been cared for at the Salpêtrière isolation has not seemed to us to be necessary. Again, it must be added, that, of the patients admitted, a certain number have been received at the hospital and naturally submitted to the discipline which belongs to an isolation ward much more for humanitarian and social reasons than because absolute isolation seemed to be formally indicated.

Rest, like isolation, is not such a simple idea but that it would be useful to analyze it. It seems to be the simplest thing in the world to advise a patient to take a rest. As a matter of fact, there are very few therapeutic agents which are as badly handled as that. Rest implies elements of various kinds. There is physical rest, and psychic rest, and moral rest, which are not necessarily associated.

Let us glance first of all at physical rest. Its maximum is evidently realized by keeping the patient in bed altogether for a considerable time. Under certain circumstances it may be necessary to impose it absolutely, but it is chiefly indicated because outside of absolute rest it is extremely difficult to attain any definite amount of comparative rest. It would seem, on first looking at it, that one might grade the rest by ordering patients to remain in bed for twelve, fourteen, eighteen, or twenty hours; but the thing that must be considered then is, not the time which the patient passes in bed or lying down, but the use that he makes of the moments when he is permitted to move about. Here, for example, is an asthenic, convinced of his physical helplessness, who when walking makes all kinds of movements which are disharmonic, and who in a few moments really tires himself out as much as a normal man would tire in ten or twenty times the length of time. Of what use is it to prescribe for him any very long period of rest if in the interval between he loses all the benefit of it? On the other hand, one sees patients who are always moving about in bed, who are restless and continually changing their position or altering the arrangement of their covers, who change the position of their pillow a hundred times. Where in such cases does the physical rest which you want to get for them come in?

Another one will lie perfectly still in his bed, but he will hold himself in a wrong position which after a short time will bring about a feeling of numbness in one of his limbs, or congestion of the head, or cold in the feet, from all of which symptoms he will suffer distress and become exasperated, and which by a different mechanism will make him lose the benefit of his rest.

All of which means that to put a patient through a course of treatment requiring absolute or comparative rest is not only to command him to lie physically still for a certain number of hours, but it also means to lay down a course of discipline for the intervals of rest, and to assure those very conditions under which the rest will be realized. In the case of absolute rest, how much time will it be necessary to keep the patient continually in bed? Here, again, it is a question of particular cases. Among those who are very much exhausted, or very much emaciated, and, above all, in those where absolute rest is indicated, complete confinement to one's bed may vary from several weeks to several months. In a general way we estimate that the physician must be guided chiefly by the patient's increase in weight. The faster he gains weight the shorter will be the time that he has to stay in bed, and by degrees he can be brought back to the times and seasons of normal life.

Now to pass on to the question of mental rest. The formula consists in prohibiting all brain work for the patient. Our subject must give up all his business occupations, leave his office, get away from his library. He will not improve any more quickly for that, but rather otherwise, if he continues to think about things, and if a thousand ideas surge through his agitated brain. It is necessary, therefore, for the prescription of mental rest to be accompanied by a certain number of points to be observed. We are in the habit of telling a great many of our patients to try to put themselves all the time into the condition of the subject who is trying to go to sleep. Certain patients revolt because they find that in this way the day seems to be interminable to them. Then make them understand that this appearance corresponds to a therapeutic reality, and that if the day seems to them to have forty-eight hours it is really, from the point of view of the withdrawing of pathological phenomena and from the forgetting of the symptoms presented, as if it had lasted the apparent time. In some cases, and among those patients who cannot seem to get to the point of checking their thoughts in this way, one can bring about a state of intellectual repose by means of work, paradoxical as this may seem. You can occupy your patients with intellectual work of some mechanical nature.

It would seem as though the blissful game of patience of our youth had been rejuvenated under the form of puzzles for the special benefit of neurasthenics. Sometimes reading some light novel will offer sufficient intellectual rest. But for mental rest, as well as for physical rest, the important thing to take into consideration is this fact,—namely, that the chief factor of fatigue in all normal sick individuals is neither movement nor work, but rather agitation or cerebral tension.

When it comes to be a question of moral rest, certain physicians think that they have solved the whole problem by saying to their patients, "Do something to distract yourself; take a journey." There are some who are content to say simply, "Don't dwell upon the things that trouble you." The advice is excellent, but often not at all easy to follow! Here the physician's help should be much more direct. It is necessary for him, having learned something about the patient's life, to direct his manner of living, temporarily, at least for the time necessary for his cure. If the patient occupies some particular social position, he must be relieved of it in such a way that, concerning that thing at least, he is perfectly tranquil. If he has children, he must intrust them to some relative in whom he has absolute confidence. The physician must think about all these things, and plan for them, in order to be sure that the moral rest, which he considers necessary, may be effectively accomplished, and that the patient, feeling a sense of security as regards the present, has only to forget the past and to strengthen himself for the future. All these ideas are evidently simply an expression of good sense, but, if we are to believe what we have seen, they are very seldom put into practice. As a matter of fact, we have seen a great many patients to whom excellent advice has been given, but not the means of following it.

Absolute rest can practically be accomplished only by strict isolation. The patient who has been promised, and who has confidence in the word of the speaker, that if anything happens to any of his family he will be told of it immediately, but who does not receive any kind of excitement whatsoever of an outside origin, will naturally find himself in the best situation to acquire internal calmness, which is the ideal form of repose.

This should apply to every degree of rest. It is a question of making arrangements and taking the minutest care on the part of the physician.

Overfeeding is an adjunct which, when one finds that it is indicated, should be applied in a much more systematic way. In the great majority of cases we still find that a partial or absolute milk diet gives the best results.

Cases where milk cannot be tolerated are met with only in the smallest numbers. An intolerance which lasts sufficiently long and is so marked that one is obliged to give up a milk diet has not been met with by us in more than the proportion of one in two or three hundred cases, in an experience of dealing with thousands of patients. What one sees most often are patients who complain of bitterness or distention, clamminess of the mouth, diarrhœa, or constipation. These phenomena, which last as a rule for only a few days, are not necessary to be considered.

It is our custom to make our patients take milk from hour to hour in increasing quantities twelve times a day. We begin by making them take three quarts the first day, perhaps two hundred and fifty drachms an hour; then we increase the hourly dose in such a way as to attain the quantity of three and a half to four quarts, and finally get up to the amount of five quarts a day, beyond which we rarely go. We get up to this last quantity in eight or ten days.

The great advantage of this milk diet is that it does not require any very great effort to take it. A cup of milk is easily swallowed. Patients will readily consent to such a diet of overfeeding who would refuse to eat bountiful or frequent meals.

It must not be forgotten that, as a matter of fact, our patients are most often apt to be in a state of very marked and sometimes extremely pronounced denutrition. Now, as they have more or less lost their appetite, and under these conditions, if at the beginning of their treatment it is difficult and perhaps almost impossible for them to take solid food in sufficient quantity not only to nourish them, but, more than that, to increase their weight, it is, however, always easy for them to drink. The practice of milk régime from the start of the treatment is, moreover, the only process which can give such remarkable—we might almost say such unbelievable—increase in weight as we are constantly obtaining, and which, as almost a regular thing, amounts to from 1500 to 1800 grammes (3 to 3.5 pounds) a week, and goes up in cases which are rare but not exceptional to as high as 6 or 8 or even 10 pounds during the first week. Do we mean by this that we attach any doctrinal value to the practice of overfeeding on a milk diet? By no means. Our experience has simply proved that this is the easiest method and the one that is surest and most efficacious.

Other methods of overfeeding, apart from the fact that they are not always free from danger to the liver and kidneys of the patient, hardly ever give the same results.

Let us add, finally, that in a certain number of cases, and particularly in those where overfeeding does not necessarily seem to be urgent as a therapeutic measure, we are perfectly willing to confine these rules for overfeeding to heartier and more frequent meals, without any other régime.

Physical and mental rest as well as overfeeding are, however, not absolutely necessary elements of the treatment of a psychoneurosis, any more than isolation. It all depends on the nature of the case, for the indications are determined by the existence of this or that functional manifestation. The only thing that seems to us absolutely and always necessary is the moral rest,—that is, the effort made by the physician and by the patient to avoid the onset of new emotions which are liable to upset the patient again and to interrupt the psychotherapeutic action. It is impossible to give the patient's mind a new direction, to lay down for him new paths of thought, so to speak, in any given direction, if he is constantly subjected to the continual action of real preoccupations corresponding to some effective cause. Naturally, in many cases these matters are not easy to arrange. One has to ask the patient to temporarily lose his interest in a whole series of facts which are apt to add their depressing influence to his preoccupation and to the old emotions which originally brought on his disease. In holding before his eyes the hope of a cure, one is often able to obtain from him this sacrifice, which elsewhere is practically brought about by isolation, which is the only thing that makes it possible to really lose interest in oneself.

There are many other helps in the therapy of a psychoneurosis. We shall have occasion to point them out as we go along, when in a little while we shall take up the study of the treatment of the functional manifestations. But the thing that we hope will be retained from the preceding pages is that in the treatment of a psychoneurosis, without this psychotherapeutic action which is the only absolutely fundamental thing, and which is always necessary to employ, there is no possible therapeutic systematization.

If we have devoted a whole chapter to the study of isolation, rest, and overfeeding, it is because these agents are employed under a great number of circumstances. They in themselves never constitute a sufficient psychotherapy, while, inversely, the psychotherapeutic treatment may, without any other aid, cure a comparatively great number of patients.

No independent treatment, such as dietetic treatment alone or isolation or rest based on some systematic method, or any such common formula, can fill the varied and multiple requirements of the treatment of our patients.

CHAPTER XXIV.

SPECIAL THERAPY OF THE VARIOUS FUNCTIONAL MANIFESTATIONS.

If general psychotherapy of the mental and moral status of the neurasthenic consists in a single therapy common to all patients afflicted with psychoneuroses, and if the same principles of treatment for the functional manifestations are susceptible to a general application, it is no less true that each particular functional manifestation calls forth indications for special treatment. This is particularly the case with the processes of re-education, which evidently cannot be the same when one is treating the case of an asthenic, or a false gastropath, or a false urinary.

Taking up the whole series of functional manifestations as we have described them in the first part of this work, let us glance successively at those particular therapeutic agents which have seemed to us to be beneficial. It goes without saying that any treatment of a functional trouble must be accompanied by treatment of the underlying moral and mental condition on which the symptom has been grafted.

I. Functional Manifestations in the Digestive Organs.

A. Disturbances of the Appetite.—Of all the functional manifestations of which the digestive apparatus is the seat, the most serious and that which requires the most prompt and specialized treatment is undoubtedly mental anorexia. This is because, although mental anorexia is a psychoneurosis as far as its cause is concerned, its results express themselves in one of the most serious organic conditions. Whether one has to treat a patient who is extremely emaciated, or whether the anorexia be primary or secondary, before any other kind of psychotherapeutic treatment can be begun, it is extremely important to isolate the patient and to feed him.

We do not hesitate to say emphatically that it is impossible to treat mental anorexia in the family circle, and that to attempt it is to run the risk of certain failure, of which the patient's death may be the outcome. This is because the family give in too easily to their patient, and do not know how to insist upon the kind of feeding that is necessary. Furthermore, it often happens that the anorexic patient seems to get a great deal of satisfaction out of complaining about his food, and of getting his family to intercede for him, and this, when the treatment is not sufficiently well systematized, leads to a continuous loss of weight which he will look upon with a sense of triumph. Isolation is, therefore, imperative, and in such cases it must be strict isolation. The desire to shorten its duration may sometimes of itself be enough to induce the patient to consent all the sooner to take food.

As far as the alimentation itself is concerned, there are two classes of patients who may be met with. Some are so feeble that one hardly dares to disturb them. Here it is necessary to carry on the feeding in a very slow and progressive manner. One may sometimes not be able to give during the first day more than a few teaspoonfuls of milk every five or ten minutes, or every quarter of an hour, and to increase little by little, but in a way which is nevertheless rapid, the amount of each feeding. If on the first day it was only possible to give the patient from six to nine ounces of milk, on the second day one ought to be able to get him to take a pint and a half, on the third three pints, and finally get to the point in eight or ten days where he will take a regular quantity of five quarts of milk, which amount should be maintained until the patient has regained his normal weight,—that is to say, during a number of weeks, which, of course, would vary in different cases. At this point one may, any day, put him upon an ordinary regular diet.

Among patients who are still vigorous, as are the majority of the primary anorexias, one manages in three or four days to get to the point where one can give the classic amount to what constitutes overfeeding in a milk diet. If necessary,—that is, if the patient refuses to take the quantity of milk which is prescribed,—one should proceed energetically. One may threaten the patient with the feeding-tube, and if necessary use it. If he makes himself vomit afterward, as often happens, one must simply begin the gavage over again as soon as he is through. The very important thing is not to give in. As a matter of fact, however, when the physician's authority is sufficiently well established, it is very seldom that one is obliged to have recourse to such extreme measures, because, when he feels that he has to do with somebody who is stronger than himself, the patient generally submits.

It may happen that, among certain patients who are extremely weak, one is obliged to seek for aid from ordinary medical therapy; one may thus have to give injections of serum, or hypodermics of caffeine, or camphor oil, to warm the patient by artificial means. These are urgent therapeutic measures such as are applied to people in the last stages of starvation and subjects who are at the point of death.

In such patients psychotherapy must not be omitted at the start if the patients are strong enough, or if they have passed the most serious point in the disease where the danger of an unfortunate outcome has been avoided; it is necessary then to try to find out, in the different ways that we have indicated, the emotional, moral, or psychical causes of the anorexic conditions. We do not insist on this point. It is the general psychotherapy of the psychoneurosis which is here in question.

But the psychic therapy of anorexics demands some special indications. These patients must be made to understand that just as long as they try to practise deceptions concerning their food they will not be cured. We are accustomed to tell our patients that the triumph for them lies not in merely succeeding to take the least little bit from the plate of meat set before them, but rather in making up their mind, by an effort of will at first and then spontaneously later, to choose if not the largest piece at least one of fairly good size.

If the patients have really understood the mechanism of their disease, which at some time you must have explained to them, if you have succeeded by an emotional reaction in penetrating sufficiently into their mentality, it is rare if they do not rapidly comprehend your point of view. At first with effort, but later quite naturally, they will eat heartily and in sufficient quantities.

Under these conditions one has no need to fear a relapse. It would, however, be almost fatal if after having made your patient gain a certain number of pounds you should leave him without having modified his mentality.

When you send such patients home to their families, you must warn them that no matter what happens, and no matter how much advice is given to them on the subject, they must never, except of course in very serious illness, consent to go upon a restricted diet.

Outside of the mental anorexias which are sharply defined, there are a great number of cases of minor anorexia where almost imperceptibly, and by very easy stages by the slow but progressive restriction of their diet, subjects are gradually in the way of developing a characteristic anorexia. Here a very rigid therapy is not necessary, at least at the start, and it is generally enough to make the patient understand the danger which threatens him, and to put him upon a hearty diet, in order for him to regain rapidly the few pounds which he has lost.

As far as unnatural cravings for certain foods and over-voracious appetites and elective anorexias are concerned, they do not demand any special indications except in so far as re-education is concerned, which ought to be carried on progressively. One must limit those with a voracious appetite to a certain quantity of food to be taken at each meal. Then one must diminish the number of meals. As for the elective anorexias, one must ask that the patients should add to their diet, which has been restricted as regards kind, at first a few and a small quantity and then a greater number and a greater quantity of the foods which they have been accustomed to refuse.

B. Disturbances of the First Three Stages of Digestion.—We have seen that in this class of functional manifestations there are two marked classes of patients. One, which is by far the most numerous, is composed of true phobics of deglutition, who do not dare to swallow. The other includes a very much smaller number of patients who after having swallowed their food are seized with spasm of the œsophagus. We may divide the first group of patients into three classes. It may happen that the alimentary restriction in relation to the phobic phenomena has been sufficiently great to bring the patient into a state of true mental anorexia. The isolation and the process of treatment applied to this last manifestation are then imposed.

Under other circumstances isolation will often be indicated because in his environment the patient will find elements which will bring back and call up and encourage the functional manifestation. Until he is cured, it will be necessary for him to avoid the daily life in which his first symptoms were called forth. Finally, in a certain number of cases in which these conditions are not realized, simple psychotherapeutic treatment will be found to be sufficient.

It is clear that, the nature of the symptoms in question having been brought out by the examination and questioning, the first work of the psychotherapeutist will be to reassure the patient by explaining to him very carefully the nature of the symptoms which he presents. He will then have to experimentally confirm this conviction, which he has induced the patient to accept, concerning the psychic nature of the phenomena which he has experienced. The best method consists in being present at one of the patient's meals, so that he may feel a sense of absolute safety that if any accident happens to him he will have immediate help. But here one must be careful not to think that he ought continually to urge the patient and encourage him. It more often happens that by doing this the emotional phenomena are recalled, and that the patient shows more hesitation than ever before swallowing anything. The encouragements and all questions concerning the emotional element which might upset the patient ought to be before or after the experimental meal. If during this repast, however, one can succeed in distracting the patient's attention in such a way that he swallows without thinking, this will be the best way of completely reassuring him. It will not always be convenient, and if one does not succeed in this way one must be content to make the patient take a certain amount of food in a given time. On the following day, and so on progressively, one will increase the amount of food while at the same time one will diminish the allotted time. In some cases one can, during this process of re-education, recommend a rather varied diet. There is, as a matter of fact, a certain number of such patients who can easily swallow liquid or soft food and who only have difficulty with solid food. There are others in whom the opposite phenomena are true. One can for several days, and during the time when one is carrying on the most energetic psychotherapy, only give the patient the kind of food which does not excite any phobic symptom in him. One will thus give his emotional condition time to calm down. One will permit the patient in this way to forget, so to speak, his functional phenomena. Normal feeding may then be taken up without any transition, and will often be readily borne.

At all events, the treatment could not be considered as finished until, either by psychotherapeutic or experimental conviction, the swallowing can be accomplished quite spontaneously.

Concerning spasms of the œsophagus a very important distinction must be made. They are not all directly and exclusively amenable to psychotherapy. There are very serious spasms (Guisez) in which organic modifications, consisting essentially of dilatation of the hypopharynx or of the œsophagus, with a more or less acute inflammatory condition, follow the functional trouble and make it worse. In such cases, when the organic modifications have not yielded to appropriate treatment which belongs to the work of a specialist, it is useless to try a psychic treatment, which by itself would be wholly inefficacious. Progressive dilatation may be indicated, and psychotherapy would only come in as a secondary element to reassure the patient and to avoid relapses.

In recent or mild cases psychotherapy and methods of re-education would, on the other hand, be enough to assure the disappearance of the functional trouble. Here again, following the circumstances which have preceded the appearance of the trouble and those which seem to be persistent, isolation may or may not be indicated.

It is rather rare in such cases that all foods should cause a spasm. However, in the case of serious spasms, when the spasm which is increased by local symptoms has become permanent, it has occurred only as a consequence of a psychic impression. When a patient has taken some food concerning which he has felt perfectly safe, no symptom is produced. One should remember this fact, as it is an aid in re-education. One should allow the patient time to feel the general psychotherapeutic influence by feeding him at first only with what he can tolerate, in order not to encourage a susceptibility which is going to diminish gradually under psychotherapeutic influence.

There are even some subjects whose attack is so slight that a single psychotherapeutic conversation may cause all their troubles to disappear, and the patient can go home and eat like anybody else.

C. Gastric Manifestations of Nervous People.—The course to be pursued varies according to whether the patient has the simple dyspeptic troubles of a neurasthenic, or gastric phobias, or characteristic pseudo-gastropathy, or neuropathic vomiting.

The *simple dyspeptic disturbances* of the neurasthenic do not require any special therapy. Moreover, they generally form merely an accessory in the symptomatic ensemble. All that we have said of the general psychotherapy of the neurasthenic and the general psychotherapy of a functional manifestation may be applied without comment to these disturbances.

Two different therapies may be applied, according to circumstances, to the *stomach phobias.* If a physician has sufficient authority over his patient, he may at the outset of a single conversation so stir him up that he can get him to throw over all his purely subjective fears. But it often happens that a physician's influence is not at first sufficiently strong, or that the patient's systematization has been too long established and too crowded with all kinds of associations. One must then go more slowly, and take up progressively the alimentary re-education of the patient. At the start, one must be prudent, and must commence by the diet which the patient thinks is the only one that he can tolerate, and must make only very slight additions. But, just in proportion as the mentality of the patient changes in response to the experiment, one may become a little bolder. The patient who would have cried out a little while before at any slight change in his food régime, "Oh, my stomach could never stand all that," is already at the point where he no longer feels astonished at having you propose an almost radical transformation of his usual diet. There are even great numbers of patients who, having been made happy at their first trial of the general psychotherapeutic action, have themselves gone upon a regular diet. Either at the start or after a little time, which rarely exceeds a fortnight or three weeks, such patients are cured.

The therapeutic action is by no means so easy to obtain in cases of characteristic *pseudo-gastropathies.* The systematizaticn of the patient in general, which is, moreover, reinforced by former therapeutic measures, is extremely strong. The symptomatology is loaded with phenomena which, as we have already seen, have an objective reality, and make a great impression on the patient. A whole series of associations of all kinds is formed, and the pathological idea is hung, as it were, upon all the constituent elements of the patient's condition due to his surroundings. More often isolation—and very rigorous isolation—is distinctly indicated. It is all the more apt to be the case with those patients who are very much morally or physically depressed, and in the state of subcontinuous emotionalism, and who are in real need of that absolute rest which can be assured only by isolation.

For such patients the part of re-education, which, however, is effective, does not appear to us to be less necessary, but rather secondary. Their moral and mental condition is generally so bad, and such a great number of symptoms presented by them might be considered as emotional gastric fixations, that in their treatment general psychotherapy must play the most important part. In proportion as the moral condition of these patients is improved there is a marked quieting down of their gastric troubles. If one makes a simultaneous attack upon the psychic conditions which have directed the patient to turn his attention upon his stomach, it is not an unusual thing for one to be able to work a rather rapid cure. It goes without saying that one will find certain phenomena persisting for a rather long time, such as those phenomena which like atony are due to poor general condition resulting from lack of food, or troubles which depend, if one might put it so, upon the bad secretory or motor habits which have become fastened upon the patient for months or years under some psychic influence. However, the persistence of these manifestations, expressing themselves by a certain bitterness or feeling of heaviness or gas, etc., is never prolonged for any length of time. It is all the more apt to be less when the general condition of the patient has been improved by having sufficient nourishment.

The restoration of the patient to normal nourishment does not always take place without some set-backs, and it is then that one must resort to dietetic re-education. This ought to be based upon the exact knowledge of the mechanism which was present at the time when the patient began to choose or suppress certain articles in his dietary régime (see Part I, Chapter I, p. 10).

It is quite certain that, in a very large majority of cases, it would be imprudent, at least, to expect to get false gastropaths, whose psychism has been for long years centred upon their stomach, suddenly to give up altogether the dietetic régime which they have followed until that day. It would be no more reasonable than to ask an hysterical hemiplegic or astasia-abasic to recover instantaneously his movements or his equilibrium. One must gradually change the patient's food régime; conquests must be made day by day and the progress be slow but regular. Under this condition only will the results obtained be definite. And although, in some cases, physicians who have considerable influence over their patients have been able to induce them to change suddenly their alimentary hygiene, we have been able to establish the fact for ourselves that, although some brilliant results have been obtained, they are very apt to be followed by set-backs, of which the most serious consequence is to fix the patient's mind still more firmly upon his disease, to anchor the conviction of his gastropathy still more firmly, and to make it more difficult to get back to a normal life.

We might add, however, that patients who have suffered sometimes for years—and we have seen those whose affection dated back for twenty-five or thirty years—do not care much whether the treatment takes several weeks more or less. Furthermore, we must frankly say that when the cure has been slow and difficult to obtain there is more chance of its lasting. The chief thing is that the patient ought to be told beforehand about how much time it will take to bring him back to his original condition, so that one may avoid in this way any possibility of disappointing him.

It is very certain that the first thing of all to combat is the actual insufficiency of food, regardless of its quality. It is necessary to induce the patient to go upon such a régime that his weight, instead of steadily diminishing as it has done hitherto, will perceptibly increase. This is the first end which one must have in view before anything else.

But, in order not to multiply one's difficulties, it will be absolutely useless to give the patient many different foods at once. At this period, at the start of the treatment, in the greatest number of cases, milk taken in small repeated doses is the thing which will fill the greatest number of requirements. Starting with a dose of three quarts, in a few days one can increase it to four or five quarts. This exclusive milk diet in large quantities ought to be kept up from a week to a month, sometimes longer, according to the manner in which the patient has been able to tolerate it, and according to the psychic modification which has been obtained by contemporaneous psychotherapeutic treatment.

The practical result, from our point of view, of this whole period is to show the patient that he can digest a large quantity of food, a quantity which in any case is enough to make him gain weight (from eight to fifteen pounds at least in three or four weeks). He will not refrain from telling you that this food has been digested by him, because it was nothing but milk and liquid diet. After the quantitative re-education has been accomplished, we insist that it must be followed by qualitative re-education, and just here, when we come to struggle against all the notions concerning the quality of food, we must proceed with more or less circumspection, because it is often just at this point that one is apt to meet the greatest difficulties.

In regard to the individual variations which one may observe and to which one should lend the greatest consideration, the attitude to take in the conduct of reconstruction of normal alimentation should be based on the exact knowledge of the psychical mechanism according to which in the particular case the progressive restriction of diet has been brought about. It is no less true that, as a rule, the ideas which have been developed from what we have said in the first part of our book are practically sufficient. That is to say, in other words, that one should avoid letting the patient be conscious of any effort in the matter of taking food. For the constituent elements of psychic sensation of the effort of eating have already been enumerated by us. They are all rather active sensorial impressions. All these mechanical difficulties of mastication or of deglutition are rather vivid sensorial impressions.

Therefore, in this progressive, systematic re-education which we are pursuing, we must begin with semi-liquid food that is not at all greasy nor highly seasoned. From this point of view, eggs, milk toast, vegetables, and minced meats that are not highly seasoned fill the need. It may be a matter of some days before one can work up to a beefsteak or a lamb chop every other day. A week or perhaps a fortnight later you will have been able progressively to re-accustom your patient to an ordinary diet. He will eat, without any fear and without any pain, absolutely everything set before him. There are cases—and they are not rare—where one has been able from one day to another, without any transition whatever, to make the patient pass from his milk diet over to an ordinary diet.

And if you have been careful to make your patient grasp the nature and the reason of the progress which he has made from the start of the treatment, or possibly later, when you have gained his confidence by your first success, you may consider the cure as completely established and absolutely definite in the great majority of cases.

During the course of this re-education of the stomach, it sometimes happens that a relapse occurs, and that some food which is well tolerated at first will be refused another time. One must then find out what are the psychic reasons which determined this refusal, and what is the exact nature of the accident which has produced it. Often it is a question of preconceived ideas concerning the digestibility of such and such a food, against which one must sometimes struggle. Sometimes one can get over the difficulty by making the patient take the same food under a different form, and to use the favorable result obtained as an argument for psychotherapy.

We might report a very great number of cures obtained by following such a method, and continued for long years. Simply to fix these ideas we will quote the case of just one man fifty-two years of age, who had suffered from his stomach for fifteen years, and who was extremely emaciated, in whom the diagnosis of neoplasm had been made.

Here are the successive dietary régimes which we prescribed for him:

First week, four quarts of milk.

Second week, five quarts of milk.

Third week, four quarts of milk, four eggs; morning and evening 100 grams of raw meat in bouillon.

Fourth week, three quarts of milk. The re-establishment of regular meals at noon and evening, with roast meat, purée of vegetables, simple desserts, eggs, and stewed fruits.

Fifth week, regular diet.

At the end of two months this patient was able to take up the work by which he and his family lived. For four years, on account of a gastropathy which had no existence, he had been obliged to give up his work altogether.

Thus, as we have already said, it is not necessary to believe that one must always proceed very slowly in the re-education of the stomach once the milk diet has been given up. There are cases, which are rather frequent, where in twenty-four hours, without any transition, the patient has been made to pass from a milk diet to an ordinary diet.

We want to insist still further on one point,—namely, that this establishment of progressive dietary régime or a sudden return to ordinary nourishment is only one part of the treatment of these patients.

Psychotherapy practised during isolation, and basing its results upon re-education, forms quite as important, if not a more important, part. It is none the less true that we have been led to ask ourselves whether many of the results which have been obtained by the aid of diet, and the treatment of patients who were considered to be suffering from organic affections of the stomach when in reality they only had functional troubles, did not spring purely and simply from a kind of unconscious re-education practised by the isolation of the patient, and also, we should not neglect to say, the isolation of the physician. And if the immediate results of such treatment may seem good, their great defect lies in the fact that they do not modify the psychic soil, which is quite ready for the cultivation of a new and energetic gastropathy the moment that there occur the same causes of a moral nature which created the initial state.

In so far as *neuropathic vomiting* is concerned, it is very certain that those particular forms among them which are the consequences of emotional reactions in certain subjects, are not susceptible to psychotherapy as far as any direct action is concerned. Nevertheless, it may diminish the great frequency of these manifestations by the superaction of phenomena of suggestibility. But here the true therapy lies in the psychological substratum of the patient himself. It is a true prophylactic therapy.

The kind of patient in whom the vomitings are due to an exaggeration of peripherical sensibilities is susceptible of education. But, as a matter of fact, these patients do not take care of themselves, because, while thus afflicted with accidental manifestations which only slightly inconvenience them, they do not pay much attention to them. It happens, however, that by unfortunate therapeutic intervention, and by the addition of phenomena of all kinds, they may secondarily become false gastropaths, with the vomiting as the most marked symptom. They will then respond to the same treatment which is applied to false gastropaths.

As for uncontrollable vomiting and habitual vomitings, whether associated or not with anuria, they come under the heading of hysterical symptoms, to which we apply a common therapeutic study.

It remains for us to glance at, in this first series of functional manifestations, two troubles, merycism and aerophagy, which present rather peculiar and somewhat analogous characteristics. While, as a matter of fact, in all preceding cases, we have seen that the rôle of the physician consisted chiefly in distracting the patient from his functional manifestations, yet here nothing of the kind is true, for these are neuropathic disturbances acquired by habit, but which are often unperceived by the patient, or to which at least he pays only the slightest attention; dwelling rather on the secondary phenomena which may follow them. A patient attacked by merycism or aerophagy is not cured by forgetting; he is cured by attention. This is, as a matter of fact, although there are a great number of functional manifestations which result from the intervention of the psychism into the automatism, and which it is logical to cure by the distraction of the psychism; there are others which, being true habits, that have become unconscious, voluntary, and automatic, can only disappear if, by the intervention of his attention, the patient will grasp the conscious mechanism. Still further, we must frankly say that under the action of the attention alone the habit tends to disappear and be modified, and behaves, as a matter of fact, like a phenomenon of normal automatism which would disturb the action of the psychism.

If, therefore, a subject suffering from merycism will be careful about his regurgitations after a meal and will make an effort to inhibit them by his will, he will succeed at first in putting them off for a time, and finally in making them disappear altogether.

As for the aerophagist, he must be made to understand how and when he swallows air, and asked to avoid all those actions which might lead to such a result. There are all sorts of classic proceedings to hold the attention of the patients, such as that which consists in putting a ribbon tightly around the neck, which, because it interferes slightly with swallowing, reminds these patients of what they ought to avoid, or of placing a cork between the teeth, holding the mouth slightly open, and thus hindering the swallowing movement.

D. Intestinal Manifestations of Neuropaths: Diarrhœa and Constipation.—We shall say only a few words concerning the treatment of the phobias of diarrhœa or constipation to which general psychotherapeutic methods pertain almost exclusively. It will be enough to reassure these patients, and to show them how the interruptions in their life are altogether out of proportion to the accident itself which they dread. One must persuade them to assume an indifferent attitude to the possible occurrence of an imperative diarrhœa or an obstinate constipation. "The only inconvenience," tell them, "will be to change your linen, or take a purgative," but assure them that there is really no reason whatsoever for leading the life of a recluse. One runs no risk in guaranteeing them that the accident will not occur again, for that is really in accord with the truth. Here, again, one must use distraction, the word being taken here in its true etymological sense.

For the whole class of educated constipations and diarrhœas it is evident that what has been accomplished by education and habit may be undone by re-education. To persuade the latter to lengthen progressively the time between their visits to the toilet, and to induce the former to "meditate" regularly and lengthily upon the result, constitutes, as a matter of fact, the whole therapy of these patients. But it would be illogical for the physician, as well as the patient, to hope to get rid, in a few days, of a symptomatology which has been increasing sometimes for years. Nevertheless, with a little patience and hearty endeavor, there is nothing to prevent one from obtaining good results under all circumstances.

The atonic constipation of those who are extremely exhausted by insufficient food and emotional fatigue carries with it no psychotherapeutic indications, except those which concern its possible persistence after the patients have recovered their general state of health. This phenomenon is not rare, especially if one permits such subjects to form bad habits along these lines while by isolation, rest, and overfeeding one is trying to bring them back to their general state of health. One only needs to be warned of the danger.

We now come to spasmodic constipation due to mental representation and the mucomembranous enterocolitis which is the direct result of it. This last affection includes so many different elements that it is not astonishing that many physicians refuse to admit that it may be purely neuropathic in its origin. They do not consider it possible to cure it by having recourse alone to psychotherapy and re-education. This is why, we think, it so often happens that when they do turn to such a therapy it is inefficacious, because it is incomplete, and because the physician has not sufficiently taken into consideration the different elements which start and encourage psychic fixation.

The psychism of the patient is, as a matter of fact, completely centred upon his intestines, and the phenomena which recall either continuously or intermittently this fixation are numerous. Here one must pay a great deal of attention to the morale of the subject, which is generally very bad. Every depressing idea, by the very force of circumstances, brings the patient's mind back again to his intestines. Then, very often, being put upon the most extraordinary diet, whose food value is wholly insufficient, these patients become extremely emaciated if not cachectic. Their strength is uncertain, and every time that they have any work whatever to accomplish their general feeling of weakness which is brought about directs their ideas to the intestinal trouble which they hold responsible for it.

On the other hand, having been thoroughly educated by the reverse psychotherapy which consists in teaching the patient to count and catalogue his symptoms, a certain patient formed a habit of watching himself and noticing particularly all his intestinal phenomena. He would feel his abdomen and try to place the intestines, and look with the most minute care to see if there was any mucus or possibly some sign of a false membrane in his stools.

Having fixed ideas concerning their diet, such subjects become more and more phobic concerning their food. Every dish which is thought to be dangerous or not properly prepared turns the patient's mind toward his intestines. Finally patients who have been ill for months and sometimes years find their condition complicated by a whole series of phenomena due to habit,—educated constipation, false diarrhœa, with tenesmus, due to frequent visits to the toilet, etc.

All these phenomena ought to be carefully gone over, for they furnish all the special therapeutic indications. To neglect any one among them is to run the risk of set-backs, whose frequency, if one is not sufficiently alert concerning them, seems to us at present quite comprehensible. In order to bring up the general condition as well as the moral tone of the subject by appropriate measures, one must not hesitate, if the case demands it, to put the patient into either comparative or absolute isolation on the one hand, and to explain to him the exact nature of all his symptoms, and to get him out of the habit of watching himself at any time or in any way; and, on the other hand, to re-educate the patient concerning his food in the way that we have described in connection with the treatment of false gastropaths; and finally to assure him that all these phenomena of education and habit will disappear: such are the various elements of the treatment. The cure will only be obtained when the patient restored physically and morally will no longer think of his intestines, and will no longer have any reason to think of them.

It would be preposterous to think that cases of long standing, complicated by an extremely strong systematization of multiple origin, could be cured in a few days. Psychotherapy can do many things, but, quite contrary to direct suggestion, it does not pretend to perform miracles, and it will not be rare for the physician to ask a patient to grant him several weeks, and sometimes three or four months, in order to bring about an absolute and definite cure. The main thing is that the patient should be warned of the duration of his treatment, and that he should know, what is nothing more than the truth, that his cure will be accomplished in the end.

There are some subjects who are so slightly affected that a few explanations and a few statements made by a physician in whom they have placed their confidence are enough to cure them. But it would be perfect folly to say to a patient with an old established enterocolitis, "There is nothing the matter with your intestine, don't pay any attention to it," and then be astonished to find that he was not cured, but was going about proclaiming the inefficacy of psychotherapy, and insisting upon the true organic nature of his mucomembranous enterocolitis.

We have now finished the particular therapy to be applied to the functional manifestations that are centred about the digestive tract. It is unquestionably true that a great number of peculiar cases have been left out of our descriptions, which are of necessity rather schematic; this is because in psychoneurotic material the individual symptomatic variability is considerable. We think, nevertheless, that we have pointed out with sufficient clearness what are the usual elements of treating the psychoneuroses and their functional manifestations. They may be summed up as follows: General psychotherapy of the moral condition of the subject. Psychotherapy of the psychic fixations by re-education or by distraction.[1] Psychotherapy of disturbances due to habit by the voluntary re-education of the patient, or what we might call auto-reëducation. Improvement, if there is occasion for it, of the general condition. These four elements, which suppose, on the other hand, the frequent intervention of the adjuncts of psychotherapy, will be found constantly in the therapeutic studies which follow.

II. Functional Manifestations in the Urinary Apparatus.

The floating kidney which is so often found in the course of the psychoneuroses as a direct consequence of emaciation would furnish no other therapeutic indications than that of putting flesh upon the patient if it did not so often become the starting-point of phobic phenomena and persistent pains. These last troubles only disappear when, under psychotherapy, the patient has grasped the true nature of the symptoms of which he complains, and when thus warned he will consent to turn his attention away from them. We shall postpone the study of the processes by which one can find "distraction" from a painful symptom until we come to the paragraph devoted to the treatment of pains, and shall now take up modifications of urinary secretion.

A. Disturbances of the Urinary Secretion.—We have seen that two classes of persistent polyuria exist, apart from accidental emotional polyuria, which is a common phenomenon without any therapeutic importance. There are polyurias which may be very reasonably explained, up to a certain point, as habit, or as due to taking a very large amount of liquid daily. Such a polyuria is amenable to the process of auto-reëducation. The patients will progressively reduce the amount that they drink until it has become normal again. If their habit has been established for some time, they will often experience considerable difficulty, especially if this reduction is made too rapidly. It will happen that they will feel an imperative desire to drink, to which if they wish to be cured, and to be cured quickly, they must not give in. In certain cases, and especially when dealing with rather

[1] The word "distraction," which comes naturally to our pen during the course of this work, ought always to be taken in its true etymological sense,—namely, "All kinds of diversion which turn the mind or the spirit to other things" (Littré).

weak-willed people, it is better to reduce very slowly the amount of liquid swallowed, and to allow weeks and even months for obtaining the cure, rather than to run any risk of a set-back. It is a very bad system to attempt to beguile the patient's thirst by the use of candy drops or by taking sips of some refreshing liquid, etc. In this way one only fixes more decidedly the psychic idea of the need of drinking, an idea to which under such conditions the patient nearly always ends by giving in.

It is needless to say that it will always be necessary to explain to the patient the nature of his condition, and that, if he can succeed by various processes in keeping his attention for a greater or less length of time on something else, which will make him forget for a time his need of drinking, the most favorable psychic mobilization will be obtained.

We shall study the treatment of hysterical polyurias, the second class of persistent polyurias, at the same time as that of the symptoms which properly belong to this psychoneurosis. To this chapter also we shall postpone the therapeutic study of hysterical anuria.

Ischuria by adipsia does not need any very long commentary. It is a mental anorexia which refuses certain drinks. Its treatment, which often cannot be accomplished except by means of isolation, consists in making the subject take a normal amount of drink when he is commanded to do so. If one explains to the patient, at the same time, the origin of his sitiophobia, one will cure him rapidly and surely.

B. Disturbances of Urination or Micturition. False Urinaries.— When one finds that one has to deal with a patient presenting a very complete symptomatology of a false urinary, the situation is practically the same as that which is offered by a pronounced enterocolitic. The moral condition is deplorable, the psychic depression often very marked, with considerably exaggerated emotionalism, localized spasmodic phenomena of the sphincter of the membranous urethra, habit symptoms, increased frequency in particular, with or without consecutive polyuria,—all the elements, in fact, *mutatis mutandis,* which we have found in the condition of the enterocolitides are found again here.

To like symptomatology is applied a similar therapy. It will be necessary to concern one's self with the moral condition of the false urinary, to build up his physical condition, to destroy the psychic fixations which are the starting-point of his spasm, and to make him lose by re-education all the bad habits which he has formed. But, before anything else, one must assure one's self that the psychic fixation is not fostered by any organic elements. A preliminary examination will be absolutely necessary for that. It alone will permit one to state, when knowing the cause, the functional nature of the symptoms presented. If one is not equipped for this examination, or if one is not perfectly competent to make this kind of an exploration, before beginning any psychic treatment one must send the patient to a specialist, indicating to him (but only to him) the very strong suspicion that the patient may be a pure neuropath. Before such a local examination was made it would be difficult to make the patient admit that we had any right to treat him as a nervous case, after so often refusing to consider himself as such. Acting in such a way, one would lose his confidence, and as the result the psychotherapy would have no effect. And this would happen all the more because very often the patient has been before to physicians who, although they have examined him, have thought that they ought to treat him as they would an organic, or at least have practised enough local therapy upon him to confirm his fixations. We have seen only too many cases of this kind.

It goes without saying that, once the neuropathic nature of the disturbances has been proved, there is no place for local therapy, which should be rigorously interdicted. General psychic actions alone are able to exert favorable action.

It will sometimes happen that the persuasive action of the physician is enough for the patient, who after a single conversation is convinced to give up all his pathological convictions. It may happen also that the therapy may be much more difficult, and that, to avoid pathological reorientations and recollections and memories of all kinds, one may find it advisable to prescribe isolation.

One may meet all degrees between the most characteristic false urinary, who is depressed and exhausted, and the patient who only presents a few functional troubles, to which he attaches a greater or less importance.

Thus, one may meet subjects suffering from simple increase in urination, who, after a few explanations, accompanied by a little advice about allowing a greater length of time between their micturitions, will be rapidly cured.

With a single conversation also one will be able to cure women who have the idea that they are suffering from an incontinence which is partially true. It will be enough to explain to them how common this symptom is, and how wrong it is for them to pay such serious attention to it.

It is simply a question of re-education, on the other hand, to accomplish the cure of patients who, for one reason or another, have, by degrees, more or less completely inhibited their sensation of need for urination, and who are suffering from a relative retention.

It is quite a different matter when one has to do with any kind of pain, urethral, vesical, or perineal, which one may find among certain patients, and which requires a very intense kind of psychotherapy, with recourse sometimes to isolation. We shall refer to these phenomena again when we take up the therapeutic study of pains.

Pain associated with frequency of micturition constitutes false cystitis, and the treatment of the latter ought to take into consideration these two elements, which are subjectively very closely allied one with another. It is impossible to reduce completely the frequency of micturition as long as the pain in the bladder has not yielded, and the treatment by re-education of the frequent micturition cannot be carried on unless the painful sensations can be made to disappear simultaneously.

False prostatics, who, as a matter of fact, are only patients with phobias concerning their prostates, whose psychism has too often been cultivated by some unfortunate local therapy, need only to be reassured. It is necessary for the psychotherapeutic action to be strong enough for the patient to cease concerning himself so much with his prostate. It is merely a question of general psychotherapy, of arousing the patient's energy, stirring up his feelings, etc. This, moreover, is the general therapy of all functional manifestations, although, as far as the individual patient is concerned, there are many special indications.

III. Functional Manifestations in the Genital Apparatus.

A. Genital Troubles in Men.—The functional manifestations in the genital apparatus are those that more than any others offer great difficulties for psychotherapeutic treatment. There are as many particular cases as there are patients, each one of which requires appropriate therapeutic treatment, and demands that the physician should exercise all the ingenuity of which he is capable. This is because, instinctive though the function may be, yet any intervention of attention or emotion is liable to change it, and once the sexual function is disturbed it practically means that whenever it is exercised it cannot help but recall the emotions or states of attention which existed previously and which have every chance to be reproduced. The custom of not talking about sexual manifestations makes it almost impossible to discuss the subject, and, as may easily be understood, it is extremely difficult, outside of a few particular cases, to teach a patient how to re-educate himself. We must also add that we have no intention here of doing more than indicating the general rules by which physicians may be guided in particular cases.

First of all, in such patients—whose moral condition is generally deplorable, more so than perhaps in any other functional manifestation—general psychotherapy of the moral and mental condition is very definitely indicated. If, on the other hand, one explains to the patient the exact nature of the phenomena which disturb him, and if in this manner one succeeds in reassuring him, one will evidently have accomplished a very useful service. But it is infinitely rare that by these proceedings alone one can succeed in conquering the patient's apprehensions and the emotional phenomena to which they give rise, and as a result the local inhibitions which follow.

A certain number of classes of patients seem to us to be established, each one presenting several special indications.

The first category consists of the chaste, who, by one of the mechanisms which we have already studied, have become afflicted by sexual phobias, and imagine themselves attacked by an impotence which they have never experienced. These patients, although their situation seems so illogical, are extremely numerous. Their condition usually arises from a conflict which exists in them between the sexual instincts which make themselves felt, and certain scruples which make them consider not only the thing itself but even the idea as shameful and blameworthy. Being obsessed with sexual phobia on the one hand, these patients, on the other hand, by reason of the multiplicity of sexual representations which throng their mind, frequently experience repeated seminal losses.

If the patient under consideration is old enough, after having reassured him, one ought to advise him to marry. In marriage, as a matter of fact, the sexual excitement may be satisfied and quieted down without raising any scruples. On the other hand, it is very comforting for the sexual phobic to feel himself in the presence of a partner whom he knows, or at least believes, to be very ignorant concerning matters of the sexual life, and incapable of judging weaknesses which under these conditions, however, one might almost say never occur.

If, for reasons of position or youth, marriage is impossible or must be too indefinitely postponed, the task of the physician becomes much more delicate. The question will naturally be raised whether one is right under such circumstances to advise a young man to avail himself of professional amours. From the point of view of pure morality it is quite certain that such conduct could not be defended. But what we also believe is this, that, still remaining within the medical domain, such indications would only offer dangers of various kinds. Suppose even that it was a choice of running one or the other "risk," there would be not the slightest doubt that one would eventually find the patient uneasy and overcome with scruples, reproaching himself over the act which he had committed and which he considers degrading and immoral. He would once more become chaste, but chaste through disgust, and not through principle. His moral condition, on the contrary, would be in no way improved. On the other hand, if it is usual for the sexual imagination of the chaste to be singularly exaggerated, it is also true that, more especially on account of their being capable of very definite images, the imagination of the "initiated" chaste is passionate in the extreme.

What then is to be done? It would seem to us that the best way to act, in connection with such a patient, is to make him thoroughly understand all the phenomena which concern the sexual life, and to let him know that the disturbances which he feels result from errors of interpretation, and that, as a matter of fact, he is experiencing perfectly natural physiological phenomena, over which he has no need to be disturbed, and concerning which he has no right to reproach himself. One must make the patient grasp the fact that his dreams and his imaginations torment morally, and that it is they which have drawn him into his obsessions and sexual phobias; one must also make him realize, we insist, that, although man is nearly always master of his actions, he is by no means master, in the same degree, of ideas which may invade his field of consciousness, and which proceed from the psychological automatism. One must then, in fact, turn one's attention chiefly to the moral condition, to reassure and tranquillize, and to turn away from the sexual sphere the attention which scruples, reproaches, and uneasiness have brought to bear upon it. If the patient has seminal losses, one must prove to him that in continent men this is a normal phenomenon, and that the exaggeration of this may be due exclusively to the introduction into his conscience of too many mental representations of a sexual nature, which of themselves give rise to that feeling of scruple which he is nursing in his mind.

On the whole, it would be much better to advise him to remain chaste until the day when he can satisfy his needs in a legitimate way.

In the same class of subjects one also finds patients who are afflicted in a very peculiar way, and who on the contrary complain of being cold, and of not experiencing any of the physical manifestations of the sexual instinct. This physical frigidity is quite often complicated by a very marked psychic excitation.

In this class of patients there are some who are chaste only because their first—and consequently their last—attempts were wholly negative in results. Here again one must make a distinction. There is a whole series of patients whose sexual affection is, as a matter of fact, constitutional, who are major psychasthenics, sexual inverts who may or not, at the time when one sees them, be still unaware of their own state. Such patients are mental cases, and, if they are capable of secondary psychoneuroses, a real mental disturbance or degenerative disturbance of a quasi-organic nature is at the bottom of things. The prognosis of such is not at all apt to be good, and the therapy is too often deficient. The psychic and moral education of the subject must be taken up, for there is a whole psychological domain lacking, which one must endeavor to recreate. It sometimes happens that one is obliged to ask these patients to accept their frigidity, and completely and definitely to renounce all sexual life. But to counsel such to marry would be to court disaster. If, at the end of a very long psychical reëducation whose effects are expressed by the appearance of physical and psychophysical phenomena so that one might consider them cured, we think that in the case of these subjects, but these subjects only, an "experiment" might be attempted before marriage.

Along with these who are naturally frigid there are others who are frigid by persuasion. These are subjects who, by religious, moral, or philosophical conviction, have been turned away in a very decided manner from the sexual life. They are those who have too assiduously read the "Kreutzer Sonata," who have become, if one might so express it, regular sexual anorexics. Let them in some particular instance, or in general, experience the desire of living the sexual life again, and they are obliged to admit that it is somewhat late, and that the psycho-physical associations are broken. Intense obsessions then arise. The patient runs from one confessional to another, risks the most hazardous practices, without any other result than that of becoming morally depressed.

It is seldom that a little reasoning, moral rest, and the abandoning of any new attempts does not lead to a cure. For such patients marriage is also a solution, but at a period which must be a little more remote than for the subject which we have just been considering.

A second large class of facts include all cases of accidental impotence. By one of the mechanisms which we have studied in the first part of our work, subjects who have hitherto been normal become absolutely—or rather, if we might say so, comparatively—incapable of practising the sexual act. This is because, as a general rule, all the psychic phenomena which intervene in the course of the sexual act tend to excite it; but in these people psychological or emotional disturbances come in to interfere and exert an inhibiting influence. As a rule, in fact, all the ideas which may be associated with the sexual act do not belong to the act in itself, but to its ulterior purposes, its causes, or its better utilization. A man in the act of coitus will think of his pleasure or the ultimate consequences of it. If he thinks of his erection it will be in a purely objective manner, and not, as the patient does, in a questioning manner. The individual, in fact, who can be obsessed, and who accidentally, from some emotional cause, has found himself unable to complete the act, or the man who in some way has been made impotent by distraction, each time that he practices coitus in the future will find awakened in him, accompanied by a very marked emotional state, a dubious questioning over the very possibility of this coitus. The subjective fear of trouble is rapidly translated into an objective weakness. And again he will fail to get his orgasm.

To illustrate the therapeutic point of view, I will describe three types of cases, which require very different handling, in order to obtain the necessary and satisfactory condition to treatment,—viz., *re-education* and *distraction.*

It is necessary to get the patient in some way or other to turn his attention away from the manner in which he is conducting himself while he is practising coitus, or else not to be disturbed by it.

First case: The patient is a celibate but marriageable.

Here the course to pursue is very simple. One should advise him to marry some one very young, where the ignorance of his companion would offer, as in the case of the chaste man of whom we have just spoken, the best element of security. It may happen sometimes that the patient's first attempts are not wholly successful, but, as there is no occasion to hurry, and as with a modest and innocent virgin masculine pride has nothing to suffer from a failure which, if it occurs, will remain a secret, matters generally end by arranging themselves. But, on the other hand, marriage with a widow should not be advised.

Second case: The subject is married, and he is unable to play the part of a husband.

It is first necessary to inquire into the conditions which preside over the psychic feeling, or the emotional inhibition. Then one reassures the patient, and begs him before submitting to any treatment to bring his wife with him. It is she who in the treatment must play the principal rôle. She must arrange to stimulate him to desire her, under such conditions that the coitus would be quite unexpected, and in consequence there would be no apprehension previous to the act itself. In order to make this possible, one must prescribe a certain period of complete abstinence, during which time the obsession will have had better chance to quiet down, as it will not have been kept in mind by repeated failures. This naturally is the only way in which an unexpected coitus could be accomplished. On the other hand, in every way that it is possible, all external circumstances which are likely to recall the emotional idea must be changed. A coitus which, for example, cannot be stimulated or accomplished successfully in the conjugal chamber or in the light may succeed if it is attempted in the dark, or in another room, or in another house.

One can see that the key to therapeutic success lies entirely in a complete analysis of the causes of the functional phenomenon, and that with the help of the wife one can succeed in suppressing the majority of the causes, and therefore the majority of the effects. Once a favorable result has been obtained, and the husband has regained his competence and self-respect, the cure may be considered as definite.

Third case: Here we have a celibate, or a married man who deceives his wife, and who cannot present his companion.

One may then avail one's self of various proceedings which sometimes one is led to use successively on the same subject. According to the degree of the phobia and sexual obsessions it will be best, first of all, for this is the simplest measure, to try the effect of simple abstinence during a greater or less length of time. If the subject is very much affected, the duration of this abstinence may be prolonged for two or three months. It frequently happens that, during a period as long as this, forgetfulness occurs, and the patient recovers the integrity of his sexual functions.

It will sometimes happen, however, that one can cure the patient psychically, by convincing him, for example, of what may be quite true, —viz., that his impotence may be a proof of the strength of his love. Armed with this doctrine, which he will develop to suit his own needs, he may acquire an idea concerning his impotence which is comforting and flattering to his pride, and almost immediately obtain favorable results. But one must be assured that he will not be so illogical as to come to the conclusion that his love has diminished because of it.

Under other circumstances one may be led to give the patient advice, the ethics of which may be questionable, but which is sometimes imposed by the situation. One might ask him to change his companion, and to provide himself, if possible, with a transient partner. It is not rare to find that the feeling of security springs up in the presence of a professional, to whom the patient is quite indifferent sentimentally, and who, on the other hand,—and this should be carefully explained to him,—is not likely to wound his masculine pride. The patient with his self-confidence restored may then return to his usual customs.

Finally, and although as a matter of principle the method seems harmful to us, there are nevertheless cases where one must have recourse to indirect suggestion. One could even be led to recommend the patient to take various treatments, of which the suggestive action would be enough, always, however, with this condition, that during the course of the treatment abstinence should be maintained.

We have glanced at several kinds of cases which the physician may be apt to meet. We have by no means taken up all of them. Here, for example, is an old man whose sexual weaknesses may easily be interpreted as due to senile involution. It is very evident that this situation demands special indications. It will be necessary to make the patient understand that at his age continence is the rule. But, if when first seen the patient is very strongly obsessed about his sexual desires, it will not always be quite prudent to ask him definitely to renounce their indulgence. For the moment his personality is tremendously bound up in his sexual functions, and one may run the risk of bringing on a very profound state of depression if one gives him any idea of the necessary and complete abandonment of what seems to him one of the vital elements of his existence. The tactful psychotherapeutist will take such steps that, first counselling a slight abstinence, he will profit by this period to modify progressively his patient's mentality. He will speak of the physical, moral, and material dangers of senile amours, so persuasively that the idea of definite continence instead of transitory abstinence will finally be grasped by him.

Let us suppose, again, the case of a subject in whom partial impotence, such, for instance, as tardy ejaculation, has been the result of Malthusian practices. It is very certain that, before any treatment is undertaken, one must disabuse the patient's mind of the ideas which he holds, for if he persists in them his functional disturbances will become permanent.

Then there are subjects who, without being impotent,—and the case is frequent among neurasthenics with otherwise diffused symptoms,—have a too rapid ejaculation. In such cases one can teach them to re-educate themselves by advising them to practise intermittent coitus, in which the prolongation of the pleasure will form the surprise.

Finally, there are other patients whose position is peculiarly lamentable. These are the degenerates with slowly developing symptoms, in whom, whether accompanied or not by sexual perversions, impotence has become established. When obliged to deal with such patients, the physician is helpless. He can hardly do more than be profuse in his consolations, and try to get them to accept what cannot be cured. It is very rare, moreover, that such subjects do not have mental disturbances of all kinds arising to complicate the situation. Such patients, who are ill mentally, but who are not afflicted with a psychoneurosis, have, however, nothing to do with our classification, except as we have indicated.

In a general way the psychotherapy of sexual manifestations in men is beset with difficulties in its special applications. But it has always seemed to us that the best chance for obtaining good results lay in interesting one's self especially in the patient's mental and still more in his moral condition. It is principally due to the lack of this part of the treatment that one must attribute the set-backs, which, however, taking it all in all, occur but rarely, when one knows how to take all the special aspects of these manifestations into consideration along with their very general conditions.

B. Sexual Manifestations of Women.—Here the mechanisms are not so various. While the sexual manifestations of women are not expressed by any objective phenomenon, they are much more likely than those of man to yield to general psychotherapy. It is none the less true, that, in order to comprehend clearly the therapeutic processes to be applied to them, we shall be obliged again to glance at a certain number of particular cases.

There is no doubt whatever that there exist a certain number of young girls who are haunted by the idea of the sexual act, that there are others who reproach themselves violently in a way that amounts to an obsession over the voluptuous satisfaction which they have been able to obtain artificially. But these troubles are much more usually cared for by the confessor than by the physician. Nevertheless, they sometimes turn to the physician, who under such circumstances has only one course to pursue,—namely, to advise them to marry as soon as possible.

The physician is much more often consulted for all those phenomena which either closely or remotely bear upon vaginismus. Here the therapeutic indications, while being very definite, are of various kinds. The first thing that is necessary to do by direct psychotherapeutic action is to struggle against all the fears with which the patient is afflicted. Without being too afraid to shock her delicacy, one must explain clearly, and if necessary anatomically, to the patient just what the sexual act consists of, and make her understand that there is no reason why she, more than any other woman, should not lend herself to it. On the other hand, according to the peculiar mental condition of the patient, there would be an opportunity of awakening the sexual desire in her by telling her that the sexual act is the very condition of maternity; under other circumstances, on the contrary, where the vaginismus is due to the fear of fecundation, one must attack the phenomenon by making the woman understand how necessary maternity is to her future physical as well as her future material and moral benefit. Finally, as is the case where the vaginismus is due to too marked sexual excitation and to too vivid mental representations, the rôle of the psychotherapeutist will be sometimes to morally and psychically inhibit an excessive sexuality.

A second series of indications concerns the husband, whose clumsiness or brutality may have been the starting-point of the functional manifestations observed. Sometimes it will happen that the best treatment for vaginismus consists in educating the husband, and in cautioning him to be more patient. The wife, knowing that she will not have to dread the rather rude treatment which had made her suffer in the sexual act, will lose her fear and with it the vaginismus itself. Many women owe their vaginismus solely to a mismanaged wedding night.

In the case of a patient being extremely phobic, with a distinct fixation on her sexual organs, it may perhaps be wise to advise her to remain continent for a time, sometimes as long as the period which one would prescribe for a man afflicted with functional sexual manifestations. Before permitting her to attempt any new experiences, one ought to allow her time to recover from those which previously had had such unfortunate consequences.

At other times, and one of us has, as a matter of fact, observed numerous examples of this, vaginismus is the consequence of incomplete coitus. Either from the beginning of marriage, which is rather unusual, or, as is ordinarily the case, after the birth of the number of children that the couple have desired to have, they practise incomplete coitus. There is no longer any synchronism in the voluptuous sensations. The wife, obsessed with the fear of a pregnancy, will not abandon herself to pleasure as before; she waits, and watches for the moment which is supreme in her husband. The latter, on his side, doing the same thing, generally withdraws before he and his wife have experienced their pleasure, and the ejaculation takes place outside of the genitals. The only therapeutic measure here of any value is to give over such practices, which for the man himself are far from being free from danger, so true is it that one must never transgress the laws of nature.

Finally, there are cases where it is necessary to undertake the actual objective re-education of the patient, where it is necessary to dilate the vagina, by making her introduce into it bougies or sounds of increasing size, until she is quite convinced that it shows sufficient receptivity for the act for which it was intended. This method has given success in cases of very long standing.

There are, however, women in whom everything fails,—direct psychotherapeutic action, prolonged abstinence, and progressive dilation. This is when it is a question of vaginal pain, which is entirely subjective and profoundly fixed, for which the therapy must be the same as for the general treatment of all the algias. But these cases are exceptional, and, whether isolated or associated, the different processes which we have just mentioned are almost always able to re-establish things in their regular way.

The contraction of the adductors, if it seems to be permanent, forms an hysterical manifestation amenable to general treatment of this very peculiar kind of functional disturbance. If, on the other hand, it is only an accidental diffusion of vaginismus, it yields at the same time as the latter to the same therapeutic intervention.

We have now come to the very special difficulty which is constituted by female frigidity. A certain number of causes may create it. It may happen that it is purely relative, and that only the husband is to blame. And if, under these conditions, the synchronism of voluptuous sexual sensations is disturbed, it is not because the woman is slower or tardy; it is because the man is too quick, if we might use this comparison. It is very evident that under these conditions it is the one at fault who should be advised, while at the same time the innocent one should be reassured. More often female frigidity results from all kinds of inhibitions, moral or religious scruples, fear of fecundation, etc. The rôle of the physician in these cases does not need to go any further than to calm fears which have no grounds, or fears which they hesitate to express.

On the other hand, one should realize that in women the voluptuous phenomena are susceptible of much greater development than in men. There are women,—a very small number, however,—for whom education in this matter accomplishes nothing, and who pass their whole life without realizing any sexual pleasure, or without even being disturbed by the fact. There are many others in whom the pains of defloration prevent and inhibit any voluptuous sensations. It is then not until after a greater or less length of experience that the woman learns to share the sexual pleasure. Such a phenomenon, which is in fact subnormal, ought not to be considered as a pathological phenomenon. When dealing with such cases, the physician must be content to reassure a husband who is disturbed, or a woman who has hitherto been unmoved except by the sorry expression of her husband on seeing her accept passively the passion which she does not share. It happens, nevertheless, as we have seen, that by a mechanism of this kind a lasting frigidity is often established. It is the very desire for voluptuous sensations which have hitherto not been experienced which prevents this kind of sensation from being produced. The wife, hurt by her husband's reproaches, feels that she must be lacking in sensation, and imagines that she is abnormal or badly formed, and at each new sexual relation there springs up a new emotional state which is peculiarly inhibitive. If the physician is consulted in time, he may, by pointing out a healthier point of view, re-establish conjugal harmony, which sooner or later will satisfy their sexual relations with the voluptuous feelings which belong to it. Here medical intervention is prophylactic rather than curative, since they ask the physician to make a phenomenon appear whose absence is at the time quasi-normal. But the lack of medical intervention, or any ill-advised direction upon his part, would cause a state which was only temporary to become lasting. When the disturbance has been established for a long time, its therapy is much more difficult, and here again, as in the case of men, it may happen that one can get results from an indirect suggestion where psychotherapeutic action of the most persuasive kind would remain wholly inefficacious.

As a matter of fact, and to analyze things thoroughly, women are much less apt than men to have what might properly be called sexual fixations; but what is much more apt to happen to her than to him are states of moral depression and serious neurasthenia, of which the starting-point is of sexual origin. Reproaches, remorse, regrets, impressions of some special failure, affecting by means of sex the vast domains of sentimentality which are so often excited in women,—these are enough, if the mechanism of preoccupations continues to give rise to serious neurasthenic conditions whose origin one must know how to trace out. But then the therapy is of a general order, and does not draw any special indications from the special origin of the troubles presented.

It happens very commonly that functional disturbances of a sexual nature are passed on from one of the couple to the other. If sterility be the cause, so that the disharmony of the sexual act becomes for both the occasion for reciprocal reproaches, for it may happen that each one of them assumes or refuses to assume the entire responsibility, the whole conjugal sexual life, encumbered by auto- and hetero-observation, may be peculiarly disturbed by it.

The intervention of the physician would be of benefit if he could explain, direct, and arrange matters; but there is no need to dwell upon this. All this therapy for sexual functional disturbances may seem rather delicate. It is, nevertheless, indispensable to know it, partly on account of the frequency of such symptoms, as well as the difficulty which one has in curing them if one is only half aware of them.

We feel that we have only given a few rules which point to the paths which must be followed in the treatment of these patients, who are often so unhappy, so obsessed, so ashamed and depressed, that more than one will not hesitate to escape by means of suicide, from an existence which such troubles make unbearable. There is, therefore, no place for ridicule or irony in the treatment of sexual functional disturbances, however Rabelaisian they may sometimes be. One must look upon them as exceedingly serious, and often very grave conditions, because the very life of the patient may depend upon their persistence or their disappearance.

In the treatment of a false genital fixation it is very essential, however material may be the nature of the phenomena that are met with, not to make fun of them. If in a theoretical description one may be justified in using circumlocution, with the patient one must use the right word, the physiological or anatomical term. He must be made to understand that the sexual functions, for a physician at least, are nothing to be ashamed of, or nothing to joke about. And if it sometimes happens that the patient jokes about his own symptoms, do not follow him in this line. He laughs perhaps because he thinks "that it is manly to laugh," while all the time he is much more inclined to weep.

C. Gynæcological Pseudo-manifestations do not offer any special therapeutic indications. The physician's chief work consists in stating to the patient, after a sufficiently thorough examination, that she is perfectly healthy, in reassuring her concerning each of the special manifestations which she presents, in getting her to turn her attention away from her genital organs, and in insisting that she give up all treatment and stop watching herself. This is very simple theoretically, but it often runs up against a most firmly established systematization which has been encouraged and developed by a long-drawn-out local therapy. It is not a rare thing, under these conditions, for the neurologist to be obliged to call in the help of a gynæcologist, who in his turn tells the patient that her fears are foolish and there is no necessity for treatment. The successive convictions which one thus tries to implant in the mind are not only added to one another but become multiplied, giving the patient a feeling of perfect security, which permits her to do, what is the one thing that one is trying to accomplish, —namely, to forget the functional manifestations with which she has been afflicted and the phobias which have deceived her.

To speak frankly, these manifestations require a certain therapy, but this therapy is prophylactic, and to be addressed to physicians and not to patients. It is not that we wish to deny the value of certain conservative practices in gynæcology. But for a certain number of cases where pessaries, tampons, glycerin, ichthyol, etc., are found to be of value, how many others are there where the physician knows perfectly well that his patient is in good health, nevertheless believes it to be right, in order to satisfy her, to make her undergo a more or less lengthy treatment. He thinks that it will calm her, but he only exasperates her. She was merely nervous, but she becomes a neuropath, with fixed obsessions concerning her genital organs. The physician is responsible if he has been weak enough to look at things from the patient's point of view, and has not had sufficient energy positively to refuse to give her the unnecessary treatment that she wanted. We cannot begin to number the women whom we have seen, as often at the hospital as in town, who have been victims of such local gynæcological treatment. The thing of which the patients must be convinced is, that, if they go on noticing and worrying themselves in this unnecessary way about their genital organs, they will develop into confirmed neuropaths, whose life will be as insupportable to themselves as to their families.

IV. Functional Manifestations in the Respiratory Apparatus.

Among the very numerous functional manifestations which may be localized in the respiratory apparatus, there are some which are purely phobic, and which do not seem to us to require any very lengthy description, as their treatment in no way differs from that of all the other fixations, which, being of a purely subjective nature and without any peripheral causes, require nothing more than a few psychotherapeutic conversations to cause them to disappear.

Other troubles, entering into the domain of hysterical phenomena or being caused by pains, will be studied with one or the other of these pathological groupings.

Only a certain number of particular indications present manifestations which, following or not some localizations of a primitive phobic nature, bring on a whole series of objective disturbances which may sometimes be rather resistant to therapy.

Of all these troubles the most important unquestionably is the decided diminution of pulmonary ventilation which one finds in such a large number of neuropaths. We have seen that the causes for these are generally of an emotional nature. We have also had occasion to note the numerous after-effects, sensations of oppression, rapid breathing playing a part in the production of certain asthenias, etc.

This phenomenon, which often passes quite unperceived, should not be neglected. There is a considerable number of subjects in whom a whole series of secondary disturbances have resulted more or less directly from bad respiratory habits which have generally been created by a subcontinuous repressed emotion. Psychotherapy is evidently not enough. If one has really found the presence of some such manifestation, it is not sufficient merely to state its existence to the patient and to explain its origin and consequences to him. It is not enough to tell a neuropath, "If you breathe too rapidly and seem to have a feeling of exhaustion, it is because you do not breathe properly;" you have to go still further, and teach him how to breathe in a normal manner; you have to undertake with him the work of respiratory re-education. This the patient ought to be taught to do while resting as well as while walking. We shall not dwell upon the technic of respiratory education. It is not a question here of acquiring a greater pulmonary capacity, which is normal but used in the wrong way; no exercises to develop strength are indicated. It will be enough to explain to the patient in what way and just where he makes a mistake by cutting short the inspiration and having too long respiratory pauses, etc., and in showing him just how a normal respiration ought to be taken, and in requiring him to practise it a certain number of times every day. If there are asthenic phenomena of a respiratory origin, when the patient begins to move about, it will be necessary for him always to pay attention and to watch his respirations. If it is conversation which causes him to be short of breath so soon, and which has so depressed and worried the patient, it will be proper for him to practise breathing in a normal way. This exercise of re-education may be carried on by making him read aloud.

If this therapy is methodically pursued, and if neither the physician nor the patient permits himself to repeat the same things, one will obtain such excellent results as even sometimes the unexpected disappearance of a whole series of phenomena, whose relation to the respiratory disturbance had in the first place been passed by unperceived.

The same kind of therapy will apply to individuals who, as a result of any real pain or thoracic algia, have immobilized a part of their chest. In such cases the patient ought to undress in order to go through his respiratory exercises, and stand in front of a mirror, and try to mobilize the region which is not sufficiently displaced in the respiratory movements. One can, if need be, at the start, mobilize this region by any movements requiring force, such as flexion or extension, moving the shoulders or the arms according to the type of the immobilization which one has to deal with.

This method of re-education will generally be very easy and often crowned with complete success in a very short time. It is also by therapeutic re-education that one gets control of troubles which, like nervous pseudo-asthma, consist really of nothing more than an emotional attack with peculiar respiratory fixation. The polypnœa of these subjects is, in fact, more apt to follow a period of apnœa of emotional origin. The simple advice to breathe deeply and profoundly, as soon as one is seized with that kind of respiratory anguish which is the forerunner of his symptoms, is sometimes sufficient to enable the patient to get entire control of his trouble, if, above all, which goes without saying, he has clearly understood the mechanism. But in such subjects one must not forget that outside of acute attacks there ordinarily exists a state of subcontinued oppression which respiratory education could quickly terminate.

Re-education will be found to dispel coughs following pulmonary phobia or laryngeal fixations, and is a mode of treatment to be used for aphonia and "lost voice." But here the indications become much more complex. One must try to force the patient to turn his attention from his functional fixation. The object of general psychotherapy, while reassuring the subject and explaining to him what is the matter with him, is evidently to render him less attentive to his fixations. On the other hand, once a patient's attention has been drawn to some symptom for one reason or another, or fixed on some phenomenon acquired by habit that has a tendency to reproduce itself, it is necessary that he should know how in some way to control his symptoms. He must try to prevent himself from coughing even when he feels the desire to cough. Even if his voice has a tendency to die away, he must force himself to speak loudly and intelligibly. One will not always obtain this result at the first attempt, and the will of the patient, which supports the condition of the neuropathic nature of the symptoms which he presents, would not be strong enough to give him the mastery. A whole series of processes could be brought in to help the patient, or to assure his progressive re-education. Drawing long breaths, making him swallow saliva, taking a book and reading aloud, will often be sufficient to inhibit the reflex habit which constitutes the nervous cough.

As for the patients afflicted with aphonia, one could require them to exercise their voices in the silence of their own rooms, or out in the open country, by pronouncing aloud the different vowels which bring the vocal cords into action. For these latter patients, if their fixation dates back for a long time, it might be useful to insist for a few days upon absolute vocal rest. During this period of rest a great many of their apprehensions disappear, and re-education becomes extremely easy.

We noted, in the course of our study of respiratory fixations, the comparative frequency of a symptom which has nothing to do with the respiratory apparatus, except that it originated there. We refer to the phobia of cold. Those patients who are afraid of catching cold, or of starting up some old pulmonary lesion which has long since been healed, often get to the point where they can no longer bear the slightest change of temperature without being extremely upset. It sometimes happens that, by the simple action of psychotherapy and authority, the physician gets his patient to the point where he has given up all his bad habits. But, in spite of the most persuasive arguments, it will also happen that, even though the patient is convinced in his mind, he, nevertheless, cannot control his fears. This is where re-education has more chance of lasting success. It might consist in asking the patient to gradually overcome his phobic preoccupations by making successive trials, or it might also be carried on in a less direct manner. We have been able to cure a patient of the phobia of cold by prescribing him douches with two jets, of which the temperature is every day a little high in one and lower in the other. The day when the patient could stand, without any emotional reaction, being sprayed first with a jet that was very warm and afterward by a jet of very cold water we considered him cured.

The study of special therapeutic indications of respiratory fixation is particularly interesting in this respect, that in it one finds the different mechanisms on which re-education may act distinctly isolated. First of all, there is the whole category of disharmonic phenomena which have been established unknown to the patient, and which are the old or recent results of disturbances which the psychism of emotion has created. For these symptoms re-education is the only therapy which will allow us to feel sure of their disappearance. There is also a whole series of disturbances which are directly engendered by emotion or attention. It is certain that pure psychotherapy can make them disappear. It is evident that a patient who is sufficiently energetic and properly informed may get to the point, by means of his own will, where he first neglects his discomforts and ends by forgetting them. But where this therapy is used by any physicians except those of a good deal of authority, it may often fail. But, if one is careful in his method, the processes which are called re-educative will prove a convenient means of turning the attention of the patient and of interrupting the diffusion of emotional phenomena. They have furthermore the advantage of suppressing all apprehension on the part of the subject, and if the latter, in spite of the general psychotherapeutic action, does not immediately feel security, re-education nevertheless enables him to get to the point of establishing this feeling of security, which, although it may come gradually, is none the less solidly established. Thus, if after explaining things to him, we tell a patient to make light of his cough or his aphonia or his pleural asthma, we may perhaps succeed in causing the immediate disappearance of these phenomena, which under sufficient psychotherapeutic influence will have lost the psychic substratum or the emotion necessary to their apparition. But it may also happen that the subject with a feeling of apprehension will say to himself, "I shall never be able to control my aphonia, or my cough, or my sense of oppression," and that he will get into a more emotional condition concerning it. The methods of re-education by asking the patient for a more frequently repeated but less intense voluntary action will not have this inconvenience. On the other hand, as we shall see further on, the choice between the therapy of gentleness which is seen in methods of re-education and the therapy of authority, bringing the patient's whole will suddenly into play, ought to be made according to the various situations in which the patient and the physician find themselves. It cannot help but be interesting to point out that re-education is a necessary element when it comes to substituting for a bad habit a new habit which is only a return to the normal, and that in such patients, in fact, much depends on it.

V. Special Therapy in Cardiovascular Manifestations.

Cardiac fixations of the psychoneuroses will not delay us long. If practically the number of heart phobias and false cardiopaths is considerable, these patients do not offer any especial therapeutic indications.

Although, on the other hand, a whole series of troubles, which we have described at some length, may result from the action of emotion on the heart, yet in such cases there is evidently no possibility of re-education working any direct effect upon this functional trouble. That which must be combated is the emotionalism itself, and the psychic convictions which encourage it, and perhaps help to narrow the emotional actions into some special physical channel. Psychotherapy alone may play a true therapeutic rôle. To explain, and reassure and re-establish the patient's confidence, to turn his attention to other things while redirecting the course of his existence, to absolutely forbid him to watch himself or to feel his pulse or listen to his heart-beats,—such would be the course of action among other things which the physician will have to put into practice and which are really after all very simple. In the great majority of cases a favorable result is obtained, once the patient's idea is "switched off." As for the patients who are afflicted with vascular disturbances, who are phobic concerning pain in their breast, or arteriosclerosis, or whose emotionalism has vasomotor expressions, they do not indicate the necessity for any particular treatment, and should be managed in the same way as the false cardiopaths.

VI. Functional Manifestations of the Skin.

Functional manifestations of the skin do not require any very long therapeutic commentary. Skin phobias are curable by ordinary methods, and the only fixation on which we need to dwell is that which is offered by those suffering from neuropathic pruritus. These are sometimes extremely difficult to cure. Patients are obsessed upon the subject to a degree that one can hardly imagine, and it is often absolutely necessary to treat them in isolation. General psychotherapeutic treatment will sometimes produce immediate results, but this is rather unusual, and it is very apt to be the case that the cure of such subjects will require a considerable length of time.

The therapeutic regulations which should be laid down are as follows: First of all, as far as possible, one must attempt to get the patient's attention away from his fixation. This, as a rule, is not an easy thing. However, by engaging in rather long conversations with him, or in getting somebody else to undertake this, one will succeed in making him forget his trouble momentarily. The fact that under the influence of a different set of ideas the patient can pass a greater or less length of time without feeling his itching will furnish an excellent psychotherapeutic argument for him to bring his will into direct play. According to circumstances, other methods of distraction than conversation could be employed, such as reading, or manual or intellectual work; the ingenuity of the physician will have to be called forth to find the best methods to use in order to turn the patient's attention away from his itching.

One must then ask the subject to resist the temptation to scratch, even if he feels the greatest need of doing so. As it often happens that patients who are very badly affected seem almost unconsciously impelled to scratch themselves, it is necessary to put some obstacle in the way to prevent them from scratching, so that, before they yield to the impulsion, the material obstacle forces them to take time to think about it. Thus, for example, in putting the patient into a bed in which the covers are very carefully tucked in or fastened down, during the time that it will require for him to free himself from his covering he will have had the opportunity of getting hold of himself and will be able to control his desires.

One can also carry on a sort of re-education at the same time by asking the patient to allow a longer and longer time between the periods when he must relieve himself by scratching. This method seems to us dangerous, because during the whole interval in which the patient is forbidden to scratch himself he will probably think of nothing else than of the moment when it will be allowed him, and, however strong may be his self-mastery and the power of his will, the obsession will have every chance to increase.

In fact, to prove to the patient experimentally, and by distraction, that he can allow a considerable time to pass without feeling the need of scratching, and to interpose, on the other hand, mechanical obstacles between the idea of scratching and its realization,—such are the two essential elements of treatment. General psychotherapy naturally is as beneficial here as elsewhere.

What we have already said concerning patients afflicted with phobias of cold spares us the necessity of giving the particular treatment of these patients who have educated themselves in thermic sensibility, whom we meet so frequently, and whose troubles are either primitive, or secondary to a phobic condition connected with the respiratory apparatus.

CHAPTER XXV.

SPECIAL THERAPY OF FUNCTIONAL MANIFESTATIONS (CONTINUED).

ALL the functional manifestations which now remain for us to study from a therapeutic point of view belong in different degrees to the domain of the central nervous system or its peripheral projections. These manifestations are innumerable, but those which are of an hysterical nature will be taken up therapeutically further on. Some manifestations are purely phobic in their nature, and do not present any special indications. There are, however, many others among these disturbances which show very special and definite therapeutic indications, which it seems to us wise to develop somewhat.

Abandoning for a moment the functional classifications which we have adopted in the first part of our work, there is, first of all, a group of symptoms which we want to study, and which may be brought together under the name of symptoms of fatigue. Neurasthenics, in regard to the fatigue which they nearly always experience, may be divided into three classes. There are some subjects who are simply phobic, and who have never had any possible reason whatsoever to experience or more particularly to dread fatigue. There are, on the other hand, patients who, having originally suffered from true fatigue, have afterward remained subjectively exhausted, but in a way which is purely psychic. There are, finally,—and this is the class of patients which, for the time being, we are considering alone,—those who are really fatigued. That emotion may give rise to a real fatigue which at the same time is psychic and physical is very well known, and there is no doubt that the repeated and continuous action of any emotional preoccupation leads likewise to this result. If, on the other hand, one takes into consideration the fact that a great many neurasthenics are very much emaciated and for weeks, months, and sometimes years have been inadequately nourished, one can see that there are patients to whom it would be preposterous to attribute the feelings of fatigue of which they complain to a purely psychic origin. A therapeutic mistake which is often made consists in prescribing, for such weakened people, more or less violent exercises, which are supposed to be useful in breaking up their emotional condition and calming their irritability, or simply for the purpose of getting them in training. By this method, however, one gets nothing but physical, moral, and intellectual depression of a more pronounced type.

Although all neurasthenias are emotional in origin, as we think that we have fully proved, yet all emotional conditions do not always necessarily result in psychic phenomena, or phenomena of suggestion or inhibition due to pathological convictions. It seems to us, then, that, in the case of patients who are both physically and psychically depressed on account of continued emotional causes, the therapeutic indications point very definitely to rest and overfeeding, and if necessary, in cases of very marked depression or excessive irritability, to isolation, which is here a very essential condition of proper rest.

It is very easy to lay down such rules for patients who appear objectively to be very much exhausted. But what is much more difficult is to determine the precise moment where it seems to be right to terminate this preliminary but necessary period of treatment and to get the patient by easy progressive stages into the line of treatment which we shall indicate. It will often happen, that, if the work of psychotherapy has been normally carried on during this first phase of treatment, and if the patient has been relieved of all the moral and psychic complications of his condition, he will be able himself to give you very valuable information, and that it will happen quite naturally, when the rest has been sufficient to cause his fatigue to disappear, that he will again feel the need of entering into active life, taking up his affairs and putting forth new energy.

It will be wise for the physician to grant him any such legitimate desires, bearing in mind, however, all the time, this fact, that he has to deal with a patient who, by reason of having rested, is wholly out of training, and who finds himself in almost exactly the same situation as a convalescent who is going out for the first time. The part which the physician must then play is that of moderation; he must hold his patient back, and not permit him to make any efforts except those which are regularly progressive. Moreover, such patients, once started off and put upon the right road by general psychotherapy, very rarely present any serious therapeutic difficulties, provided, however, that they have not been allowed to retain any of their former dread of fatigue.

As a matter of fact, it will happen also, although not very often, that even after a sufficiently prolonged rest the patient will still consider himself as suffering from fatigue, and that all effort on his part will be accompanied by a greater or less feeling of apprehension. Where he was once merely fatigued he has now become phobic, or rather, though the real elements of fatigue have disappeared, the subjective elements have persisted.

Is there any objective idea whatsoever which will enable the physician to tell exactly when the time has come for him to make his patients take up their responsibilities, whatever may be their fears or their persistent convictions concerning them? For instance, what should we do when we have a patient who is afraid to put his foot on the ground but who is very restless in bed? Under such circumstances the thing which would give us the most positive light on the subject is the patient's increase in weight. Any patient who, having lost a greater or less number of pounds, has almost regained his normal weight may be restored progressively to physical activity without inconvenience. We would not be far wrong in thinking that this should also be the guide to tell us the time when he might return to intellectual activity. But here we must take into account the clinical condition of patients at the time when their treatment commenced. This is because, as a matter of fact, psychic depressions and physical depressions, however closely associated they may be, do not necessarily follow a strictly parallel course. There are many subjects whom emotional fatigue has affected more in the domain of their psychic faculties and less in their physical activities. There is a small number of patients, on the other hand, who, although very emaciated, have nevertheless preserved the ability to accomplish a certain amount of intellectual work. The disappearance of the phenomena of irritation at noise will be of importance; but what perhaps can better guide the practitioner, and enable him to divert all the subjective elements of the persistence of an intellectual fatigue, is the manner in which the patient behaves during the course of psychotherapeutic conversations. The subject whose brain is truly fatigued reasons very little if at all. From the moment he begins to discuss and reply, and from the moment that you see that in the interval between the psychotherapeutic conversations he has been reflecting upon things of his own accord, you may without fear let him go back to some intellectual work, of which, however, you must measure the quantity to be permitted at a time.

In other words, a return to normal ways and a spontaneous return of intellectual activity which is in some degree unpremeditated: these are the elements which permit one to consider that the preliminary treatment of the various aids to psychotherapy has been sufficient.

The time which, as a matter of fact, will be devoted to such treatment must evidently vary according to the degree in which particular cases are affected. In the majority of cases from six weeks to two months are sufficient, and the cases are less frequent where this part of the treatment must be prolonged for several months. It will more often be found that this time has by no means been lost, because it will have given a very excellent opportunity for psychotherapeutic treatment.

Let us hasten to add that cases of neurasthenia, with or without functional manifestations, which require a very prolonged rest, are rare, and that the important thing is not to confuse real fatigue with subjective fatigue.

Now that we have explained ourselves concerning those facts which we are inclined to consider as exceptional, we can continue the therapeutic study of the functional manifestations to which there is no physical substratum, which has not been the case in those thus referred to.

I. The Therapy of Functional Disturbances in the Neuro-muscular Apparatus.

For the moment we shall leave untouched all hysterical manifestations, contractures, paralyses, choreas, and tremblings, and shall take up only physical asthenia on the one hand and disturbances of equilibrium on the other.

A. Physical Asthenia.—Setting aside all the exceptions which we made in the cases which we considered in the preceding paragraphs, we shall now consider only those subjects whose fatigue is purely objective, or who, having originally been greatly fatigued, have remained so and do not seem to be able by means of rest to get back their old strength, and who, as a matter of fact, are really suffering from secondary phobias.

The asthenia of these patients is made up under such circumstances of two different phenomena, psychic phenomena on the one hand, consisting of conviction of helplessness and of apprehension concerning all kinds of tire, and disharmonic phenomena on the other hand, which are the more or less direct results of that very apprehensiveness from which the patient suffers. We dwelt for a long time upon these points in the first part of our work, so that it is not necessary to go over them again.

What therapy shall one bring to bear upon these manifestations? Psychotherapy will undoubtedly do the work, but it must be experimentally demonstrated to the patient that he is capable of making physical efforts. It is very evident that one must work his training. But here one encounters a series of small practical difficulties which one must know how to handle. It is by no means enough to say to a patient, "To-day you must walk for two, three, four, or five minutes; and every day hereafter you must increase by a given time your walking and any other exercise which may have been prescribed." If his training is outlined in such a manner, there will be great likelihood that it will amount to nothing, or have but indifferent results, and will only succeed in strengthening in the patient the psychic conviction of his physical helplessness.

Anything which is apt, in any kind of training, to fix the patient's attention on the probable appearance of fatigue is dangerous; because, as a matter of fact, the moment the attention is fixed upon the idea, subjective fatigue will immediately appear, and from that will come disharmonic phenomena which will make the fatigue effective.

Hence, from the moment the training is begun, a certain number of precautions should be laid down. Later, when the patient has made a certain amount of progress, he will be convinced that he can get back his old physical activity in this way, and then they will be unnecessary, for the subject, being reassured and more confident, will carry on his training alone.

These precautions are of various kinds. First of all, it is evident that one must avoid the occurrence of any disharmonic phenomena which might become habits, such as rapid breathing due to insufficient respiration, or walking stiffly, which will bring on rapid fatigue. One must, therefore, tell the patient to walk in such a way that he can accomplish it slowly and easily, to try "to keep step," as we are accustomed to tell him, and to stop frequently and breathe deeply. It is not always wise—but that depends upon particular cases—to give the patient a set time during which he should walk, and then a fixed time during which he should rest. It will often happen, if this is the case, that the patient with his watch in his hand will fix his attention upon his walking, and will feel subjective fatigue coming on quickly. The best way certainly would be for this kind of training to be undertaken with a physician. It would then be he who would take all the responsibility, and who would determine according to the patient's mental condition the times to rest and the time to walk, while at the same time by means of conversation he would keep the patient from all auto-observations; but it is evident that this is far from being always possible. One must then manage things differently, and the surest method seems to us to be the following. It consists not in giving the patient a minimum, but a maximum time to walk. "To-day," you will tell him, "you will walk not more than half an hour during the day." In this way, the patient is not haunted with anxiety if he does not fulfil the conditions of his task. On the other hand, the time he is to watch is not that devoted to walking, but that which is to be given to rest. He leaves at a given time, armed with his camp-chair, if he is in a place where there are not apt to be any seats. He walks for a certain length of time along the road,—no matter where, provided that it is a distance that he thinks he can accomplish without fatigue and which will not cause him any apprehension. He sits down, looks at his watch, and rests as long as it seems to him necessary. The moment he starts again, he looks at the time and calculates how long he has rested; and by this method, by the simple act of subtraction, he will at the end know the exact time that he has been walking. At no time in this way is his attention fixed upon his walking, not even during the time when he is actually doing it.

One will be astonished, if one proceeds in this way, at the rapidity with which the patient in most cases will completely lose his sense of fear, and will reach the point where, subjectively as well as practically, he will behave like a normal individual.

It is very evident that walking is not the only kind of training and development which the physician will be called upon to regulate. All forms of physical activity may be affected, either simultaneously or—what is much more curious—one at a time. One sees patients who say that they are quite able to walk for an hour, but unable to stand still for five minutes.

Now, the training which is necessary to enable one to stand is one of those which offers the greatest difficulties. Here, again, disharmonic phenomena come in. One must be very particular to make the patient understand that standing upright does not mean to hold one's self absolutely rigid and fix one's self in a position which may not be changed even to draw a breath. It will often be easy to give him some direct proof that it is quite possible for him to remain standing much longer than he thinks he can. All that is necessary to do this is to change the trend of his ideas by means of conversation, and to attack his pathological convictions as it were by surprise. You may let this duty devolve upon some friend of the patient or some one who is in his household. It may happen that in your presence the patient will be somewhat defiant, and that he will try to give you some objective proof of his subjective incapacity. It happens in the same way in some circumstances for walking as well as for standing, and also for any other kind of particular physical incapacity, that one will have to break through the pathological convictions in which the patient has bound himself up by surprising him. You can adopt this method as well whether it is a case of general asthenia or one or other of the localized asthenias that we have studied.

But in a general way, all this therapy ought to be summed up at the beginning in these words,—re-education without drawing attention to it.

It will happen, however, that in a great many cases so many precautions will be quite unnecessary, and that, having fully penetrated the psychism of your patient, you will have been able to awaken in him a sufficient desire for new activity and a sufficiently strong conviction of a possibility of such activity as to make his training take place as naturally as if there were nothing more serious the matter than is the case in the convalescence of any individual who, having been inactive for a long time, for any reason whatsoever, independent of his psychism and his will, is anxious to get back his customary activity.

B. Disturbances of Equilibrium.—Many of these disturbances belong largely to hysteria, but they are far from being rare in neurasthenics, as a result of phobic phenomena. These are the subjects who, believing or fearing that they are afflicted with some disease of the brain or of the spinal cord, or experiencing some form of vertigo, think that their kinetic or static equilibrium is no longer true. By making a series of false movements in order to maintain equilibrium, which is really in no danger of being disturbed, they get to the point by disharmonic troubles where they sometimes make it still more uncertain. To explain this, and convince them, and re-educate them are three steps of treatment for these cases. Their re-education will consist simply in making the patient walk with somebody near him—it is very rarely necessary to support him—so that he has a sense of security, then to ask him to go on to the point where he will simply hold a stick in his hand to preserve his equilibrium in case he feels that he is going to lose it, and finally in making him walk alone without any aid.

In a general way, the therapy of these disturbances in neurasthenics is very easy, and does not require any lengthy consideration. But here, naturally, one must at the same time try to make over the patient's mental state.

II. Special Therapy of Disturbances of Sensibility. Pains.

We will not dwell upon the objective disturbances of sensibility which for the most part spring from hysteria. The only phenomenon which one may come across, also, among neurasthenics, is generalized hyperæsthesia due to psychic irritability. This trouble stands in relation to the subcontinuous emotional state in which the patient finds himself. As such, it is susceptible to general psychotherapy. When it is very marked, it may be necessary to isolate the patient, who, as soon as he receives only the minimum of sensations and excitations, will quite soon forget the hyperexcitability which was preoccupying him.

From the special point of view with which we are concerned, the pains are much more interesting. They are nervous manifestations, which, as a matter of fact, are extremely difficult to cure in many circumstances. Certain patients are so systematized, the pains which they feel create such violent impressions upon them, that in certain cases it is almost impossible to draw their attention away from them by any method whatsoever. The pain sometimes occurs under the form of a type of obsessive pain, and one will find almost as great a difficulty in getting anything to quiet it as one would experience in helping a mental case to get rid of a real obsession. One must not, however, simply pronounce the patient incurable. Although the pain phenomena which are associated with the functional manifestations of different organs, and which as a rule are only of mild or moderate intensity, are often very quickly cured, the same is not true when one has to deal with serious algias whose starting-point lies in some bodily phenomena which cannot be made to disappear with any ordinary method of therapy.

Everything here depends on bringing the energy into play and arousing the patient's will by bringing to bear the proper general psychotherapy. It is necessary for the subject to be not only told, but convinced, of the neuropathic nature of his pain, and for him to awake to the fact that he must control it himself. Whoever the physician may be and whoever the patient may be, this rule is for all, and we do not know of any other therapeutic method.

Here, for example, is a patient who is suffering from a painful symptom which appears in the form of a boring sensation localized in the pit of the stomach. This pain is almost continuous, but between the times when it is practically bearable there occur in each day several hours when it is very much worse, and when, as the patient will say, it becomes practically insupportable. Whether he is sitting down or whether he is in bed, he will leap up and begin to stride about his room, clasping his abdomen with both hands and uttering deep groans. The perspiration will break out on his forehead, and he will get into a state of intense emotion, will find life unbearable and plan to get out of it. It may sometimes happen that such a patient may be cured in a few days, even though he may have suffered for months or possibly for years. We could quote a great many examples of such cures.

In the majority of cases isolation is distinctly indicated. It is not always absolutely necessary, but the thing which is indispensable is that the patient must put forth a tremendous amount of energy. When the painful symptoms are starting in, it is necessary for him to force himself absolutely to keep still. He must take a book and compel himself to read aloud, or, more simply, to recall what has been told him,—namely, that his pain will surely disappear if he knows how to get the mastery over it. He must then calmly, and with something of heroic tranquillity, wait for it to pass. From this first effort he will gain something, because from the very start the duration of the painful attack will be considerably lessened. At the end of a few weeks, sometimes only of a few days, nothing will remain of those manifestations which disturbed the patient's life for so many months or years but a very disagreeable memory, which the patient who is now wrapped up in his cure must not go back to any more often than is unavoidable.

An algia is the type of functional manifestation which can be cured only by stoical contempt. It is also necessary, however, for the patient to receive from a vigorous dose of psychotherapy sufficient faith and strength to work him up to the point of making an effort which requires that all his will and all his energy should be bent upon his cure. To try to cure an algia by slow and gentle methods is almost certain to run the risk of a set-back from which the patient will emerge completely hopeless. It is almost the only functional manifestation whose therapy needs be so sharp, and the only one where methods of reeducation, of distraction by surprise, etc., are unable to supplement the patient's deficient will or the insufficient authority of the physician. This does not apply, it is of course understood, to any but the great central algias, which are more often found in neurasthenics under the title of monosymptomatic functional manifestations.

All pains of phobic origin, due to fixation of the patient's attention on some point of his body, and by the sub-continuous calling forth of a pain whose cause has long since disappeared, may be treated in the same way. But other processes, such as distraction, turning the attention away from the trouble, and the simple psychotherapeutic action of explanation, may often be sufficient to cause a disappearance of phenomena which, as a matter of fact, occupy only a small place in the symptomatic ensemble. In a similar way precordial, abdominal, genital, or perigenital pains can be made to disappear at the start, if the patient is reassured concerning their cause, and if one is able to get the patient's mind off of the possible disease with which he believes himself attacked, and to arrive by re-education at the point where any functional trouble that has presented itself may be made to disappear. In cases like this the pain is for the patient, or becomes for him, nothing more than a psychic justification of a pathological conviction; the disappearance of the pathological conviction brings about the disappearance of the pain, even though the latter has been the origin of all the symptoms.

III. Therapy of the Functional Manifestations of the Organs of Sense.

These fixations will not detain us long. Sometimes consisting of pure phobic manifestations, sometimes resulting, as in the case of irritability to noise, from a condition of fatigue or an emotional state, sometimes caused by disharmonic disturbances, such as a deafness of attention in those patients who do not hear because they do not even attempt to listen, they do not furnish any special therapeutic indications. And the patient whose faith is established, and who has been made to understand the real cause of the troubles which he presents, concerning which we have already sufficiently expatiated, will easily rid himself of them.

IV. Therapy of Nervous and Psychic Manifestations Properly So Called.

Here, on the other hand, there are numerous special therapeutic indications, and, even though we eliminate from our actual study all the disturbances which have any connection with hysteria, there will still remain much to do if we mention all the processes and all the therapeutic precautions which belong to these very specialized localizations.

A. Disturbances of Sleep.—In the first part of this work we set forth our ideas concerning disturbances of sleep. We have shown that there are insomnias due to education in subjects who, either accidentally or on account of the way their lives are arranged, have formed a habit of doing with very little sleep; insomnias of phobic origin in patients whose fear of not sleeping has made them restless and chased away their sleep; insomnias due to the obsessive action of some emotional cause which exists spontaneously in the patient's consciousness, or which he voluntarily keeps recalling. Finally we recall that there is a whole series of sleep disturbances resulting from a less marked state of preoccupation or which are due to pure auto-suggestion. These are not expressed objectively in the form of insomnia, but are brought home to the patient in the form of simple subjective impressions.

Of all these manifestations insomnia due to education is undoubtedly the one which is most difficult to treat. Among those patients who have formed a habit of not sleeping more than an hour or two each night, or going to sleep at the start but wakening at a given hour, the reestablishment of normal sleep is often extremely difficult. We have seen patients who without any question have been suffering from severe neurasthenia, but in whom, with a physical and moral symptomatology which was sometimes extremely complex, their insomnia would be the only thing left at the end of a given time that would refuse to yield to any treatment. We do not hesitate to confess that as far as this manifestation is concerned we have had some therapeutic failures, but we have also had a certain amount of success, which enables us to lay down certain conditions by means of which one has the chance to obtain favorable therapeutic results.

There are, first of all, a rather large number of people who have become accustomed to their insomnia and who have planned their lives accordingly, knowing that, whatever they do, their sleep comes rhythmically, with a rhythm, it is true, that is insufficient, but nevertheless is perfectly regular. These patients busy themselves until the time when their regular hour of sleep is at hand. They read or do something with their hands. If, in their case, it is the waking hour which comes too early, and not the fact that the hour for going to sleep is delayed, they plan to fill the hours which must pass before it is time to get up. In itself this method of living is legitimate, for one must remember that they are wide awake and feel no need of sleep, and absolute inactivity seems to them peculiarly distressing and something which they try to avoid. But one must also realize that in this way their habit is encouraged and strengthened, and the first therapeutic indication which must be given to these patients is to tell them to give up doing anything whatsoever during the hours which should normally be devoted to sleep. Not only must they cut off any occupation, but, still further, they must try not to think about anything whatsoever. They must behave exactly as if they were going to sleep again naturally, but, above all, they must not think anything about their sleep.

This advice given alone is very rarely followed by any immediate result, but if the patient has the courage to force himself to follow this prescription for a sufficient length of time, and if he will be content to wait for some weeks, it may have a favorable result, and then again it may happen that it will be inefficacious.

One should then try, if we may use the expression, to throw the patient's habits off their track. In order to accomplish this, one must make him go to bed at all sorts of hours, and encroach upon his regular hours of sleep in different ways. If, for example, he is accustomed to fall asleep at about eleven o'clock at night and wake at one in the morning, one would tell him to go to bed at any hour during those of his customary sleep.

If, on the contrary, we have to deal with a patient who does not sleep until far on in the night, one would go to work differently. For example, if the patient sleeps between four and six o'clock, one would waken him after he had slept a half an hour or an hour. It might then happen that he would fall asleep again, and perhaps sleep for a very long time.

Even in this way one is not always sure of success. Certain physicians in these cases have recourse to hypnotics, and think to take advantage of their action in such a way as to cause sleep before the usual hour or to prolong it by this means. They then prescribe for the patient veronal, trional, or sulphonal. But the chief thing is not to give an hypnotic of a given dose at a given time. Still further is it necessary that the patient should not form a habit of being able to go to sleep only by such an artificial aid, and that one should not be obliged to prolong indefinitely the use of any drug which will finally lose its effect. In this lies the danger of such a proceeding, and it is for this reason that we do not recommend it, having too often seen in our practice subjects who for years have not been able to sleep without the aid of drugs, of which they have naturally grown to take larger and larger quantities. We much prefer in these cases of rebellious insomnia to advise sponging off with tepid water, or prolonged tepid baths, from which treatment we have more than once had very good results.

At all events, we think it extremely dangerous in dealing with such insomnias to practise such devices as obliging the patients to take violent and long physical exercise, with the end in view of tiring them out, and fairly forcing them, as it were, to sleep. As a matter of fact, the effect which is most often produced is, that the patient reacts to his fatigue by absolute insomnia, and that by such practices he loses what little sleep he had, which, although it may not have been sufficient, yet was comparatively restful.

Quite to the contrary, in very obstinate cases, we think that it is much better to have recourse to absolute rest, even to isolation, which has sometimes succeeded in overcoming insomnias which hitherto had resisted all the therapeutic measures which had been employed.

The treatment of patients whose insomnia is of phobic origin is also not without some difficulties. If there are some subjects who, for fear of not getting enough sleep, get to the point where they sleep more than they need to, and whose insomnia is, as a matter of fact, purely subjective, there are others whose insomnia is absolutely real. Through their restlessness, and the irritated state that they work themselves into while waiting to fall asleep, they are constantly repelling the sleep which only asks to be allowed to come. The rôle of the physician must evidently be to reassure his patient, and to explain to him the causes of his insomnia, which in themselves have nothing to do with sleep. But that is not always enough, and the patient often clings to his fear of insomnia so strongly that the bad habits which he has formed are frequently kept up in spite of all psychotherapeutic intervention.

The treatment which consists in requiring the patient to lie perfectly still in bed while waiting for sleep to come, or of requiring him to employ some mechanical device, such as counting indefinitely in a low voice, so as to permit sleep to steal upon him unawares, etc., seems to us poor, for it only keeps the patient's mind either upon his craving for sleep or (what amounts to the same thing) upon the fear that it will not come to him.

One has to be a little more subtle in handling the therapy for this symptom. If simple therapeutic action has had no results, or if, in other words, in spite of all one has said to him, the patient cannot get to the point of paying no attention to his theoretic or real insomnia, one must resort to some more circuitous method.

Here is one method which has sometimes succeeded for us. After having made our patient understand that the restless condition into which he worked himself was the only cause of his insomnia, we have asked him to go to bed at some time before his usual hour, telling him not to try to go to sleep then, but simply to give himself time to allow the excitement caused by his day to quiet down. He may get up, we tell him, half an hour later, and not go to bed again until his accustomed time. Now, during this period, when the patient, thinking that he is simply resting, is not trying to go to sleep, it frequently happens that he falls asleep and does not wake up until morning. From that time on, being reassured, he will go to sleep normally.

In fact, in such cases the methods of distraction are those which are most likely to succeed. The physician will have to exercise all the ingenuity of which he is capable to make them fit the particular circumstances. But here again he will fall into a series of therapeutic errors if he thinks that by tiring his patient physically, or putting him through a severe hydrotherapeutic treatment, he will get a good result. The insomnia will, as a rule, only become more pronounced, and will have a natural cause, for we know that excessive fatigue is apt, even in many people who are perfectly well, to drive away sleep.

Now that we are ready to take up the insomnias which arise from the fact that the patient, whatever he may do, is pursued by an obsessive preoccupation, or those which encourage the voluntary persistence of such preoccupations in consciousness, the therapy is quite a different thing. The insomnia is only a secondary phenomenon, and its disappearance will be brought about by the disappearance of the causes which created it.

Rest, isolation, and overfeeding, which permit the subject to get hold of himself more easily, and which cause the disappearance of all those troubles which emotional fatigue, itself the cause of insomnia, has brought about, with the addition of psychotherapy, with its reconstructive and liberating action, will be enough, without resorting to any indirect processes, to bring back sleep to such patients, who sometimes have been without it for a long time. All those subjects who do not sleep because they are thinking about things are much more preoccupied by their thoughts themselves than by the insomnia which follows them.

In the great majority of cases, such subjects have no phobias concerning sleep. However, it may happen that the mechanisms will combine, and that even in these cases methods of distraction and even those of re-education may be found useful. As a matter of fact this is rather rare. It is necessary, however, to point out the possible existence of such an association.

As for the functional disturbances of sleep, restless sleep, sleep which leaves one still tired, etc., which may result either from a pure suggestion, or in the case of a patient who is much preoccupied by reason of the repeated invasions of the psychological automatism into the domain of consciousness, their treatment evidently requires general psychotherapeutic methods, and has no special indications.

B. Headache.—The headache of neurasthenics has a double origin. Often it is a question of a true headache,—a headache due to fatigue, which disappears spontaneously with rest in isolation, or even sometimes by the simple action of rest alone, under the conditions, it must be understood, that emotional fatigue is not kept up by any persistent preoccupation. This first form of neurasthenic headache yields to the action of psychotherapy combined with its supplementary adjuncts.

Under other circumstances, the headache is only a subjective phenomenon, which by a sort of instinctive logic the patient associates with all his psychic weaknesses, whether real or theoretical. He will translate under the form of headache the impossibility which he feels, for example, of doing any work. It is along the same line of reasoning, or perhaps more conscious, that so many young people or young girls, make a headache their pretext to excuse themselves from some duty which they had not performed or which had not been finished. Between an impression of helplessness and an impression of pain, the subjective margin is not very great,—not great enough in any case to prevent neurasthenics from quickly taking advantage of it.

It goes without saying that, therapeutically speaking, the fate of this kind of headache is directly associated with the diminution or the disappearance of the psychic asthenia with which it is associated. Psychotherapy is all that is needed here, and in itself it will be sufficient.

C. Psychic Disturbances.—The disturbances of psychological functions which we observed in neurasthenics spring, as we have seen, from a certain number of different mechanisms. True psychic asthenia, due to emotional fatigue; false psychic asthenia, occurring more often in patients who are preoccupied and who cannot succeed in turning their attention to outside things, or who are put to considerable strain to obtain such a result; phobic symptoms or obsessions: these, in short, constitute the disturbances which are most frequently observed.

True psychic asthenia, due to fatigue, yields to rest, whether or not accompanied by isolation. It ought to be relieved in a comparatively short time, and we have already indicated the way in which one can tell about how much time must be allowed for a curative rest.

False psychic asthenia may follow a true asthenia. It occurs in patients who during a period of fatigue have become absolutely convinced of their mental weakness, and who are so convinced of their inability that they refuse to make any efforts, which, from the start, they think would be quite useless. False asthenia may also be established alone as a result of the patient's really finding considerable difficulty in performing any intellectual work. These difficulties have nothing to do with any lack or psychic deficiency whatever, but are only the natural expression of the impossibility which a preoccupied patient will find of fixing his attention on anything but that which is preoccupying him.

Evidently, in the presence of such troubles, general psychotherapy will be all that is required. The moment the preoccupations disappear, the symptoms which were secondary to them will have every chance of disappearing also. It is no less true that attention is a psychological function which educates itself, and which to a certain extent, if it is not used, can be brought into play later only with some difficulty. This is an idea which the physician ought continually to bear in mind, for it will often be necessary for him progressively to re-educate the attention of his patient.

There is no lack of means of accomplishing this; from simple arithmetical calculations to the most complex problems, there is a whole series of gradations in the attention necessary to solve them. One can employ these if the patient who is to be re-educated has any idea of mathematics.

The habit of making a summary of what one has read, and increasing the amount and the difficulty of the subject, is something which is possible for any patient to do. One may along these lines find a thousand ways of requiring patients to sustain their attention more and more until they themselves recognize the fact that they are capable of normal work. Some precautions, however, must be observed. For instance, it is not wise at the start to ask a subject who is still convinced of his helplessness, and whose outlook on life is pessimistic, to fasten his attention on any intellectual work which is at all like that which he was used to doing in his normal state. Under these conditions there would be too great a chance that the patient by comparison with his former facility would exaggerate his actual incapacity. Also in laying out the daily amount of intellectual work to be accomplished, one must be careful to limit the amount and to plan it in such a way that the impression of fatigue may not arise and bring with it a whole series of depressing ideas. It seems to us that the best way is to act exactly as in the treatment of psychic asthenia, to which, *mutatis mutandis,* and to avoid too much repetition, we refer the reader.

How should one act in the presence of a patient who is affected by various phobic symptoms? These, from the therapeutic point of view, are of two kinds. Sometimes the phobia refers to something objective, and is in consequence, such as is the case with agoraphobia,—we refer here to that of the neurasthenic, and not of the major psychasthenic,—susceptible to re-education. To reassure the patient, show him experimentally that he may be master of his phobia by progressively making him accustomed to the various elements of which it is composed. This is the rule to follow in such cases. It means practically that one must therapeutically organize and direct the struggle which the patient must make against his phobia.

But when it is a case of phobias which depend purely upon ideas, such as the phobia of suicide or of doing harm to some one else, where any objective re-education is quite evidently impossible, how can one then proceed? This is an important matter, for these phobic symptoms are bound up with intense emotional states, and it is most essential, in order that a neurasthenic should be cured, that they should disappear at the same time as the emotion, which can be (as we have seen) both the cause and the consequence at one and the same time.

Something is already accomplished when one has reassured the patient and shown him the nature of the symptom from which he is suffering, and established the difference that there is between this symptom and the impulsion which is the only thing that could lead to suicide or crime. By such steps one will get to the point where he will be convinced that he is running no risk, and where he will assure himself that he will never commit suicide and never do any harm to any one unless voluntarily and for some given reason. He will take less precaution, for instance, to avoid passing an open window or seeing or touching fire-arms. He cannot help having an involuntary apprehension, and here we are in the domain of the subconscious and psychological automatism. It is evident, that, every time the memory of his phobic symptom is called forth by the association of ideas, it will produce in the patient's mind a very disagreeable impression, accompanied by this feeling of apprehension, which is a minor type of phobia, purely involuntary and quite subconscious, against which the patient may struggle, but whose apparition is none the less quite independent of his will.

It seems to us, that, when we have to deal with symptoms which bring the psychological automatism into play, we must take into consideration the condition which attends its most frequent and most intense occurrence. It is very certain that any idea whatsoever will have all the more chance of crossing the threshold of consciousness if it has been recently associated with a great number of facts or things. In the presence, therefore, of phobic symptoms of the kind which we have just been considering, we do not always advise starting out to make a sort of experimental struggle against the phobia. If we are in the room of a patient who is afraid that he will sometime throw himself out of the window, if we open the casement wide to prove to him how certain it is that he runs no risk, and to base our argument on the very fact that instead of throwing himself toward the window he draws back into the room, it seems to us that such a proceeding is very good to try *once*. Nevertheless, we would not think it wise, especially if one could not have continuous psychotherapy going on at the same time, to ask the patient at the start to sleep with his windows wide open; nor would we advise those who are afraid of naked weapons or firearms always to have a set of razors or a six-barrelled revolver and a number of guns lying about. Such methods *may* give excellent results. They may cause the almost instantaneous disappearance of phobias, sometimes of long standing, by the feeling of security which they give to the patients. But they may also encourage a state of unintermittent emotionalism, and, by multiplying the association of ideas, work the phobia into a much more continuous though possibly less violent condition. It has often seemed to us that it was more prudent at first, and sometimes for a considerable time, to be silent concerning these phobic symptoms. It seems to us that it is often more necessary to teach the patient how to forget than how to struggle. To withdraw the patient from his daily surroundings both of people and of things in which the phobia was started, to avoid everything that may recall it to him, to avoid even mentioning it, in short to get as far away from it as possible, is perhaps a cowardly proceeding, but one which, nevertheless, often succeeds very well, when the patient, it is understood, has been previously reassured concerning his condition.

When new ideas have been born, and a different association of ideas has come, so to speak, to overlay and blot out the old phobic associations, they will be called forth much more faintly. The struggle will then be, but only then, comparatively easy for the patient, and will take place without the aid of any emotional phenomena, which are often dangerous because they are depressing.

As to the disturbance of the will which, according to certain authors, is characteristic of neurasthenia, we do not believe in it. Quite evidently, in people who are greatly fatigued by emotion, the will is secondarily deficient, as it might be in any one who was ill or convalescing; but it is found to be virtually intact after sufficient rest. The thing that is lacking in the neurasthenic is not, as we have so repeatedly said, his will, but it is a point of application that will make his will persistent. We have laid sufficient stress upon this in our chapter on the general psychotherapy of the moral and mental condition of the neurasthenic, on the necessity there is for the physician to redirect his patient's mind for the very purpose of furnishing his will with a point of application. It does not seem to us necessary to return to the subject.

V. Special Therapy of Hysterical Symptoms.

Although contrary to the descriptive order which we have adopted in the first part of this work, we have thought that it would be interesting, from the point of view of the therapeutic study, to treat all the hysterical symptoms together, because, as a matter of fact, some very general lines of treatment are applicable to all of them while at the same time some require very special treatment,—very special because they apply only to hysterical symptoms, and very general also because they apply to all these symptoms.

This is because hysteria is therapeutically, as a matter of fact, composed of two things, a mental and moral condition on the one hand and symptoms on the other. Although the moral condition of the hysteric, as well as his mental condition, may be very directly helped by the psychotherapy of persuasion, we cannot apply the same treatment with any success to the symptoms. One can reason with a person who is preoccupied or who has some localized phobia, for these phenomena have a positive psychological reason for being; but how can we reason with a person whose symptom, like that of any hysterical symptom, is merely a minus sign, a psychological lack of interest, if one might so call it, concerning the function or the organ which is affected? One could not, therefore, properly speak of persuasion as having any effect in such cases, but we might better use the words "act of recalling," or "re-education," to describe the actions to which we refer. It must, nevertheless, be understood that all that we have said concerning the action of sthenic emotions in the treatment of the psychoneuroses is true for hysterical symptoms, and that the best action of recall, the very condition under which re-evocation is possible, will be the disappearance, under the action of sthenic emotions, of all those ideas and emotional memories of every kind which could be continued by inhibition.

But, outside of the very special rôle of sthenic emotion,—which, however, cannot always be voluntarily produced,—it has always seemed to us that the therapy of all hysterical symptoms might be summed up in this formula—re-education in isolation.

If it is a question of contractures, of paralysis, or of disturbance of general or special sensibilities, there is no treatment for the hysterical symptom other than isolation. It has been experimentally proved as a fact, and a fact which must be admitted, even though the reason for it often escapes us. It may be that isolation acts by suppressing all outside causes for emotion, or that it acts by encouraging the patient to forget the inhibitive emotional cause, or it may be that the action is due rather to the concentration of the patient's psychism, which when not in isolation is readily dissipated, but which in solitude is concentrated sufficiently to recall the forgotten functions. It may be that isolation exercises an action of constraint upon patients whose symptoms may in some cases, though certainly not in all, have arisen from suggestion, and that in order to be free from their solitary confinement they are willing by auto-suggestion to throw off their symptoms. It is quite certain that with patients whose character is difficult to manage and with children and young people this mechanism may be very frequently used. Isolation then acts in the same way that a more or less strong emotion will act, producing the effect of a moral shock upon the patient, which is capable of "letting loose" his constraint. When in hysteria, for example, one sees the attacks which have been uninterrupted, such as contracture or paralysis, disappearing within twenty-four or forty-eight hours, it is perfectly evident that isolation acts as a moral shock would in such cases.

At other times it is possible that isolation has an element of conviction which acts upon the patient's mind, and that in this way the idea becomes more firmly fixed in the patient that he can be cured and must be cured, and that he will not be restored to liberty until the symptoms which have troubled him have disappeared. The one thing that we must not forget is that in such cases isolation is an imperative necessity, and that, whatever may be the way in which it acts, its action is at least favorable, and generally sufficient.

The second element of treatment consists in re-education. It is by means of re-education that all the special psychotherapeutic action has its effect. This re-education includes two elements, according to whether the loss of voluntary action is associated or not with the persistence of automatic action. Here, for instance, is a subject who is suffering from an hysterical hemiplegia,—that is to say, he is incapable of any voluntary motor action in one half of his body. The process of re-educating him consists simply in asking him to bring his will to bear upon his voluntary movements, making an effort to perform some of them partially at first, and then to make them more completely. Another patient is anæsthetic. Re-education in this case will teach the patient to fix his attention on his sensibility until the mental representations will again correspond to the stimuli.

Re-education in cases of this kind is only an act of recalling or an act of reconstitution.

Here, on the other hand, is a patient suffering from an hysterical contracture. As far as phenomena of consciousness and will are concerned, he is practically paralytic, as he has lost all capacity for voluntary movement. His contracture is only due to the persistence of an automatic action, which, as we have seen, is practically but the continuation of the impulsion received at the moment when the dislocation was established. Here the action of re-education will be twofold: it will be passive in a large degree, and will consist of appropriate movements to break the existing contracture, while, on the other hand, the patient will be asked to put forth his will directly to produce the movements in the contracted limb.

As for the way in which this re-educative will can put forth its solicitations, it ought to be directed toward opposing the convictions of helplessness which the patients have experienced, an inverse conviction which expresses itself in affirmations and authoritative deeds. One should not hesitate to encourage these solicitations of the will in some practical form. The patients who do not make any progress should be punished in some way, and those who do improve should be rewarded. The gradation in more or less complete or more or less severe isolation will give steps in this ladder of punishments and rewards, which may be used with advantage. The permission to receive letters, and visits, or the privilege of going out for a walk if one wishes, etc., will constitute, for example, motive influences which will often have much more effect than the most subtle persuasion in determining the patient's efforts.

What we have called "punishments" must be limited to this, and this only. We absolutely disapprove of all processes of intimidation, which are more or less brutal, in the treatment of hysterical symptoms. The method which we employ is that of absolute firmness, under which the patient, however, can see that we have his interest at heart. It is what we might describe as an iron hand gloved in velvet, and, according to our way of thinking, it is the only thing which is truly logical, for we have been convinced for a long time that an hysteric is not a person who imagines himself ill for the fun of the thing, but that he is quite as much to be pitied as the neurasthenic.

There are no hysterical symptoms which will hold out against this therapy, whose details we shall not dwell upon, because what we have just said seems to us to be sufficient to direct re-education according to each particular case. But it must not be imagined that, because it happens so frequently, the cure always takes place rapidly. In a great many cases one cannot predict the length of time that will be required for the treatment. There does not even seem to be any definite relation between the long standing of the symptoms and the time that will be required to make them disappear. But in a general way we might say that the symptom is either cured very quickly or it is cured very slowly. Intermediate cases are, as a matter of fact, rather rare.

While one is carrying on the treatment of the symptoms, one must at the same time put forth the strongest pedagogic influence upon the mental condition which has allowed it to become established. This action ought always to be prolonged, even after the symptom has disappeared. For in it lies the prophylactic therapy which we shall refer to further on.

CHAPTER XXVI.

PSYCHOTHERAPY AS REGARDED BY PHYSICIANS AND PATIENTS.

We have now taken up the majority of functional manifestations which seem to us to require some special treatment. In one case it is struggle and endeavor, in another it is psychological forgetfulness, in still another it is distraction in the etymological sense of the word, that is changing the course of ideas. Elsewhere it is the re-education of the patient, sometimes voluntary and sometimes carried on without the patient's knowledge, which must be thought out and directed according to each particular case. One sees how great a diversity there may be in psychotherapeutic work. When people say that psychotherapy has always existed, and when physicians state—remembering how they are wont to comfort and encourage their patients by patting them affectionately on the back—that they have always practised it, we feel that they have not taken the subject very seriously. Undoubtedly it is psychotherapy, and one of the best forms of psychotherapy, to take an interest in the moral welfare of a patient. But it is not enough to be interested in it as a whole, or *en masse,* if we might so express it; one must concern one's self with every detail, with its intimate and sometimes very remote causes, and chiefly in all the different consequences which the moral condition of a patient is apt to result in under emotion as well, and, above all, in all the different consequences which are apt to occur to the patient's moral condition when in a state of emotion.

We shall have finished with our therapeutic study when we have pointed out a few of the particular ways in which psychotherapy is indicated to the physicians who practise it, or to the patients who put themselves under such treatment.

In order to practise good psychotherapy, it is absolutely necessary to know one's patients through and through in every part of their personality. This is a necessary condition, but it alone is not enough. It is also necessary to know one's self, and to realize whether one has sufficient tact and authority to handle a certain patient, and to what degree one is capable of inspiring his confidence.

This is because, although the psychotherapeutic result which is sought for represents a constant factor, the various methods of psychic action are variable factors depending upon the physicians and upon the patients. Given a certain symptomatic ensemble, certain psychotherapeutic processes will be successful when practised by a certain physician on a certain patient, but the same will have no value at all if practised by another physician on a different patient. His age, his position, his physique, and even the tone of his voice may lend an authority to one physician which will be wholly lacking in another, and will permit him to practise a very different psychotherapy from another man who may be obliged to confine himself to some other methods.

All the preliminary endeavors of the physician should be to gain his patient's confidence, but this confidence should in no wise be forced, lest he experience a rebuff.

Take, for example, the act of confession, upon whose liberating action we have dwelt at such length. To try to force the patient's confidence, and to urge him to make an absolute and unrestrained confession, without having first been able to inspire him with a feeling of sufficient security, is to run the risk that the patient will not wholly unbosom himself. Later, if you have succeeded in completely winning his confidence, it would be apt to be the case that, having become entangled in his denials and reticences and former fibs, he would not like to acknowledge them.

All therapeutic work which is lacking in patience is apt, in some way, to be compromised. This confidence, which a young and inexperienced physician can win only after a long time, will very often be called forth immediately by a physician who has more presence and authority.

Take again, for example, the assurance of cure, which is so comforting and strengthening. It is very certain that the physician who does not impress the patient will not be able to make him see this possibility, but that when such a statement is made by an expert it will be regarded as a certainty by the patient, when he would have considered it merely as a possibility if a less experienced man had uttered it.

Let us take, for instance, a patient suffering from some functional disturbance. A physician would tell such a subject to pay no attention to this disturbance, and to treat it as though it were of no consequence, assuring him that it is purely negative in its effect. He will be believed if he says this with a sufficient tone of authority, and the patient will rapidly get over it without any other treatment, but the same patient would receive the same advice with much less conviction if it were given by a physician whom he did not consider so well informed.

Often, however, in order to avoid a set-back, one would be obliged in some particular case to have recourse to methods which are much slower and more certain, such, for example, as treatment by re-education or distraction.

But the authority which one may enjoy and the confidence which one can inspire are things of an extremely personal nature, and cannot easily be expressed in values. Is there any way for a physician to know just how much power he possesses in this direction, especially as the effect of such power varies in different patients and with individual affinities? It is simply a question of the way that one impresses a patient, and is purely a matter of tact. The manner in which the patient behaves, and in which he gives his replies, the manner in which he listens, the nature of the objections which he raises, his attitude of doubt toward medical statements, are all just so many elements which enable one to a very great degree to determine just what are the best measures to adopt in order to gain control over a given subject. One will always succeed in inspiring confidence in a patient and acquiring a sufficient authority over him, under the conditions which we have just given; but this does not necessarily happen immediately, and the confidence thus gained is liable to be shaken by various influences. You must know how to feel and understand the attitude of the patient himself toward you. This will reveal new psychotherapeutic needs in the patient. To regain a confidence or authority that has been shaken requires a certain delicacy of touch.

All of which amounts to the same thing as saying that psychotherapy cannot be practised unless the physician is in perfect sympathy with his patient. When it is a case of the moral treatment or psychotherapy of functional symptoms, this is always an indispensable condition. One should be able to perceive this feeling of fellowship or sympathy the moment it is established, for it is only when it comes that it is possible to obtain a complete confession, and to start in upon the work of reorientation in the personality. One must also be able to know just how far it goes, and whether the patient is capable of accepting, for certain of these functional manifestations, the conception which the physician has and which is generally quite different from his own. Tact, moderation, and observation must all come into play, but, as a matter of fact, it is simply a question of an impression which is always easily felt when this indispensable bond of sympathy is created between the physician and his patient.

Although when the physician is not armed with sufficient authority he is obliged to proceed cautiously with all his patients, there are, on the other hand, subjects whose treatment necessitates a certain manner of conduct particularly adapted to their cases, on the part of all physicians. Although the psychotherapeutic action may vary with physicians, it varies still more in connection with the patients, their age, sex, characteristics, education, and even their religion.

First of all, age furnishes a certain number of special indications. One would not, as a matter of course, dream of employing the same psychotherapeutic methods with an old man, or a patient well on in years, as with a young person or a child.

There is no doubt that in the case of a child, or even of a youth, the most profitable psychotherapeutic action may be practised upon the parents, who are, in the majority of cases, responsible for the symptoms which their offspring display. Although the action to be brought to bear upon the older people be that of persuasion and reasoning, in the majority of cases that which is appropriate to the various symptoms occurring in younger subjects is the action of authority. Neither the child nor the young person is able to reason. It is very rare to find that education, which is nothing more than a long-continued suggestion, has developed a critical spirit in them. What one finds in these subjects, on the other hand, is a spirit of contradiction, the common reaction of the weak and the young to the suggestion of others. To attempt to reason with a child or a young person is to run great risk of seeing the symptom grow worse, and, far from being cured, to plunge them into a much more complex and intense symptomatology. That one should take advantage of childish sentimentalities is naturally to be understood; one may ask a child to try to act in this manner or that, for example, in order to please his parents,—that goes without saying; but to explain to him the why and the wherefore of his symptoms will often be to lose valuable time. Only one form of therapy is called for here. It is that which consists in using appropriate measures to oblige or constrain the child, or youthful patient, to give up his symptoms. Isolation is often indicated in just such cases as a somewhat coercive measure, and ought not to be abandoned until the subject makes up his mind to give up the various symptoms which he presents. Simple statements and suggestions while awake are, we feel, practically the only things that are indicated in such cases. Still, it must be understood that, among young children who are very emotional, the action of sthenic emotion should by no means be neglected. But one should always be on one's guard against more or less conscious tendency to simulation, and to more or less marked auto- and hetero-suggestibility which so frequently characterizes the infantile mentality. If we may be allowed the expression, children are much more apt than grown people to lead their physician a dance, and if the latter does not take this into account the therapeutic result will often be curiously compromised.

Precautions of the opposite nature must be taken with self-centred old people who are fixed in their systematizations. Any determined statement or conviction too emphatically expressed which is opposite to their own way of thinking is sometimes quite enough to destroy the certain value of all consecutive psychotherapeutic treatment. One must slowly and gradually penetrate the systematizations of the old. At least, it must be understood if he is a little weak, and has at the end of the long road of life returned to an infantile stage in which, credulous and suggestible, he will pay no attention to reasonings which he only vaguely understands, but will, on the contrary, not be able to stand out against plain distinct statements.

In a general way and without reference to any particular cases, we find we have to treat patients of each sex in a different way. The critical spirit is rarely much developed in woman. Her sentimentality, however, is usually exaggerated. The beauties of a syllogism and the fine points of a subtle or possibly specious argument will leave her unmoved; she will perhaps be carried away by the harmony of sound, but rarely by the harmony of ideas. But to make up for this, all the chords of sentiment are ready to vibrate, and the physician who does not take advantage of the fact and play upon them will lose his best and surest mode of action. A woman more than a man needs repeated and almost uninterrupted psychotherapy. She is by nature more variable. Her psychic conditions follow one another quickly and without much coördination. When a man is away from his physician he reflects; a woman forgets much more quickly what he has told her, at least if what he has said has not touched her in the vital part of her sentimentality; but, although in a man the sentimental emotion disappears very soon, to give way to logical thought, in a woman, though the action of the reason is somewhat fugitive, the action of sentiment lasts a long time. It is very important to take these ideas into consideration in practising psychotherapy.

Other indications, which are often very important, may be drawn from the character of the patient,—not his artificial character, or that mask, one might call it, which his sickness gives to him, but his previous character. The methods to be employed with a patient who has always been weak and cowardly will by no means be suitable to a person who has hitherto been full of energy but is temporarily down. To ask the latter to make the same effort of will that one would demand of the former would often be imprudent. For the latter it is often enough merely to point out the way; but with the feeble individual, on the contrary, we have to guide his every step, as he hesitates at trifles, and even when he is set upon the right road he loses sight of his destination and sees nothing but the obstacles in the way.

There are other elements of character which are also very essential if one is to succeed in directing the patient by psychotherapy.

We have said a great deal about the liberative action of confession, but it is more or less difficult to obtain, not only on account of the nature of the thing which the patient may have hidden in his heart, but also on account of the habit, which he may or may not have formed, of wrapping himself up in an impenetrable personality, which he considers unapproachable. The influence of education plays a very weighty part in matters of this kind, and especially religious education.

It is a certain fact that we keep during our whole lives the mentality of the religion in which we are brought up, whether we have remained faithful to our religion or not. This mentality is of great importance in the formation—we might almost say in the essential characteristics—of character, and, even with a person who has become a freethinker, a monotheist, or an atheist, it does not require a very long conversation in order to know what religious beliefs he formerly adhered to.

It is by no means our intention to make any profession of faith whatsoever, but this does not hinder us from saying, that, from the stand-point of physicians, they are obliged to recognize that it is very much more difficult to produce any psychotherapeutic action upon a Protestant than upon a Catholic, and this, we repeat, is true whether or not the one or the other has remained faithful to the religious conceptions of his youth. The Catholic, accustomed through confession to disclose the most secret depths of his intimate personality, acts with infinitely less reserve in the presence of the physician than the Protestant. He shows the psychotherapeutist nothing of that instinctive and irrational defiance of the latter, who considers his personality inviolable, and who meets any one who tries to get at the depths of his being with a stone wall, and often rather a rough one. Those unfortunates whose disease or isolation or unsympathetic environment have forced upon them the solitary worship of their own personality show a very similar mentality. It is positively painful for all temperaments like these to acknowledge their mistakes, or to even let any one know their convictions or their profound aspirations. They raise a little altar within themselves, the searching of their conscience forms the sacrifice of this worship, but no one else may approach this altar, no one else may be present at the sacrifice, under pain of being accused of persecution or sacrilege. One sees that in such subjects it may be very difficult to practise psychotherapy. Accustomed to examine and to reason about things that cannot be reasoned about, to know their impressions and feelings, it is hard to reach them in any of the strong emotions. As for reasoning with them, which in fact is somewhat difficult in all individuals, they are so set that they consider it as an attack upon their personal dignity. What precautions one has to take with invalids like this! One must proceed by insinuations, by questions with implications; one must guess what they do not confess, get the patient in such a mood that he will think that he is drawing from his own inner consciousness ideas which, as a matter of fact, come to him only at second hand; and even that is often not enough. As a rule, all these "shut-in" personalities take two or three times as long to cure as those who, also having their secret gardens, yet are more willing to allow their confessor, their friend, or even, if the case demands it, their physician, to enter it.

It seems illogical to admit that there may be neuropaths who do not second the efforts of the psychotherapeutist, and who accept with very ill grace, which they barely disguise, all the efforts which he makes upon their behalf. The fact is, however, very rarely observed. When it is the case of minors isolated by the family authority, the matter is of not much importance, and isolation very quickly rights these faults in their characters. But when one has to deal with adults, the question of how to conduct one's self is much more delicate. It must not be forgotten that these are patients, and that consequently the physician's self-respect is not to be considered here. He must not depart from his usual manner, unless he finds himself dealing with a subject who is inclined to "take his physician's head off." In such a case two solutions are possible. Either one can send the patient away and have nothing more to do with him, which is evidently not at all humane, or else one can render him most energetic aid and give him a good sound rating. The last proceeding is the one to which we generally have recourse, and it has always given excellent results.

Finally it may happen, but the thing is rather rare, that one has to do with subjects who are so convinced of the incurability of their condition that, while they do not show any ill will, but are extremely grateful, and even moved by all the trouble that they give to other people, they will none the less make no attempt to pass out of "the jelly-fish stage." In such cases one must try to find some strong emotion or some moral shock which is capable of vitalizing them. We have several times succeeded in curing such patients by making them give, more or less by force, their word of honor to take hold of themselves and improve. This method succeeds chiefly among those psycho-neurotics who have some monosymptomatic form, and, we repeat, among those subjects who have chiefly lost all hope of being cured. This was how, in a case of complete aphonia which had lasted for four years, coming on in a woman thirty years of age, after extreme emotion due to the death of her mother, a case in which all psychotherapeutic methods had come to nothing for four months, the return of her speech was finally obtained by making the patient sign an agreement, upon her word of honor, to speak at a fixed date. It is evident that in this case the reason that this method gave such a good result was because it was addressed to a person whose nature, we happened to know, was upright, and to whom, as the patient told us more than once afterward, the idea of breaking her promise produced extreme moral suffering.

It is only by considering the social environment and the education that the patient has received, that the physician can plan his methods of psychotherapy. This man with severe asthenia, who says that he is incapable of any intellectual work, will have read, when he comes to consult his physician, nearly all the neurological literature which might interest him. However fatigued he may be, being accustomed to discussion and criticism, he will already have laid down in his mind a parallel between whatever one might have said to him and what he has read. He will have some answer ready to give a physician on every subject, and if the latter is taken unawares and does not know how to give him a ready answer in return, his influence will become decidedly weak. Nevertheless, when one meets patients who are really very well educated, and who are intelligent, they will lend themselves readily to your reason. The situation, however, is quite otherwise when one has to deal with people who are only semi-educated, and who are conceited by what they know, which, though sometimes covering a great many subjects, is rarely profound. Proud of their knowledge, but often with very limited comprehension, their minds are like a glassy surface, which the psychotherapeutist finds it almost impossible to gain a hold on. Among these we find the systematists and the ultra-scientists who are as firm in their pathological convictions as they are in their political ideas. If "Monsieur Homais" had been neurasthenic, he would no doubt have been incurable.

Such patients are very difficult to treat. It is a loss of time to reason with them. Proof even does not convince them. Moreover, they are often so sentimentally atrophied that the action of their sthenic emotions becomes effective only when it has to do with their pride, or ambition, or their own good opinion of themselves. With these patients one has to say, apparently quite impressed and convinced of the truth of their first proposition, "Now, you are an intelligent and well-educated man . . . and you will understand that . . ." One can often win them by flattering when it would be impossible to make any appeal to their feelings.

Such cases are, fortunately, rare, for such subjects possess almost none of the qualities that are necessary for one to become neurasthenic. One, however, meets some who are very emotional and depressed, because they consider themselves to be shamefully misunderstood. Being such, which is quite the contrary to the great majority, and the almost universal condition of the patient which we have to deal with, they are very seldom interesting because they are seldom sympathetic. To tell the truth, it is not their fault alone, but rather and above all the fault of the environment in which they have lived. They are the result of erroneous principles of education, of which our actual state of society shows perhaps only too great a tendency to multiply applications. If in such patients the physician does not find a single responsive chord, and if he feels himself unable to penetrate whatever conviction they may hold, one last resource remains for them,—namely, to enforce his authority by simply giving orders and commands. One will often be surprised to see how these shallow, undisciplined characters will often accept a statement or consent to obey when they merely have to do it passively. If one lets them argue or reason, one is lost.

It is very different, on the other hand, with patients who come from the class of people living nearer to a state of nature, who have along with their lesser education a better developed sentimentality, great spontaneity of feeling, and often very good sense, which is far from being a detriment. With them all that one needs to do is to get into touch with them, to talk to them simply, and not to try to dazzle them with any scientific jargon that they do not understand. It is not necessary for the physician to give them all of this external knowledge, at least as far as anything concerning the pathological situation, which, as we have just seen, is merely a therapeutic threshold. They have hearts. One can talk to them about their feelings. They have good sense, and a straightforward, almost self-evident argument will always strike them more than subtle reasoning. Along this line success will be certain. As far as the treatment of the psychoneuroses is concerned, one might say, more than under any other circumstances, "Blessed are the simple-hearted, for they will be cured."

CHAPTER XXVII.

PROPHYLAXIS OF THE PSYCHONEUROSES. THE MORAL RÔLE OF THE PHYSICIAN. CONCLUSIONS.

It is a very commonplace aphorism to say that prevention is better than cure. Prevention simply means to practise hygiene, and, if a hundred years from now an historian should try to give the most characteristic medical work of our present century, it is very probable that the thing that would strike him most in the medical evolution of our period would be the development of the science of hygiene. It is a subject which deals with the masses. It lays down the measures to be taken to avoid epidemics or endemics. It is also interested in the individual, looks for hereditary defects, and outlines the best method of living and the best form of nourishment that could combat their possible tendencies. But the same historian, who will describe our century as a century of hygiene, will not fail to express his astonishment that physicians seem to be so firmly convinced that their preventive action should be limited exclusively to physical life. Is it possible, however, to dissociate in any being a physical organism on the one hand which will function autonomously and in some degree spontaneously, and on the other hand a psychic organism which will think and feel in space? It is true that physicians are willing to concede that the physical may exert some action upon the moral part of the being. But is there any living thing or relationship in life which is so one-sided? We do not think so. It is the very essence of life to be composed of phenomena which are at the same time both cause and effect. It is hardly necessary to soar into metaphysical abstractions to show that it is by that very thing that life goes on. We can hardly mention the action of the physical and the moral without in the same breath stating the reciprocal action of the moral upon the physical, and if, in the course of the preceding pages, we have made our thought clear, the reader must have seen that, according to our way of thinking, all the functional manifestations of the psychoneuroses are the direct result of pathological deviations of this action of the mental upon the physical. Why then, as we have a physical hygiene, should we not have a mental hygiene, whose care it is to prevent diseases of the psychism just as physical hygiene tries to prevent diseases of the body? Why, if the physician is interested in treating diseases of the morals and the deviations which occur between the psychophysical relations, should he leave the work of correcting and avoiding defects, whose causes he cannot exactly determine or whose consequences foresee, to the exclusive care of spiritual directors and pedagogues? That certain great educators, whether inspired or not by religious and philosophical principles, have been able to lay down precepts which will, empirically at least, help one to realize moral hygiene and health, is a fact which we should be the last to discredit or to fail to acknowledge. This does not prevent us, however, from seeing that, if we want to find definite cause of this extraordinary modern increase in neuropathic manifestations, we cannot attribute it to anything else but the modern lack of moral education. The rôle that others have not filled satisfactorily or have left unnoticed the physician has the right to adopt. Knowing the importance of hereditary defects and being able to determine the constitutional element of a psychic situation, acquainted through long experience with all the woes of human mentality, knowing how these are constituted and what have been their natural consequences, why should he not have the right, or rather would it not be his duty, to go on still further, and lay down certain generalizations and essentials which should serve as moral principles of life? Unquestionably such ideas would only draw forth raillery from some, indifference from others, and scepticism from the majority. Moral hygiene is not yet taught by any chair in the faculty of medicine, and the physician would be thought to have lost standing who made a practice of palpating a patient's sentiments or auscultating his conscience. There are orthopædics for irregularities in the spinal column or the limbs, but there are not (at least not yet) any orthopædics for irregularities of the psychism or the morale. Would people really believe that a physician went beyond his province if he consented to become an educator, and if, knowing why and how a moral malady is apt to start, he should try by counsel and warning to strengthen the patient's resistance against it, and teach him how to avoid those factors which predispose him to it?

This function, which we insist is right for the physician, would never under any circumstances be denied him when he has to do with patients whom he has cured. Does he not warn a neurasthenic who has regained his health to avoid any strong emotions, and to lead a very regular life, so that by suppressing causes he may ward off effects? Emotion, we have seen, is the great factor of the psychoneuroses. To do everything one can to avoid emotional upsets would be the surest guarantee against relapse. But the very essence of emotions is just the fact that they overwhelm one when one is not expecting them, and the patient who has given way so to sentimentality, and shown so much personality, and has been so emotional as to become a neurasthenic, would not know how, without much discomfort and emotional conflict, to lessen the demands upon his life. Therefore, does it not seem that, from this point of view, one ought to practise prophylaxis?

It is of no use to try to escape from one's emotions; the chief thing is to learn to judge them. But, in order that such judgment may be possible, it is necessary that the whole personality of the patient should have been oriented in a monoideistic sense, and turned toward some practical philosophical or religious end. It seems almost elementary to refer every happening whatsoever to its general effect upon life, and to the halt or the retardation which it may cause in one's journey to a given goal. Nevertheless, there are very few persons who judge things according to their absolute value in relation to life taken as a whole. However, if one should act in this way, one would avoid many of the great climaxes which result from trifling causes. If one could teach a patient in this way to judge the value of his emotions, and not to be too much affected by things which are going on in the fields along his way, but which offer no barrier nor even a trifling obstacle to his path, one will have rendered him the greatest possible service.

But it is not only facts in outside life which are apt to hinder the general onward march of our subject's life; he is held back by the depths of his own nature, by his previous education, by all the bad habits which he has formed during the course of his disease, which cause him frequently to halt or go more slowly. Physical and moral auto-examination, with the inhibition of the will which necessarily belongs to such a habit, seems to us to play a very important rôle from this point of view. It must be understood that this auto-examination may be the natural result of the absolute lack of confidence in himself which the patient has contracted during the course of his disease. But, even when his self-confidence has been more or less restored to the patient, the habits which he acquired previously are very apt to remain with him. It is the physician's duty to show him his danger, and to point out to him the way to avoid it or to protect himself from it. Here his advice will vary according to different personalities as well as to circumstances. There are some subjects whom one will have to advise to change wholly the direction to which they have been accustomed. Such would only be the case with those who are constitutionally scrupulous. One would ask others to give up absolutely, without any question, the habit of examining themselves physically, and to refuse to attach any importance whatsoever to any symptom that was not very severe or that had a logical cause. And, although one would hardly have the right to tell any person not to examine his conscience or to weigh all his resolutions, yet one might at least ask him to proportion the time spent upon his self-examinations to the importance of their object.

If, as we think we have shown, one becomes neurasthenic because emotion gains the upper hand over reason, one will remain normal for all time after one is once cured, if one can only learn to use his reason, and to have it always on hand and in working order for every happening in life, and if one knows how to take advantage of it, to correct bad habits which are already formed.

We have had a great many subjects to treat who were extremely neurasthenic. We have been able to follow several of them during a good part of their lives. There are some who have sustained great shocks, and others who have gone through many lesser emotional phases, but they have always known how to withstand them. The essential thing in well-ordered psychotherapy is to give the patient a greater moral and psychic resistance than he had before the attack of weakness which made him come to you.

Is it possible to practise a prophylactic therapy for hysteria and its symptoms? This seems to develop naturally from the explanations given concerning the nature of these symptoms. One must teach the patient how to establish a more resistant intellectual control, as well as to distrust his impressions and sensations, chiefly those which have to do with his own special emotional reaction. But in such cases the most important thing seems to us to be the re-orientation of his personality. Any person who is striving toward a given end, whose thoughts and actions are coördinated by it, loses at once that mentality which is so peculiar to hysterics, and which is due, as we have seen, to all kinds of incoördinations. When one really wants to go anywhere, is one apt to be overcome by any great emotion on the way, or to be stopped by an attack of hysterical hemiplegia?

There are still other subjects than confirmed invalids for whom the prophylactic care of the physician can be of peculiar value. We refer to children whose constitutional emotionalism is seen from their earliest years, and who are in a position to become candidates for eventual neuropathic disturbances, but which could be prevented by well-managed psychic and moral hygiene. Little things who flush or turn pale and who start or tremble at nothing, who are alternately sad or exuberant, who fear new faces, but who cling desperately to those in whom they have confidence,—these show in such manner their physical emotionalism, as well as their moral emotionalism. That this emotionalism is taken advantage of in bringing them up is too often the case, and mothers who are somewhat sentimental develop this sentimentality still more in their children, and we find them becoming timid, overscrupulous, and restless. They will have an absolute lack of confidence in themselves, considerable self-esteem, and very great susceptibility. They will have their affections excessively developed, understanding nothing of the need of sharing with others. They will not dare to do anything, but will suffer from everything; although they will need to find some rational direction outside of themselves, yet they will not submit to any but sentimental guidance. They will be in a perpetual state of agitated excitement, but it will be purely internal and have no application to anything. The most sensible person who tries to educate them, unless he appeals to them through their pride and sentiment, will only make them exasperated and rebellious.

And when they go out into the world and are obliged to shift for themselves, by reason of their over-emotionalism and their poor equipment for the struggle, they will run all the more risk of failing, because their very inferiority multiplies the opportunity for emotional disturbances. They will only take a half-hearted interest in their career, which they have chosen without knowing why. They will fear reproach and will not stand any criticism. Let anything happen to upset them in their sentimental life, and they will immediately sink into a state of depression and will become neurasthenics.

But, if their education had been better directed, if they had been taught to feel less and to be more discriminating in their judgment, such unfortunate consequences could have been avoided. All that would have been necessary would be to teach them whenever they felt a wave of emotion to look for the cause of it, and to get hold of themselves by examining it, as it were, from an intellectual point of view. Later on, it would have been enough to teach them that all feeling or sentiment is dangerous when it impedes action, and that, on the other hand, one cannot demand absolute reciprocity in all affairs of sentiment. When they were quite young they ought to have been accustomed to making prompt decisions, and, if one had been able by the wise comprehension of their personality to start them off along certain given lines, one could undoubtedly have avoided what otherwise had been the almost fatal failure of their existence.

Among men of science there are few who, like the physician, are made by the very nature of their studies so opposed to all metaphysical abstraction. The mathematician reasons concerning time and space, the physicist and the chemist are obliged to come to abstract opinions which are beyond physical or chemical reasoning concerning the formation of matter, the physician, who deals only with concrete material in its most complex and highest forms, has no tendency to indulge in abstract conceptions which take him away from practical realities. A great mathematician or physicist must of necessity be at the same time a philosopher and a metaphysician. Medicine and metaphysics, however, are two terms so diametrically opposed to each other that they can hardly ever be brought together. The physician who is a positivist, sceptical, indifferent, and still further very apt to be ignorant, absolutely refuses to let his mind wander off into the realm of abstractions.

But, although one can see how the physician who is interested only in the body may show the greatest indifference to all the problems of life, in the metaphysical sense of the word, the same thing is by no means true for him who desires to be a physician of the mind. This is the case of the psychotherapeutist.

We are certainly most strongly opposed to any systematic psychotherapy which, starting from any particular philosophical or ethical system, will impose a point of view which is often quite opposite to all their previous conceptions upon patients who are still lacking in control and incapable of discussion. We hold that psychotherapy must appeal first of all to the feelings and to sentiment. We do not mean by that that it should be practised upon the automatic psychic functions; quite the contrary, it should, from the very start, be addressed to the personality of the patient on those points which are the most secret as well as the most quivering and responsive. It is not until much later, however, that the psychotherapeutist may dare to dwell upon abstract ideas, without running the risk of doing the patient more harm than good, by introducing, into a mentality which is already diffuse, additional elements of uncertainty and disorientation. We have already said,—and we do not hesitate to repeat it,—the first work of the psychotherapeutist is to let daylight into the mentality, the morality, and the personality of his patient, and to bring to bear upon him whatever arguments may help to build up his former personality according to whatever intrinsic value his personality may have had.

But one can never attack psychotherapy without knowing that the patient, once he is cured, will ask his physician for moral support and general directions concerning his life. He will consult him as if he expected him to lay down some rule which will henceforward definitely protect him from any new moral failures in the future; he will also try to find out just why it is that he fell ill, and how he was cured. He will have been shown that what he must try, before anything else, to do is to regain his self-control, and to establish moral control over his physique. However slight may be his intelligence and instruction, he is going to call upon you to settle this double problem of free will and responsibility on the one hand, and relations between the physique and the morale on the other.

According to our ideas it would be very ill advised for a psychotherapeutist to refuse to enter into a discussion upon these points, and to draw back into a narrow positivism by denying the principles which, whether metaphysical or not, justify and warrant his methods of procedure.

There is one case, however, where the physician must be silent. If he has to deal with a patient who has very strong religious convictions, what need has he for metaphysics? Faith is enough, and serves the purpose much better than any amount of reasoning. Whether the physician be sceptic or atheist, he has no right to attack beliefs which, as experience has shown, form the firmest prop and the surest support. Do you think you can replace by any deterministic doctrine or monistic conception what constitutes the very framework of their personality in patients who, from their infancy, have been accustomed to believe, possibly without reason, but nevertheless with faith and feeling, and accustomed to find in their faith a motive in life, and a directing purpose? By no means. Such a procedure would seem to us most dangerous, and almost immoral. It would be much better for the patient to think—and there is nothing to be ridiculed in this—that you are a believer like himself, rather than to deprive him of this moral foundation, formed by the idealistic conviction that lies so deep in his heart.

Does this mean to say that we think that elsewhere determinism and monism are good theories to uphold in patients for whom psychotherapy by persuasion has accomplished its work? It must be understood that we do not intend to discuss the intrinsic value of these philosophic doctrines. But how can one help seeing that these metaphysical systems carry with them the denial of any possibility of psychotherapy by persuasion?

If we have been able to make ourselves clear in the pages which have preceded, one must have grasped the fact that we hold that the whole work of psychotherapy ought to be to give back, to the subject who has lost it, the full strength of his intellectual control, and to restore to him the possibility of following a given line and full consciousness of his responsibility, as well as to disentangle in him the phenomena of the physical life from those of the moral life. Now, it is very certain that any such work would be theoretically impossible if one admitted a narrow determinism of things, if one denied the existence of any responsibility whatever, and if one refused to man, either wholly or in part, the liberty of self-guidance.

How, on the other hand, can one assure in any individual the ascendency of the moral and psychic life over the physical if he does not first admit that there is a relative independence between—to employ the usual phrases—the body and the soul?

How, in other words, can one be a psychotherapeutist if one is a determinist or a monist? Although, pushing the conception to its limit, one may see how a therapeutist by pure suggestion may introduce new factors into a patient's mind, how can one grasp the possibility of making over the subject's personality by persuasión? Yet this, however, is just what we ask our patients to do. The emotional actions which can be brought into play are to us only the means of a reawakening and recall of the conscience or the will, which are purely personal, of our subjects. We give them the desire to be cured, but it is they themselves who work the cure. This is the very thing which constitutes, we think, the great superiority of psychotherapeutic methods by persuasion. They develop in people the feeling of personality and responsibility, they increase their intellectual control, they accustom them to plan their lives and direct their energies by themselves, the reverse of all other psychotherapeutics, which, whether it is acknowledged or not, are suggestive therapeutics, acting on the human mind as on a mechanism whose machinery one tries to adjust.

The psychotherapeutist who wants to be logical with himself must, therefore, plainly tell his patients that he thoroughly believes in the free will of man. He ought also to tell him, that, although the automatic psychic functions are closely allied to the purely physical life, he does not, however, admit that there is any identity between the soul and the body, and that his function, as a psychotherapeutist, is that of awakening and exercising the power of recall over those superior psychological functions which emotion and life have rendered diffuse and which are, so to speak, thrown off their centre.

There are a great many individuals who do not share this way of thinking. They will discuss, in a logical way, which is so close as to become disconcerting, the very existence of their free will; they find in the very denial of their responsibility an excuse for their moral failures. The physician who is short of arguments and who is not able to prove the unprovable, and also is unable to persuade his subject to accept what, for him as a physician, may be an article of faith, will often have to employ the following argument, which we have frequently used:

Without the ideas of time and space, which in themselves may be contingent, there could be no possible knowledge. The philosopher who is most convinced of the relativity of knowledge must none the less make use of these elementary ideas. Now, if time and space form the framework of knowledge, responsibility and free will are the framework of action. One cannot act if one is not conscious of his free will and his responsibility. Deterministic interpretations are only interpretations *a posteriori*. They may follow actions, but they cannot demand them, quite as ideas concerning the relativism of knowledge are secondary to the knowledge itself, which in the absence of its framework would be impossible. At all events, and in all cases, we therefore have to act as if we were responsible, and as if we were enjoying our absolute free will. In the same way we get a knowledge of things just as if time and space were true realities outside of ourselves.

This manner of reasoning, which is in some way positivistic, is hardly more than an argument of despair. We have used just such when subjects were trying by their deterministic ideas to find an excuse for their fall, and eventually for their relapse.

How, otherwise, could one ask a subject to control the phenomena of his physical life, so far as his psychism has a physical basis, if one might so call it, if he does not get to the point where he can conceive that, beyond the phenomena of psychologic automatism, there is a place for the superior moral faculties, which are used, to speak truly, by the psychological automatism, but which are not wholly constituted or formed by it? How can one ask him to combat or to neglect an obsessive preoccupation, if he imagines that this preoccupation is furnished by a mechanism which nothing in his individualism can touch? How can one ask him to recover his judgment by his own strength if this judgment is practically nothing but a question of the number and quality of purely passive association of ideas? The clear explanation of the automatic and involuntary origin of so many preoccupations and slight obsessions can only serve as a starting-point of psychic therapeutics in so far as one admits in addition the independence of the superior psychic faculties.

But is it possible to prove that there is this independence between what is body, and consequently susceptible to all physical and chemical actions of the organism, and the mind, properly so called, in the sense in which the ancient idealistic philosophers used the word?

The practical demonstration of this independence is a direct result of this fact, that patients have been able, by the action of their will and their intelligence alone, to regain that full consciousness and mastery of themselves which prevented the repeated incursions of the automatism into the realm of consciousness which was more or less disturbed by emotional action. And the argument may be summed up in the following way by telling the patients: "You see that you have been able to gain the mastery over yourself since you have known how to cure yourself." We have hastened to bring to a close this paragraph, which has led us to what we must frankly confess are the cloudy heights of pure abstraction. It has, however, seemed to us that these things should be said, because we have an idea, and a very definite one, that deterministic or monistic doctrines have done a great deal of harm to a great many patients.

On the other hand, one can do much good to numerous patients by showing them that the surest guarantee against all little and even great emotions is to build up either an ethical or a philosophical or a religious ideal. This idea is one on which we have often insisted, because it has seemed to us to have the value of experience. Life shows every day that those have been the best able to stand up under anxiety, grief, or various vicissitudes who have known how to create objectively an ideal outside of themselves, no matter what it may be, but whose progressive realization has brought unity into their life. Those men, on the other hand, whose life seems to be lived day by day, as it were, without any purpose or direction, who seem always to be stopping and losing themselves or wandering into all sorts of lanes and blind alleys, are much more poorly equipped. Without any definite convictions, they have no definite reasons to go in one direction more than another, and the slightest obstacle which they meet in their path leaves them standing still upon their way.

If it is true, as we think it to be, that moral health results from the free development of the personality, how can we help but see how great an interest there is in directing this into a path which, by its very nature, offers the greatest security and an almost perfect guarantee against the accidents of existence?

Having now reached the end of our study, we feel that it would be wise to sum up in a few lines those ideas which seem to us to have the most characteristic importance.

So we shall say:

1. All the functions may be disturbed by the improper interference of the mind. It is in this way that functional manifestations are created.

2. This interference of the mind has in almost every case some emotional cause for its origin.

3. Emotion may act by repeated actions. It then creates neurasthenia—the syndrome of emotional preoccupation.

4. Emotion may act by the sudden action of dissociation. Under these conditions it results in hysterical symptoms.

5. The action of emotion which creates the psychoneuroses and their symptoms can only take place on emotional soil. But when the eventual neurasthenic is essentially obsessable and the hysteric is by definition an unstable and incoördinated personality:

6. We hold that it is wrong to have included under neurasthenia, which is an affection of psychic origin, the various asthenias of organic origin which have nothing in common with them but symptoms of fatigue.

7. Although, as far as their secondary phenomena are concerned, the psychoneuroses may be treated in various ways, there is but one etiological therapy for them,—namely, that of psychotherapy.

8. There is but one legitimate form of psychotherapy,—namely, the psychotherapy of persuasion, which should be addressed both to the symptoms and to the mental and moral make-up which has permitted them to become established.

INDEX

Classics in Psychiatry

An Arno Press Collection

American Psychiatrists Abroad. 1975

Arnold, Thomas. **Observations On The Nature, Kinds, Causes, And Prevention Of Insanity.** 1806. Two volumes in one

Austin, Thomas J. **A Practical Account Of General Paralysis, Its Mental And Physical Symptoms, Statistics, Causes, Seat, And Treatment.** 1859

Bayle, A[ntoine] L[aurent] J[esse]. **Traité Des Maladies Du Cerveau Et De Ses Membranes.** 1826

Binz, Carl. **Doctor Johann Weyer.** 1896

Blandford, G. Fielding. **Insanity And Its Treatment.** 1871

Bleuler, Eugen. **Textbook Of Psychiatry.** 1924

Braid, James. **Neurypnology.** 1843

Brierre de Boismont, A[lexandre-Jacques-François]. **Hallucinations.** 1853

Brown, Mabel Webster, compiler. **Neuropsychiatry And The War:** A Bibliography With Abstracts and **Supplement I,** October 1918. Two volumes in one

Browne, W. A. F. **What Asylums Were, Are, And Ought To Be.** 1837

Burrows, George Man. **Commentaries On The Causes, Forms, Symptoms And Treatment, Moral And Medical, Of Insanity.** 1828

Calmeil, L[ouis]-F[lorentin]. **De La Folie:** Considérée Sous Le Point De Vue Pathologique, Philosophique, Historique Et Judiciaire, Depuis La Renaissance Des Sciences En Europe Jusqu'au Dix-Neuvième Siècle. 1845. Two volumes in one

Calmeil, L[ouis] F[lorentin]. **De La Paralysie Considérée Chez Les Aliénés.** 1826

Dejerine, J[oseph Jules] and E. Gauckler. **The Psychoneuroses And Their Treatment By Psychotherapy.** [1913]

Dunbar, [Helen] Flanders. **Emotions And Bodily Changes.** 1954

Ellis, W[illiam] C[harles]. **A Treatise On The Nature, Symptoms, Causes And Treatment Of Insanity.** 1838

Emminghaus, H[ermann]. **Die Psychischen Störungen Des Kindesalters.** 1887

Esdaile, James. **Mesmerism In India,** And Its Practical Application In Surgery And Medicine. 1846

Esquirol, E[tienne]. **Des Maladies Mentales.** 1838. Three volumes in two

Feuchtersleben, Ernst [Freiherr] von. **The Principles Of Medical Psychology.** 1847

Georget, [Etienne-Jean]. **De La Folie:** Considérations Sur Cette Maladie. 1820

Haslam, John. **Observations On Madness And Melancholy.** 1809

Hill, Robert Gardiner. **Total Abolition Of Personal Restraint In The Treatment Of The Insane.** 1839

Janet, Pierre [Marie-Felix] and F. Raymond. **Les Obsessions Et La Psychasthénie.** 1903. Two volumes

Janet, Pierre [Marie-Felix]. **Psychological Healing.** 1925. Two volumes

Kempf, Edward J. Psychopathology. 1920

Kraepelin, Emil. **Manic-Depressive Insanity And Paranoia.** 1921

Kraepelin, Emil. **Psychiatrie:** Ein Lehrbuch Für Studirende Und Aerzte. 1896

Laycock, Thomas. **Mind And Brain.** 1860. Two volumes in one

Liébeault, A[mbroise]-A[uguste]. **Le Sommeil Provoqué Et Les États Analogues.** 1889

Mandeville, B[ernard] De. **A Treatise Of The Hypochondriack And Hysterick Passions.** 1711

Morel, B[enedict] A[ugustin]. **Traité Des Degénérescences Physiques, Intellectuelles Et Morales De L'Espèce Humaine.** 1857. Two volumes in one

Morison, Alexander. **The Physiognomy Of Mental Diseases.** 1843

Myerson, Abraham. **The Inheritance Of Mental Diseases.** 1925

Perfect, William. **Annals Of Insanity.** [1808]

Pinel, Ph[ilippe]. **Traité Médico-Philosophique Sur L'Aliénation Mentale.** 1809

Prince, Morton, et al. **Psychotherapeutics.** 1910

Psychiatry In Russia And Spain. 1975

Ray, I[saac]. **A Treatise On The Medical Jurisprudence Of Insanity.** 1871

Semelaigne, René. **Philippe Pinel Et Son Oeuvre Au Point De Vue De La Médecine Mentale.** 1888

Thurnam, John. **Observations And Essays On The Statistics Of Insanity.** 1845

Trotter, Thomas. **A View Of The Nervous Temperament.** 1807

Tuke, D[aniel] Hack, editor. **A Dictionary Of Psychological Medicine.** 1892. Two volumes

Wier, Jean. **Histoires, Disputes Et Discours Des Illusions Et Impostures Des Diables, Des Magiciens Infames, Sorcieres Et Empoisonneurs.** 1885. Two volumes

Winslow, Forbes. **On Obscure Diseases Of The Brain And Disorders Of The Mind.** 1860

Burdett, Henry C. **Hospitals And Asylums Of The World.** 1891-93. Five volumes. 2,740 pages on NMA standard 24x-98 page microfiche only